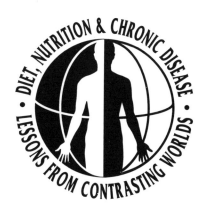

· DIET, NUTRITION & CHRONIC DISEASE ·

· LESSONS FROM CONTRASTING WORLDS ·

Also available in the Wiley Series of *London School of Hygiene & Tropical Medicine* Annual Public Health Forums...

HEALTH AT THE CROSSROADS
Transport Policy and Urban Health
Edited by TONY FLETCHER and ANTHONY J. McMICHAEL
0471 96272 4   354pp   1996
Fifth Annual Public Health Forum

VACCINATION AND WORLD HEALTH
Edited by F.T. CUTTS and P.G. SMITH
0471 95242 7   308pp 1995
Fourth Annual Public Health Forum

TUBERCULOSIS
Back to the Future
Edited by JOHN PORTER and KEITH McADAM
0471 94346 0   304pp   (pr) 1993
Third Annual Public Health Forum

EUROPE WITHOUT FRONTIERS
The Implications for Health
Edited by CHARLES E.M. NORMAND and PATRICK VAUGHAN
0471 93761 4   396pp   (pr) 1993
0471 93759 2   396pp   (cl) 1993
Second Annual Public Health Forum

MALARIA
Waiting for the Vaccine
Edited by GEOFFREY TARGETT
0471 93100 4   236pp   1991
First Annual Public Health Forum

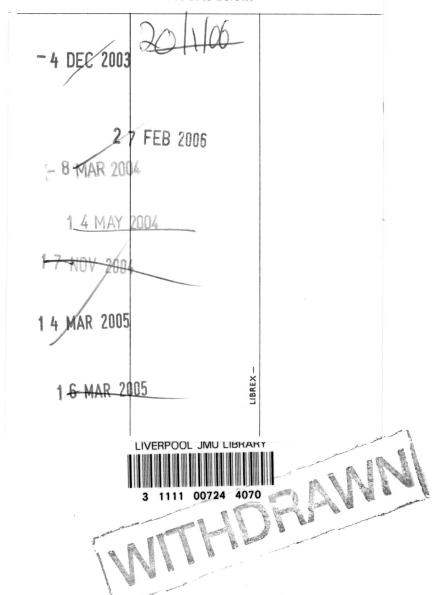

London School of Hygiene & Tropical Medicine
Sixth Annual Public Health Forum

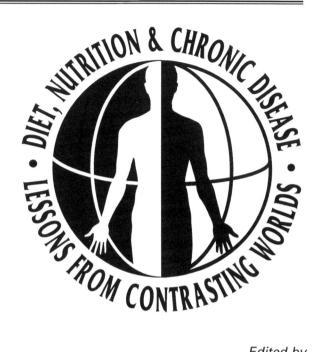

Edited by
Prakash S. Shetty and Klim McPherson

Assistant Editor
Alice Dickens

Series Editor
Barbara M. Judge

London School of Hygiene
& Tropical Medicine, London, UK

JOHN WILEY & SONS

Chichester · New York · Weinheim · Brisbane · Singapore · Toronto

Other Wiley Editorial Offices

John Wiley & Sons, Inc., 605 Third Avenue,
New York, NY 10158-0012, USA

VCH Verlagsgesellschaft mbh, Pappelallee 3,
D-69469 Weinheim, Germany

Jacaranda Wiley Ltd, 33 Park Road, Milton,
Queensland 4064, Australia

John Wiley & Sons (Asia) Pte Ltd, 2 Clementi Loop #02-01,
Jin Xing Distripark, Singapore 129809

John Wiley & Sons (Canada) Ltd, 22 Worcester Road,
Rexdale, Ontario M9W 1LI, Canada

Library of Congress Cataloging-in-Publication Data

Diet, nutrition, and chronic disease : lessons from contrasting worlds / edited by Prakash S.
   Shetty and Klim McPherson ; assistant editor, Alice Dickens ; series editor, Barbara M. Judge.
      p.   cm.
   Proceedings of the Sixth London School of Hygiene & Tropical Medicine Public Health
Forum, held Mar. 31–Apr. 3, 1996 in London.
   Includes bibliographical references and index.
   ISBN 0-471-97133-2 (cased)
      1. Nutritionally induced diseases—Congresses.   2. Chronic diseases—Congresses.
3. World health—Congresses.   I. Shetty, Prakash S.   II. McPherson, Klim.
III. London School of Hygiene & Tropical Medicine Public Health Forum (6th : 1996)
      [DNLM: 1. Chronic Disease—congresses.   2. Diet—congresses.
3. Nutrition—congresses.   4. World Health—congresses.   WT 500 D565 1997]
RA645.N87D55   1997
616.3'9—dc21
DNLM/DLC
for Library of Congress   96–50379
                                                                                          CIP

British Library Cataloguing in Publication Data

A catalogue record for this book is available from the British Library

ISBN 0-471-97133-2

Typeset in 10/12pt Times from the author's disks by Vision Typesetting, Manchester
Printed and bound in Great Britain by Biddles Ltd, Guildford and King's Lynn
This book is printed on acid-free paper responsibly manufactured from sustainable forestation,
for which at least two trees are planted for each one used for paper production.

Contents

Contents

Contributors

David J.P. Barker, MRC Environmental Epidemiology Unit, Southampton General Hospital, Southampton SO16 6YD, UK

Sheila A. Bingham, MRC Dunn Clinical Nutrition Centre, Hills Road, Cambridge CB2 2DH, UK

Bennie Bloemberg, Division of Public Health Research, RIVM, PO Box 1, 3720 BA Bilthoven, The Netherlands

George Bray, Pennington Biomedical Research Center, Louisiana State University, 6400 Perkins Road, Baton Rouge, LA 70808, USA

Eric Brunner, Department of Epidemiology and Public Health, University College London, 1–19 Torrington Place, London WC1

Francisco Cappuccio, Department of Medicine, St George's Hospital Medical School, Cranmer Terrace, London SW17 0RE

Chen Chunming, Chinese Institute of Preventive Medicine, 27 Nan Wei Road, Beijing 100050, People's Republic of China

John H. Cummings, MRC Dunn Clinical Nutrition Centre, Hills Road, Cambridge CB2 2DH, UK

Elizabeth Dowler, Human Nutrition Unit, London School of Hygiene & Tropical Medicine, Keppel Street, London WC1E 7HT, UK

Anna Ferro-Luzzi, Unit of Human Nutrition, National Institute of Nutrition, Via Ardeatina 546, 00178 Rome, Italy

C. Gopalan, The Nutrition Foundation of India, C-13 Qutab Institutional Area, New Delhi 110 016, India

Diederick Grobbee, Erasmus University Medical School, PO Box 1738, 3000 DR Rotterdam, The Netherlands

W. Philip T. James, Rowett Research Institute, Greenburn Road, Bucksburn, Aberdeen AB9 2SB, UK

Eric Jéquier, Institute of Physiology, University of Lausanne, 7 rue du Bugnon, 1005 Lausanne, Switzerland

Rudolph Kaaks, Unit of Nutrition and Cancer, International Agency for Research on Cancer, 150 Cours Albert-Thomas, 69372 Lyon Cedex 08, France

Timothy Key, ICRF Cancer Epidemiology Unit, Gibson Building, Radcliffe Infirmary, Oxford OX2 6HE, UK

Kay Tee Khaw, Clinical Gerontology Unit, University of Cambridge, Addenbrooke's Hospital, Cambridge CB2 2QQ, UK

Daan Kromhout, Division of Public Health Research, RIVM, PO Box 1, 3720 BA Bilthoven, The Netherlands

Tim Lang, Centre for Food Policy, Wolfson School of Health Sciences, Thames Valley University, 32–28 Uxbridge Road, Ealing, London W5 2BS, UK

Michael Lean, Department of Human Nutrition, University of Glasgow, Royal Infirmary, Queen Elizabeth Building, Glasgow G31 2ER, UK

David Leon, Epidemiology Unit, London School of Hygiene & Tropical Medicine, Keppel Street, London WC1E 7HT, UK

Jim Mann, Department of Human Nutrition, University of Otago, PO Box 56, Dunedin, New Zealand

Paul McKeigue, Epidemiology Unit, London School of Hygiene & Tropical Medicine, Keppel Street, London WC1E 7HT, UK

Anthony J. McMichael, Epidemiology Unit, London School of Hygiene & Tropical Medicine, Keppel Street, London WC1E 7HT, UK

Klim McPherson, Health Promotion Sciences Unit, London School of Hygiene & Tropical Medicine, Keppel Street, London WC1E 7HT, UK

Abdulrahman Musaiger, Department of Food Sciences, United Arab Emirates University, PO Box 17555, Al Ain, United Arab Emirates

Kaare R. Norum, Institute for Nutrition Research, University of Oslo, Faculty of Medicine, PO Box 146, Blindern, 0316 Oslo, Norway

Andrew M. Prentice, MRC Dunn Clinical Nutrition Centre, Hills Road, Cambridge CB2 2DH, UK

Jane Pryer, Human Nutrition Unit, London School of Hygiene & Tropical Medicine, Keppel Street, London WC1E 7HT, UK

Pekka Puska, Division of Health and Chronic Disease, National Public Health Institute, Mannerheimintie 166, 00300 Helsinki, Finland

K. Srinath Reddy, Department of Cardiology, All India Institute of Medical Sciences, Ansari Nagar, New Delhi 110 029, India

Elio Riboli, Unit of Nutrition and Cancer, International Agency for Research on

Cancer, 150 Cours Albert-Thomas, 69372 Lyon Cedex 08, France

A. Gerald Shaper, Emeritus Professor of Clinical Epidemiology, Royal Free Hospital Medical School, Rowland Hill Street, London NW3 2QG, UK

Prakash S. Shetty, Human Nutrition Unit, London School of Hygiene & Tropical Medicine, Keppel Street, London WC1E 7HT, UK

Dinesh P. Sinha, formerly of the Caribbean Food and Nutrition Institute, PO Box 140, Kingston 7, Jamaica, West Indies

Lars Sjöström, Department of Medicine, University of Göteborg, S-413 45 Göteborg, Sweden

Alison E. Tedstone, Human Nutrition Unit, London School of Hygiene & Tropical Medicine, Keppel Street, London WC1E 7HT, UK

Margaret Thorogood, Health Promotion Sciences Unit, London School of Hygiene & Tropical Medicine, Keppel Street, London WC1E 7HT, UK

Hester H. Vorster, Department of Nutrition, Potchefstroom University, Potchefstroom 2520, Republic of South Africa

Walter C. Willett, Department of Nutrition, Harvard School of Public Health, 665 Huntington Avenue, Boston MA 02115, USA

Foreword

The world is experiencing an accelerating epidemic of diet-related non-communicable diseases (NCDs). Unbalanced and excessive food and nutrient intakes, often closely associated with other changes in lifestyle that include reduced physical exercise, stress, tobacco smoking, and excessive alcohol consumption, underlie a range of these diseases, especially coronary heart disease, hypertension and stroke, various cancers, non-insulin-dependent diabetes mellitus, obesity, dental caries, gall-bladder disease and osteoporosis. In many countries such diseases have already become the leading cause of death. It is not that the tragic global burden of malnutrition has suddenly become less important. Indeed, WHO currently estimates that 174 million children under the age of five are still malnourished in terms of underweight, and the World Food Summit stressed that 841 million people worldwide are still undernourished because they are food-energy deficient. Likewise, our world still sees the health, sight, intelligence and survival of many millions of children threatened by micronutrient malnutrition, with 750 million people suffering from iodine deficiency and 250 million pre-school children vitamin A deficient. Overall, we now know that 54% of all deaths in under-fives in developing countries—a truly staggering figure of more than 6 million in all—are associated with malnutrition. Yet, even as this huge burden of malnutrition-related morbidity and mortality is carried by the developing world, it is some of the same group of low-income countries that are now having to shoulder another burden, the rapidly rising adult death and disability rates due to diet-related NCDs.

Until quite recently, it was believed that diet-related NCDs were a minor or even non-existent problem in developing countries. However, a WHO analysis in 1992 that examined mortality trends from diet-related NCDs found that over the past 30 years there have been large increases in mortality rates from diet-related NCDs in both Eastern European and developing countries. Although diet-related NCDs account for nearly 40% of all deaths worldwide—and this proportion is continuing to rise—trends in individual countries show considerable variation. Some of the established market economies, for example Australia, Canada, Finland, Japan and the USA, where diet-related NCDs already account for more than two-thirds of all deaths, are now showing a marked decrease in deaths that is associated with improving dietary patterns, medical care, and health screening. Vigorous educational efforts to influence dietary intakes—especially to limit intakes of total fat, saturated fat and salt, and to promote healthier lifestyles—have also been credited for their positive contribution. In developing countries, although diet-related NCDs still account for only a quarter of all deaths, dramatic increases in this mortality rate are occurring in a significant number of countries—particularly where development patterns are characterised by a rapidly evolving situation affecting income, urbanisation, and changing dietary patterns.

All countries' populations are ageing, but those of middle- and low-income countries, following steep declines in both fertility rates and deaths due to childhood disease, are ageing more rapidly than those in industrialised countries. Ageing is a major factor in the increasing burden of NCDs, and both the absolute number of deaths and, in many countries, the proportion of all deaths, will continue to rise for years to come. Moreover, a major concern is that although increased mortality for diet-related NCDs affects people in their later years, the influences contributing to death from these causes operate *throughout* an individual's lifetime. Since changes in diet and lifestyle can take decades to affect mortality rates, it is essential that preventive measures be implemented early in life. It is tremendously encouraging to note that, in a few countries at least, this approach seems to be succeeding in slowing and even reversing trends.

From a global health perspective, research is of paramount importance on two major fronts: epidemiological studies better to define the nature and magnitude of trends in diet-related NCDs, and intensive health policy research to identify effective options for their prevention and control. Studies and options then need to be thoughtfully combined to produce effective national policies and interventions that address this epidemic. By bringing together scientists, policy-makers, and members of the public health community from around the world, and straightforwardly addressing epidemiological, research, policy and intervention issues, I am convinced that the Sixth Annual Public Health Forum will have made a significant contribution to the much needed acceleration of action that is required to counter and reverse the accelerating global epidemic of diet-related non-communicable diseases.

Graeme Clugston
Director, Division of Nutrition,
World Health Organization, Geneva, Switzerland

Preface

Diet and lifestyle changes that follow in the wake of industrialisation, urbanisation and economic development have a significant impact on the health of populations. It is predicted that in the next millennium, the incidence of chronic non-communicable diseases will increase dramatically and replace in a large measure the problems of dietary deficits, hunger and malnutrition globally. Developing countries, in particular those that are in rapid transition and demonstrating a shift in population distribution from rural to urban areas, are likely to have to face the consequences of both nutritional deficits and excesses, that is, the double whammy of undernutrition and the growing epidemic of non-communicable diseases such as cardiovascular diseases and cancers largely determined by overnutrition. Industrialised nations with the established market economies have already made considerable progress in coming to grips with the public health and preventive aspects of non-communicable diseases. Countries belonging to the former socialist economies of Europe are currently confronting this major public health problem, while developing countries are only just beginning to recognise the early signs of the epidemic of chronic diseases that is yet to burden their fragile economies. It is therefore only appropriate that the London School of Hygiene & Tropical Medicine, a pre-eminent international school of public health, should have taken a lead in organising this, the Sixth Annual Public Health Forum to discuss the public health impact, preventive strategies and policy issues related to the problem of chronic non-communicable diseases on a global basis.

The Forum provided a platform for the sharing of current knowledge and understanding of all aspects of the problem of chronic diseases from a public health and preventive point of view. It also endeavoured for the first time to bring together contrasting interests and disciplines; those with an interest in cardiovascular disease with others only interested in cancers, epidemiologists and social scientists, clinical investigators and public health physicians, nutritionists and policy analysts.

We are grateful for the generous financial support from the following organisations, without which this meeting would not have been possible: the British Heart Foundation, the Cancer Research Campaign, Unilever plc, The Wellcome Trust, and the World Cancer Research Fund, and in particular, to Knoll Pharmaceuticals, who sponsored the symposium on obesity, and the publication of this book.

Many people contributed to the success of the Forum. We would particularly like to thank Professor Philip James for his constant encouragement and support, Dr Andrew Prentice, Mr Geoffrey Cannon and Dr Eric Brunner. From among the staff at the London School of Hygiene & Tropical Medicine, we are especially grateful to Professor Tony McMichael and to Dr David Leon, Dr Alison Tedstone and Dr Paul McKeigue.

Prakash S. Shetty
Klim McPherson
Alice Dickens

1
Overview of diet-related non-communicable diseases

1.1 Diet-related non-communicable diseases in Europe

Daan Kromhout and Bennie Bloemberg

National Institute of Public Health and the Environment, Bilthoven, The Netherlands

Within the affluent part of the world the state of health differs considerably. Life expectancy continues to increase in the United States and in Western Europe. This is, however, not the case in Eastern Europe, and in Russia life expectancy is actually decreasing. It is therefore of interest to describe the current state of health in affluent countries and to discuss the possible reasons for those differences. In this paper the description will be restricted to the European situation; this is because of the similarity between changes in the state of health in the United States of America (USA) and some Western European countries, e.g. Finland. The increase in life expectancy in these countries is mainly due to a decrease in age-standardised cardiovascular disease mortality. A recent paper from Minnesota showed that the decline in age-standardised coronary heart disease mortality in the USA that started in the mid-1960s is still continuing (McGovern *et al*, 1996). This is similar to the situation in Finland (Vartiainen *et al*, 1994).

Diet, Nutrition and Chronic Disease: Lessons from Contrasting Worlds.
Edited by P. S. Shetty and K. McPherson © 1997 John Wiley & Sons, Ltd.

Diet-related non-communicable diseases

There is a great deal of interest in the relationship between diet, lifestyle and non-communicable diseases. In recent years several comprehensive reviews on the subject have appeared. Two important recent reports emphasise the role of diet in the occurrence of these chronic diseases (US National Research Council, 1989; WHO, 1990). The most important associations between diet and chronic non-communicable disease *mortality* in Europe will be highlighted in this chapter, since comprehensive information on the state of health in Europe is only available for mortality. This overview will also be confined to cardiovascular diseases, cancer and chronic obstructive lung diseases because these are the major diet-related contributors to mortality in Europe.

Associations between diet and chronic diseases are largely but not exclusively based on observational epidemiological studies. For instance, when evaluating the role of diet in ischaemic heart disease, information is available about *in vitro* and *in vivo* studies on cholesterol metabolism, controlled metabolic studies on the influence of diet on serum cholesterol, population trials on the impact of serum cholesterol reduction and ischaemic heart disease occurrence, as well as clinical trials on the effect of diet modification on regression of coronary sclerosis (Levine *et al*, 1995). With respect to diet and cancer, most of the evidence is based on observational studies and population-based intervention trials (ATBC Prevention Study Group, 1994). A relatively new area is research on diet and the occurrence of chronic obstructive lung disease. In the two recent reviews on diet and chronic disease (US National Research Council, 1989; WHO, 1990), almost no attention was paid to the association between diet and pulmonary function. Results of recently reported observational studies suggest that diet may also be of importance in relation to respiratory disease (Sridhar, 1995).

A large number of associations have been made in observational studies on diet and chronic diseases. Only those for which consistent evidence from different types of studies is available will be reviewed here. Dietary fatty acids are important determinants of ischaemic heart disease occurrence. The Seven Countries Study has shown that population saturated fat intake levels are directly related to long-term coronary heart disease mortality rates (Kromhout *et al*, 1995). Metabolic studies have shown that saturated fatty acids, especially those with 12–16 carbon atoms, increase serum cholesterol compared with unsaturated fatty acids and carbohydrates (Keys *et al*, 1965; Mensink and Katan, 1992). Serum cholesterol levels are directly related to ischaemic heart disease occurrence, as has been shown in observational studies and intervention trials (Law *et al*, 1994). Lifestyle changes, including reductions in saturated fat, are associated with regression of coronary sclerosis (Ornish *et al*, 1990).

Trans fatty acids are formed by partial hydrogenation of oils in the production of margarines. Controlled metabolic studies have shown that these trans fatty acids increase total and LDL-cholesterol levels and decrease the protective

HDL-cholesterol fraction (Mensink and Katan, 1990). Positive associations between trans fatty acids and ischaemic heart disease have been reported in a prospective study of US women and in an ecological analysis of the data of the Seven Countries Study (Willett *et al*, 1993; Kromhout *et al*, 1995). Evidence is accumulating that, besides saturated fatty acids, trans fatty acids promote the occurrence of ischaemic heart disease. Mono- and polyunsaturated fatty acids, both of the n-6 and n-3 family, may be protective against ischaemic heart disease occurrence. However, the evidence is less strong than that for saturated and trans fatty acids (Willett, 1994).

Vegetables and fruits are rich sources of nutritive (e.g. beta-carotene, vitamin C and E) and non-nutritive (e.g. flavonoids) antioxidants. Antioxidants may play a role in the occurrence of cardiovascular diseases through their influence on atherosclerosis and thrombosis, and may also prevent binding of carcinogens to DNA and therefore have a protective effect on the occurrence of certain types of cancer. They may also prevent tissue damage in obstructive lung disease, an inflammatory phenomenon related to damage mediated by oxidants. Because of plausible mechanisms there is currently a great deal of interest in the role of vegetables and fruits in the prevention of chronic diseases.

Evidence for a protective effect of vegetables and fruits from cardiovascular diseases, such as ischaemic heart disease and stroke, was obtained in prospective studies (Kushi *et al*, 1985; Gillman *et al*, 1995). At normal levels of intake, the nutritive antioxidant beta-carotene is strongly associated with disease occurrence (Van Poppel *et al*, 1994). This association may, however, be limited to smokers. Of the non-nutritive antioxidants, flavonoids have been associated with a reduction in the occurrence of cardiovascular diseases (Hertog *et al*, 1993; 1995; Keli *et al*, 1996). Flavonoids are present in vegetables such as onions, in fruits such as apples, and in red wine and tea. Case-control studies have shown that persons consuming large amounts of vegetables and fruits were less prone to develop different types of epithelial cancers (Steinmetz and Potter, 1991). There is strong evidence for an inverse relationship between vegetable and fruit intake and lung and colon cancer, two of the most frequently occurring types of cancer in Europe. It has been suggested that the antioxidant beta-carotene is responsible for the inverse relationship between vegetable and fruit intake in lung cancer. This finding could not, however, be confirmed in either an interventional trial or an ecological study (ATBC Study Group, 1994; Ocké *et al*, 1995). The inverse relation between intakes of vegetables and fruits and the occurrence of colon cancer is probably not due to antioxidant vitamins, but dietary fibre may play a role (Greenberg *et al*, 1994; Howe *et al*, 1992). These results show that the relation between the intakes of vegetables and fruit, the responsible nutritive and non-nutritive antioxidants and the occurrence of epithelial cancers, is very complex and far from elucidated. The associations between vegetable and fruit intakes and the occurrence of the major hormone-dependent cancers such as breast and prostate cancer, are much weaker than those for epithelial cancers

(Steinmetz and Potter, 1991). Therefore, breast and prostate cancers are currently viewed as cancers in whose aetiology diet plays a minor role.

Cigarette smoking is the dominant risk factor for lung health (Sridhar, 1995). Therefore a possible role for diet in the occurrence of chronic obstructive lung disease has been neglected until recently. It has now been shown that a raised serum concentration of vitamin C has a protective effect against lung function and respiratory symptoms. Fruit consumption was also related to lung function and the occurrence of chronic obstructive lung disease. The results of these studies suggest that fruit intake or one of its major constituents, the antioxidant vitamin C, may be protective in relation to pulmonary function and health.

Patterns of mortality due to chronic disease

National mortality data from Europe have been submitted regularly to WHO for many years, and these data are used for international comparisons. Although most European countries perform analysis of mortality at the sub-national level, international analysis using sub-national data has been made only for selected diseases, e.g. cancer mortality by the International Agency for Research on Cancer (IARC), Lyon. The advantage of this type of analysis is that spatial variability in mortality patterns can be shown across borders. This may help in identifying factors responsible for this variation.

The World Health Organization European Centre for Environment and Health (WHO-ECEH) in collaboration with the United Nations Economic Commission for Europe (UN-ECE), the Central Bureau of Statistics of the Netherlands (CBS/Net) and the Dutch National Institute of Public Health and the Environment (RIVM) have conducted a project entitled *Spatial patterns of mortality at the sub-national level in Europe* (WHO-ECEH, in press). The aim of this project was to describe spatial variations by age, gender and selected cause-specific mortality rates across Europe, taking into consideration the sub-national patterns and their continuity across country borders. The results of this project are due to be published shortly, and only the methodology and results relevant to this paper are described here.

Regional data on population structure, all-cause and cause-specific mortality by age and gender, were made available by the National Statistical Offices and/or national institutes. The mortality data consisted of eight main groups of causes of death accounting for approximately 80% of all deaths as well as 17 specific diagnostic categories which constitute the most important causes of death in the European population. The boundaries for EU countries, as well as some other demographic data, were mainly provided by EUROSTAT and the boundaries for the rest of the WHO European Region were collated by WHO-ECEH.

The atlas presents maps for the combined mortality data of 1990 and 1991. These two years were combined in order to get more stable rates, and will for the sake of brevity be referred to as the 1990 data. All rates are per 100 000 population and directly standardised using the WHO European standard population of 1976. Rates are classified into the following seven categories: below 10, 10–25, 25–40, 40–60, 60–75, 75–90 and above 90th percentile. In order to draw more attention to the extreme regions the 90th and 10th percentile are used for calculating the ratio between regions with high and low mortality rates. All percentages are population weighted.

All-cause mortality

These maps also show distinct patterns in all-cause mortality rates in 1990; age-standardised mortality rates are higher in men than in women and show a clear west–east pattern. In both men and women all-cause mortality rates are almost twice as high in Eastern Europe as in Western Europe. The lowest mortality rates are observed in the Mediterranean countries while the highest is in Russia. Also, large variations can be observed within countries; for example, within the UK a distinct north–south gradient is present, with almost 50% higher all-cause mortality rates in the north compared with the south.

Ischaemic heart disease

Ischaemic heart disease mortality patterns are similar to all-cause mortality patterns. A clear west–east pattern can be noted here, with the highest mortality rates in Eastern Europe. The ratio between the 90th and the 10th percentile was, however, higher than for the all-cause mortality ratio: about 1.7 for all-cause mortality compared with about 5 for ischaemic heart disease mortality. The distribution shows that the differences in mortality rates within Western Europe are relatively small compared to those in Eastern Europe. In the UK the north–south gradient is also greater for ischaemic heart disease mortality than for all-cause mortality. Mortality patterns for stroke are comparable with those of ischaemic heart disease, with a few exceptions. Compared with the mortality for ischaemic heart disease, the mortality for stroke is higher in the Mediterranean countries and lower in Ireland.

Lung cancer, colorectal cancer and obstructive lung disease

An east–west gradient is also observed for lung cancer in males. The distribution appears to be bell-shaped, with noticeably low rates in the Nordic countries of Norway, Sweden and Iceland. For females, the rates are much lower than for males, with a more scattered picture and a much larger variation in rates. The percentile ratio in males is 2 while it is 5 in females. There is also no east–west gradient. The rates in the UK and Ireland are relatively high. For mortality from colorectal cancer, the highest rates are observed in Western Europe, with the exception of the Mediterranean countries. The picture is similar for males and females, with a percentile ratio of about 2 for both. The mortality rates for chronic obstructive lung disease are highest in the Eastern European countries and the UK for both males and females. The percentile ratio is about 3 for both sexes. It is also noticeable that in males this picture is comparable to that of lung cancer mortality rates.

The atlas shows that large differences of up to six-fold in mortality rates from chronic diseases are present within Europe. For public health purposes it is of interest to study the determinants of these population differences in chronic disease mortality rates. Regional differences may be due to socio-economic conditions, lifestyle variations including that of diet, environmental exposures, and accessibility to and effectiveness of health services. Further research on these associations is needed since it can provide important basic information for public health policy makers.

Changing ischaemic heart disease mortality patterns in Europe

Coronary heart disease mortality patterns have changed dramatically during the past 25 years in Europe. In the early 1970s, mortality rates were high in, for instance, Finland, and low in Eastern European countries like the former Yugoslavia (Uemura and Pisa, 1988; Vartiainen et al, 1994). Between 1972 and 1992 the age-standardised ischaemic heart disease mortality declined by more than 50% in men and women aged 35–64 in Finland (Vartiainen et al, 1994). However, between 1970 and 1985 increases of 65% and 36% were noted in ischaemic heart disease mortality in the former Yugoslavia in men and women, respectively, aged 35–64 (Uemura and Pisa, 1988). These data show that mortality rates from ischaemic heart disease can change very fast. From a public health point of view it is of interest to know what the determinants of these changes are. In the context of this paper, most emphasis will be put on the importance of changes in diet on the occurrence of ischaemic heart disease.

The extent to which changes in the main coronary risk factors (serum cholesterol, blood pressure and smoking) contribute to the decline in ischaemic heart disease mortality was evaluated for Finland (Vartiainen et al, 1994). Changes in all three risk factors together predicted a 44% decrease in ischaemic heart disease mortality in men and a 49% decrease in women. The actual percentage decline was 55% in men and 68% in women. These results show that reduction in risk factors is associated with a decrease in ischaemic heart disease mortality. It was estimated that a 13% decrease in serum cholesterol in Finnish men between 1972 and 1992 was responsible for a 26% decline in ischaemic heart disease mortality. The decrease in serum cholesterol is the consequence of dietary changes in Finland. Milk consumption as well as the fat content of milk decreased. The change from butter on bread to vegetable oil margarines led to a substantial reduction in saturated fat intake. The change from use of boiled to filtered coffee may also have contributed to lowering the serum cholesterol level.

These data suggest that population changes in diet are associated with a decline in serum cholesterol and consequently also of ischaemic heart disease. The decline in serum cholesterol in the Finnish population was thus responsible for more than 50% of the total decline in ischaemic heart disease mortality in Finland (Puska, this volume, Chapter 10).

Opposite trends in risk factors and ischaemic heart disease mortality were observed in the former Yugoslavia. Within the Serbian cohort of the Seven Countries Study a 1.5 mmol/l increase in serum cholesterol and a 28 mmHg increase in systolic blood pressure were noticed during 25 years of follow-up (Kromhout et al, submitted). At the start of the Seven Countries Study the serum cholesterol and systolic blood pressure level of Serbian middle-aged men were similar to those of their Japanese counterparts. Owing to substantial increases in serum cholesterol and systolic blood pressures, the 25-year mortality rate from ischaemic heart disease was more than twice as high in Serbian men as in Japanese men. At the baseline survey, the average serum cholesterol levels of Serbian and Japanese men were similar, i.e. about 4.3 mmol/l. During 10 years of follow-up the average serum cholesterol level of Serbian men increased by 1.2 mmol/l, in contrast to the serum cholesterol level of the Japanese men. Between 10 and 25 years of follow-up the average serum cholesterol level of the Serbian men increased by another 0.4 mmol/l. This meant that in 25 years the average serum cholesterol level of Serbian men increased from 4.3 mmol/l to 5.8 mmol/l. Such an increase in serum cholesterol levels has a large impact on the occurrence of ischaemic heart disease.

Based on observations around the world, it has been shown that population ischaemic heart disease mortality rates are uniformly low when average population serum cholesterol levels are below 5.2 mmol/l (Blackburn and Jacobs, 1989). Ischaemic heart disease is a major burden only in populations having a relative hypercholesterolaemia, i.e. an average serum cholesterol level of 5.7 mmol/l and above. The Serbian men shifted in 25 years from a low population average of 4.3 mmol/l to a high population average of 5.8 mmol/l. Ischaemic heart disease mortality survival curves show that differences in mortality between Serbian and Japanese men became apparent after 10 years of follow-up. Soon after the increase in the population average serum cholesterol level to above 5.2 mmol/l, the mortality rate from ischaemic heart disease started to increase. These observational data support the view based on interventional trials that the full impact of a change in serum cholesterol level is obtained after about 5 years of intervention (Law et al, 1994). Unfortunately, dietary data have only been collected during the baseline survey in Serbia. It is therefore not possible to relate the changes in serum cholesterol level to changes in the diet. It is likely that an increase in saturated fat intake in the diet occurred due to an increase in meat and animal fat consumption, as suggested by the food supply statistics (Kromhout et al, 1989).

These examples of Finland and Serbia show that changes in risk factors, including changes in diet, are related to changes in ischaemic heart disease mortality rates. This holds true both in relation to decreases and increases in the risk factors and the consequent effect on ischaemic heart disease mortality rates. Diets low in saturated and trans fatty acids and rich in vegetables and fruits may keep population chronic disease mortality rates low in low-risk cultures and will reduce chronic disease mortality risk in high-risk cultures. These dietary patterns are therefore a prerequisite for a healthy life expectancy and probably also for a good quality of life.

References

Alpha-tocopherol, Beta-carotene Cancer Prevention Study Group (ATBC). The effect of vitamin E and beta-carotene on the incidence of lung cancer and other cancers in male smokers. *New England Journal of Medicine*, 1994; **330**: 1029–1035

Blackburn H, Jacobs DR Jr. The ongoing natural experiment of cardiovascular disease in Japan. *Circulation*, 1989; **79**: 718–720

Gillman MW, Cupples LA, Gagnon D et al. Protective effects of fruits and vegetables on development of stroke in men. *Journal of the American Medical Association*, 1995; **273**: 1113–1117

Greenberg ER, Baron JA, Tosteson TD et al. A clinical trial of antioxidant vitamins to prevent colorectal adenoma. *New England Journal of Medicine*, 1994; **331**: 141–147

Hertog MG, Kromhout D, Aravanis C et al. Flavonoid intake and long-term risk of coronary heart disease and cancer mortality in the Seven Countries Study. *Archives of Internal Medicine*, 1995; **155**: 381–386

Hertog MG, Feskens EJ, Hollman PC, Katan MB, Kromhout D. Dietary antioxidant flavonoids and risk of coronary heart disease: the Zutphen Elderly Study. *Lancet*, 1993; **342**: 1007–1011

Howe GR, Benito E, Castelleto R et al. Dietary intake of fiber and decreased risk of cancers of the colon and rectum: evidence from the combined analysis of 13 case-control studies. *Journal of the National Cancer Institute*, 1992; **84**: 1887–1896

Keli SO, Hertog MG, Feskens EJ, Kromhout D. Dietary flavonoids, antioxidant vitamins and incidence of stroke. *Archives of Internal Medicine*, 1996; **154**: 637–642

Keys A, Anderson JT, Grande F. Serum cholesterol response to changes in the diet: IV Particular saturated fatty acids in the diet. *Metabolism*, 1965; **14**: 767–786

Kromhout D, Keys A, Aravanis C et al. Food consumption patterns in the 1960s in Seven Countries. *American Journal of Clinical Nutrition*, 1989; **49**: 889–894

Kromhout D, Nedeljkovic SI, Grujic MZ et al. Changes in major risk factors for cardiovascular diseases over 25 years in the Serbian cohorts of the Seven Countries Study. *International Journal of Epidemiology*, 1994; **23**: 5–11

Kromhout D, Menotti A, Bloemberg B et al. Dietary saturated and *trans* fatty acids and cholesterol and 25-year mortality from coronary heart disease: The Seven Countries Study. *Preventive Medicine*, 1995; **24**: 308–315

Kromhout D, Bloemberg B, Keys A et al. The dynamics of coronary heart disease in populations in relation to increases in risk factors. Submitted

Kushi LH, Lew RA, Stare FJ et al. Diet and 20-year mortality from coronary heart disease: The Ireland–Boston Diet-Heart Study. *New England Journal of Medicine*, 1985; **312**: 811–818

Law MR, Wald NJ, Thompson SG. By how much and how quickly does reduction in serum cholesterol concentration lower risk of ischaemic heart disease? *British Medical*

Journal, 1994; **308**: 367–372

Levine GN, Keany JF Jr, Vita JA. Cholesterol reduction in cardiovascular disease. *New England Journal of Medicine*, 1995; **332**: 512–520

McGovern PG, Pankow JS, Shahar E *et al.* Recent trends in acute coronary heart disease. Mortality, morbidity, medical care, and risk factors. *New England Journal of Medicine*, 1996; **334**: 884–890

Mensink RP, Katan MB. Effect of dietary trans fatty acids on high-density and low-density cholesterol in healthy subjects. *New England Journal of Medicine*, 1990; **323**: 439–444

Mensink RP, Katan MB. Effect of dietary fatty acids on serum lipids and lipoproteins. A meta-analysis of 27 trials. *Arteriosclerosis and Thrombosis*, 1992; **12**: 911–919

Ocké MC, Kromhout D, Menotti A *et al.* Average intake of antioxidant (pro) vitamins and subsequent cancer mortality in the 16 cohorts of the Seven Countries Study. *International Journal of Cancer*, 1995; **61**: 480–484

Ornish D, Brown SE, Sherwitz LW *et al.* Can lifestyle change reverse coronary heart disease? The Lifestyle Heart Trial. *Lancet*, 1990; **336**: 129–133

Sridhar MK. Nutrition and lung health. *British Medical Journal*, 1995; **310**: 75–76

Steinmetz KA, Potter JD. Vegetables, fruit and cancer. I. Epidemiology. *Cancer Causes and Control*, 1991; **2**: 325–357

Uemura K, Pisa Z. Trends in cardiovascular disease mortality in industrialized countries since 1950. *World Health Statistics Quarterly*, 1988; **41:** 155–178

US National Research Council. *Diet and Health. Implications for Reducing Chronic Disease Risk.* Washington, DC: National Academy Press, 1989

Van Poppel G, Kardinaal A, Princen H, Kok FJ. Antioxidant and coronary heart disease. *Annals of Medicine*, 1994; **26**: 429–434

Vartiainen E, Puska P, Pekkanen J, Tuomilehto J, Jousilahti P. Changes in risk factors explain changes in mortality from ischaemic heart disease in Finland. *British Medical Journal*, 1994; **309**: 23–27

Willett WC. Diet and health: What should we eat? *Science*, 1994; **264**: 532–537

Willett WC, Stampfer MJ, Manson JE *et al.* Intake of *trans* fatty acids and risk of coronary heart disease among women. *Lancet*, 1993; **341**: 581–585

World Health Organization (WHO). *Diet, Nutrition and the Prevention of Chronic Diseases.* WHO Technical Report Series 797. Geneva: WHO, 1990

WHO-ECEH, RIVM, UN-ECE, CBS. *Atlas of Mortality in Europe, Sub-national Patterns 1980/81 and 1990/91.* Copenhagen: WHO Scientific Publications, in press

1.2 Diet-related non-communicable diseases in South and South-East Asia

C. Gopalan

Nutrition Foundation of India, New Delhi, India

The countries of South and South-East Asia account for roughly 56% of Asia's population and about a third of the present world population (UNDP, 1995). Practically all these countries (with the exceptions of Nepal and Thailand) attained political freedom less than 50 years ago, and embarked on their developmental journeys, with the handicap of a fairly heavy backlog in different areas related to their overall social and economic development. Currently these countries are in different stages of developmental transition. According to the ranking by International Agencies (UNDP, 1995) based on a composite 'Human Development Index' derived by them from data on life expectancy, educational attainment and income, most of these countries fall in the 'medium' or 'low' categories; indeed, the only Asian countries that qualify for the 'high' category are Japan, South Korea, Singapore, Thailand and Malaysia.

Some major attributes of the developmental process to which these countries are now subject that have a bearing on the emergence and increasing rates of diet-related non-communicable diseases in these countries are: changes in dietary practices; urbanisation; demographic transition and ageing; and environmental degradation. These, along with other genetic and environmental factors that could contribute to the escalation of chronic diseases in these countries, are briefly considered here.

Changes in dietary practices

An important dietary change which has taken place among sections of the population that have moved up the socio-economic scale following on development is: the substitution of 'coarse' grains, the usual staple of the poor, by more 'prestigious' cereals—wheat and rice—which could result in a significant curtailment of the dietary fibre intake (Gopalan, 1994). Intake of green leafy vegetables, scorned as the 'poor man's food' of low social prestige, remains low. There has been a progressive increase in fat intake with a growing preference for hydrogenated fat in place of vegetable oils, a relatively high intake of ghee (clarified butter) and a higher intake of animal foods. Intake of sugars has also increased, as has overall energy consumption in relation to energy expenditure. The important beneficial dietary change has been the increased consumption of legumes, fruit and vegetables.

Urbanisation

A major attribute of developmental transition is rapid urbanisation and the growth of mega-cities. The total urban population of Asia, which was 226 million in 1950, will be nearly 1245 million by 2000 AD and it is estimated (Buch, 1991) that the population of 13 Asian cities will have exceeded 10 million by then. An important side-effect of urbanisation, and of recent policies of economic liberalisation, is the emergence of a rapidly expanding 'urban middle class' who, in India alone, number over 200 million. It is this segment of the population that seems specially prone to chronic degenerative disease because of the dietary changes, and the effects of stress and environmental pollution.

Rising affluence in the rapidly emerging middle class is being reflected in the increasing incidence of obesity. A comparison of the BMI profile for the general adult male population (largely composed of the rural poor) as reported by the Indian National Nutrition Monitoring Bureau, with the BMI profile of a group of middle-class urban male adults in Delhi in a study being carried out by the Nutrition Foundation of India highlights this point (Nutrition Foundation of India, unpublished data). The rising incidence of obesity is associated with an increase in coronary heart disease (CHD) and diabetes mellitus.

Demographic transition and ageing

An inevitable consequence of increasing life-expectancy and decreasing birth-rate incidental to development is a progressive change of age-structure of popula-tions—ageing of populations. This process is already evident in Japan, and to a lesser extent in other countries of Asia. Ageing of populations is a major factor contributing to the progressive escalation in the overall incidence of chronic degenerative disease in these populations.

Environmental degradation

Unregulated urbanisation and industrialisation appear to be responsible for considerable degradation of the environment in many parts of Asia (Gopalan, 1992). Some aspects of such environmental degradation may be expected to contribute to the escalation of degenerative diseases and cancer and include the following:

1. Depletion of soil micronutrients due to faulty and unregulated use of intensive agricultural technology as part of the Green Revolution. The heavy use of chemical fertilisers and intensive irrigation not generally accompanied by soil replenishment have resulted in the depletion of zinc, sulphur, iron and other micronutrients in the soil (Kanwar, 1990). Studies by the Food and Agriculture Organization (FAO) (1982) in several countries, including some in Asia, have revealed such micronutrient depletion, especially of zinc, reflected in poor yield and eventually in poor micronutrient content of foods grown on such soils.
2. Pollution of riverine and marine food sources by toxic industrial effluents from, for example, pulp, paper, textiles, tanneries, sugar, distilleries, coal and petrochemicals, being discharged into rivers and ponds in developing countries in the absence of a vigilant regulatory authority. The important metallic pollutants of water sources in Asian countries appear to be mercury, lead, cadmium, copper, zinc and chromium. Pesticide use, intensive and indiscriminate in agricultural operations, is an important source of contamination, as is insecticide used during the storage of foods to prevent spoilage.
3. Air pollution—urban populations in the densely crowded growing cities of Asia are particularly exposed to air pollution (Gopalan, 1995). Nearly two-thirds of the air pollution in cities such as Delhi and Bangkok is attributable to emissions from fossil fuel use. It seems reasonable to argue that at least part of the striking differences in the incidence of CHD between urban and rural Asia could be attributable to air pollution, and not merely to changes in dietary patterns. The toxic components in polluted air may be powerful pro-oxidants known to have a deleterious effect on a range of body functions and the requirement for antioxidant intake in the diet may be presumably higher in urban populations than in rural.
4. Contaminants in processed foods may also contribute. These include the use of non-permitted colours and preservatives during food-processing and highlight the lack of adequate controls and mechanisms to regulate the food industry in a rapidly expanding economy.

Other factors

The rising incidence of chronic degenerative diseases in developmental transition populations in Asia have other determinants:

Genetic factors. There is evidence of greater vulnerability of South Asian migrants to CHD and diabetes, as compared to the native populations. This increased susceptibility is reflected by the prevalence to Syndrome X characterised by abdominal obesity, hyperinsulinaemia, hypertriglyceridaemia, low concentration of high-density lipoprotein (HDL) and hypertension. Syndrome X and its associated susceptibility to CHD and diabetes mellitus may have a genetic basis. In support of this is the reported increase in LP (a) levels in Asian migrants

(Bhatnagar and Durrington, 1993; Cremer *et al*, 1994). This genetic trait may not find expression in conditions of poverty and in the absence of amplifying factors such as dietary excesses and errors. The role of genetics as determinants of plasma cholesterol and other facets of lipoprotein metabolism is now more clear, and may contribute to population differences in the prevalence of CHD and diabetes (Simopoulos, 1995). Dealing with dietary and lifestyle changes during developmental transition that may express the genetic susceptibility of specific populations becomes urgent.

Foetal undernutrition.   The fascinating studies of Barker's group (Barker, 1995) suggest a possible aetiological role for foetal undernutrition in the development of chronic degenerative diseases in adulthood (Barker, this volume, Chapter 2). Barker's group postulate that intra-uterine growth retardation (IUGR) 'programmes' the foetal tissues, such that amplifying factors associated with affluence in adult life lead to chronic degenerative diseases. Considering that the incidence of low birthweight is high in South Asian countries (Table 1.1), this hypothesis may explain the rising incidence of CHD in urban populations of Asia in transition, particularly among those born in poverty but emerging into affluence in their adulthood.

Current situation in Asian countries

Data on degenerative diseases and cancer in many South and South-East Asian countries are often incomplete. Apart from their paucity, data may not be entirely reliable because of under-reporting from deficient case detection and recording. The extent of these deficiencies may vary from country to country and from time to time, making inter-country and intra-country comparisons and time trends of limited value. Nevertheless, there are discernible trends revealed by well controlled small-scale studies, and degenerative diseases and cancer are emerging as major causes of death in some South and South-East Asian countries.

Table 1.1   Percentage of infants with low birthweight (1990)

South Asia	%	South-East Asia	%
Bangladesh	50	Cambodia	–
India	33	Indonesia	14
Nepal	26	Laos	18
Pakistan	25	Malaysia	10
Sri Lanka	25	Philippines	15
		Thailand	13
		Vietnam	17
		Fiji	18
		Papua New Guinea	23

Source: UNDP, 1993

In the interpretation of data pointing to increasing proportions of deaths from degenerative diseases and cancer in these countries, however, three factors other than a true increase in the incidence of these diseases must be borne in mind:

1. Progressive reduction in the incidence of major infectious diseases which hitherto figured as major causes of death.
2. Increasing longevity.
3. Improvements in case detection and reporting.

Such data on age-specific evidence as are available, however, do indicate a progressive increase, showing that increasing longevity may not be the major contributor to this increase. If present trends continue, within the next three decades South and South-East Asia may emerge as the region with the highest concentration of cases of diabetes mellitus and CHD.

CHD

The traditional predominantly cereal-based diets of these countries are rich in fibre and low in saturated fats, cholesterol and meat, and must be considered to favour a low incidence of CHD. Kestin and others (1989) have pointed out that, in general, vegetarians have lower serum lipid and blood pressures than omnivores, and that substitution of conventional high-fat, high-meat diets by lacto-vegetarian diets could result in a significant lowering of blood pressure, serum total cholesterol and low-density lipoproteins. With a considerable proportion of India's population being vegetarians by choice or economic compulsion, there is a strong need to foster and preserve the salutary traditional dietary practices currently in vogue amongst vast sections of the population. However, there are already indications of an escalation in the prevalence of CHD in urban areas of some Asian cities for which reports are available. Table 1.2 presents data relating to deaths due to CHD in some countries of the region, while Table 1.3 summarises the results of a community-based survey of CHD carried out by Chadha and colleagues (1990) in Delhi, India.

One can discern from Table 1.3 two distinct factors that are associated with an increased prevalence of CHD, i.e. urbanisation *per se*, and affluence. The prevalence rate (for both sexes) in the lower-income urban group was 14.0 per 1000 as compared to 5.9 per 1000 for the rural population. The rural population, although predominantly composed of low-income groups, also included a small proportion of middle- and high-income families, and the diets of the urban population, in particular that of the low-income groups, had lower energy and fat content than the rural diets. This difference must be considered as significant, and as reflecting the effects of factors attributable to the urban environment *per se*, rather than to the result of dietary change. The prevalence in the urban high-income groups, at 46.1 per 1000, is a three-fold increase over that in the low-income groups. This difference may be attributed to affluence and lifestyle

Table 1.2 Death rates from all cardiovascular diseases

Country	Year	Death rate per 100 000 persons
Brunei	1992	86.3
Japan	1992	251.4
Malaysia	1991	60.4
Philippines	1991	124.6
Singapore	1992	176.7
Thailand	1992	79.2

Source: *SEAMIC Health Statistics, 1993*

Table 1.3 CHD prevalence rate per 1000 adults (Delhi Study)

	Urban			
	All	High SES	Low SES	Rural
Male	39.5	61.0	20.0	7.4
Female	25.3	30.2	8.5	5.1
Total	31.9	46.1	14.0	5.9

SES = Socio-economic status
Source: Chadha *et al*, 1990

changes associated with sedentary occupations, and possibly other factors, such as stress. Dietary surveys in the same populations (Chadha *et al*, 1996) showed that the diets of the urban poor with a higher prevalence of CHD than the rural population provided less energy and lower levels of fat intake. The diets of the higher-income urban groups provided higher levels of energy and fat than the diets of the urban poor, but did not contain high levels of ghee (clarified butter), to the increased intake of which, because of its cholesterol oxide content (Jacobson, 1987), is attributed a higher vulnerability of Indian immigrants to CHD. The role of factors other than dietary changes in an urban environment—including lack of adequate physical exercise, stress arising from competitive occupations, and exposure to environmental pollution—may be important.

In a study of CHD factors in a randomly selected group of migrants from India living in West London, Bhatnagar *et al* (1995) found that serum LP (a) levels were similar to their siblings living in India but were significantly higher than those seen in native British populations. On the other hand, the UK migrants had higher BMIs, systolic blood pressures, serum cholesterol, triglycerides and apolipoprotein Bs, fasting blood glucose and lower HDLs with increased insulin resistance compared to their siblings in India. These data have been interpreted as indicating that 'excess CHD mortality and increased prevalence of non-insulin dependent diabetes mellitus in migrant Asians' relate to a 'conspiracy of genetically acquired risk factors that are potentiated and supplemented by Westernization'. Studies of the rural and urban differences (Chadha *et al*, 1990;

1996) suggest that internal migration from rural to urban environments may bring about marked increases in the prevalence of CHD and non-insulin-dependent diabetes mellitus (NIDDM).

Non-insulin-dependent diabetes mellitus

There are striking ethnic differences with respect to the prevalence of NIDDM in world populations, and the available evidence suggests a special vulnerability of Indian migrant populations (Ramaiya *et al*, 1990) (Table 1.4).

Several epidemiological studies carried out in different parts of India in the 1960s and 1970s had generally indicated a prevalence rate of NIDDM of about 2.4%. Because of considerable variability in sample selections, small sample size, and lack of uniformity with respect to criteria for diagnoses in these different studies, these earlier studies were of limited value. A major multi-centric study (Ahuja, 1979) of the prevalence of diabetes was carried out under the auspices of the Indian Council of Medical Research (ICMR) in the late 1970s on a large and representative sample. Reliable analytical methods were employed, using uniform standardised and statistically acceptable sampling procedures. The study revealed an overall prevalence rate of 2.1% in the urban and 1.5% in the rural population. Breakdown of the data on the basis of age, sex and location, set out in Table 1.5, indicates that the urban male over 40 years of age is the most vulnerable. It did not reveal a linear relationship between diabetes prevalence and low socio-economic status, low calorie intake and low bodyweight.

When this survey was done, almost 20 years ago, less than 20% of India's population was urban. In the 1990s, nearly 35% of India's population is urban, and the population over 40 years of age, according to recent estimates, accounts

Table 1.4 Prevalence (percentage) of NIDDM in migrant Indians compared to other ethnic groups

Country	Ethnic group						
	European	African	Melanesian	Malay	Chinese	Creole	Indian
Trinidad	4.3(M)	8.2(M)	–	–	–	–	19.5(M)
	10.2(F)	14.8(F)					21.6(F)
Fiji	–	–	3.5(M)	–	–	–	12.9(M)
			7.1(F)				11.0(F)
South Africa	–	3.6	–	6.6	–	–	10.4
Singapore	–	–	–	2.4	–	–	6.1
UK							
(Coventry)	2.8(M)	–	–	–	–	–	11.2(M)
	4.3(F)						8.9(F)
Mauritius	–	–	–	–	11.5	10.4	12.4
Tanzania	–	1.9	–	–	–	–	7.1

Source: Ramaiya *et al*, 1991

Table 1.5   Prevalence (percentage) of diabetes mellitus in India by age and place of residence (1972–1975)

Age group	Prevalence rate	
	Urban	Rural
15–29	0.9	0.7
30–39	1.0	1.0
Over 40	5.0	2.8
Total M + F	2.1	1.5
M	2.6	1.8
F	1.5	1.4

Source: Ahuja, 1979

for 22.2% of the total population. Using the prevalence rates reported in the ICMR study (Ahuja, 1979) it may be estimated that the number of subjects with diabetes in India would exceed 20 million in 1996. In recent population studies in South India consisting of smaller sample sizes, Ramachandran et al (1992) have claimed that the age-adjusted prevalence of diabetes was as high as 8.2% in urban areas and 2.4% in rural areas. If this finding is generalised, it would imply that, in the years between the two surveys, both the overall prevalence rate and the urban–rural differences have further increased, and that the prevalence rate among Indians in urban India is just as high as that reported among South Asian migrants in the UK.

The predominant type of diabetes in India is the non-insulin-dependent variety, i.e. NIDDM. Obesity, using BMI as criterion, appears to be a much less common feature of NIDDM in India than it is in Europe and the USA. Only 22% and 47% of men and women diabetics respectively in a study in India (Yajnik, 1995) were obese, compared with about 80% of cases of NIDDM in the West. On the other hand, the Indian diabetics exhibit features of the insulin resistance syndrome and higher waist/hip ratios, i.e. abdominal obesity.

There are ethnic and regional differences even within Asian countries with respect to susceptibility to CHD and NIDDM. It is not yet clear whether these differences are of genetic origin, or whether they can be explained on the basis of Hales and Barker's 'thrifty phenotype' hypothesis (1992). Even within South Asia, Bangladeshis are less prone to CHD than Sindhis (Shaukat, 1995), possibly due to their higher levels of fish consumption. Properly conducted epidemiological studies among populations of South and South-East Asia may help tease out the possible genetic, dietary and environmental factors involved in the escalation of incidence of CHD and NIDDM in South Asia.

Cancer

Food and dietary practices, lifestyle and cultural differences apparently play an important role, and if international epidemiological studies on cancer reveal large differences in the incidence rates between different geographic and ethnic groups. Doll and Peto (1981) estimated that 35% of cancers in the USA may be diet-related. It has been estimated (*World Health Report 1995*; WHO, 1995) that there are 9 million new cases of cancer occurring every year in the world. Cancer accounts for 6 million, or 12%, of total global deaths, some 58% of them in the developing world (Doll and Peto, 1981). In India alone, 6–700 000 new cases of cancer are estimated to occur with an estimated prevalence of 1.5 to 1.8 million. The age-adjusted incidence rates for all types of cancers in India are currently estimated at about 130 in males and 120 in females per 100 000 population (Table 1.6).

The overall age-specific incidence of cancer in males exceeds that in females in the age groups < 25 years and > 55 years; the picture is reversed in the age groups 25 to 55 years, with females showing a higher incidence (NCRP, 1988). Table 1.7 shows that the death rates due to cancer are well below 50 per 100 000 in the countries of South and South-East Asia, with the exception of Singapore. Among Asian countries, the highest cancer death rate in Asia is recorded in Japan, the most affluent. This picture could change rapidly within the next few decades.

There are apparently some differences with respect to the sites of cancer occurrence between South and South-East Asian countries, and the USA and European countries. The percentage distribution of cancer incidence by site and sex in India (Table 1.8) suggests that 35–40% of cancers in India are related to tobacco chewing, and the sites of occurrence are the oral cavity, oesophagus and stomach and larynx in men (NCRP, 1988). In women, cancers of the cervix predominate. The incidence of breast cancer in women (Table 1.9), though not infrequent, appears to be less than in Europe and the USA. Lung cancer also appears to be less frequent in Asian countries than in Europe and the USA, but

Table 1.6 International comparison of age-adjusted (world population) incidence rate (AAR) of cancer per 100 000 persons

Year studied	Registry		AAR Male	AAR Female
1978–1982	USA	White	318.1	263.0
		Black	381.1	240.4
1979–1982	UK	Birmingham	235.1	188.8
		Oxford	245.3	203.7
1978–1981	Japan (Miyanzi)		215.1	144.8
1978–1982	Singapore (Indian)		153.7	171.2
1989	India	Bombay	130.4	120.4
		Delhi	118.8	140.7
		Madras	118.5	135.0
		Barshi (rural)	57.6	52.2

Sources: International Agency for Research on Cancer (1987); NCRP (1989)

Table 1.7   Death rates per 100 000 due to malignant neoplasms (1991–1993)

Country	Male	Female	Total
Malaysia[a]	–	–	23.2
India[b]	25.7	24.5	25.2
Philippines[a]	37.5	32.5	35.0
Brunei[a]	37.5	37.2	37.3
Thailand[a]	51.2	35.7	43.5
Singapore[a]	135.1	98.1	116.1
Hong Kong[c]	192.1	121.2	157.3
Japan[a]	230.5	146.7	187.8
USA[c]	221.5	187.5	204.1
France[c]	307.6	187.0	245.7
Germany[c]	273.4	254.6	263.7
World[d]	–	–	108.2

Sources:
[a] *SEAMIC Health Statistics, 1993*
[b] Based on resident cancer deaths and resident population in selected areas (NCRP, 1989)
[c] *World Health Statistics Annual, 1994* (WHO, 1995)
[d] *The World Health Report, 1995* (WHO, 1995) (estimated)

Table 1.8   Percentage distribution of cancers in India by site and sex

Site	Male	Female
Oral cavity	10	6
Pharynx and larynx	13	–
Breast	–	20
Lung	9	–
Oesophagus	7	5
Stomach	7	3
Other digestive organs	10	7
Urogenital	11	–
Ovary	–	5
Cervix	–	24
Leukaemia and lymphomas	12	6
Others	21	24
Total	100	100

Estimates based on crude incidence rates for Bangalore, Bombay, Madras, Delhi (NCRP, 1989)

this picture could change rapidly because of increasing air pollution in Asian countries, increasing trends in smoking among the young, and heavy addiction to smoking in some of these countries.

The possible effect of prevailing food and diet practices in Asian countries on cancer risk may be seen. While in the case of cancer of the breast, colon, rectum,

Table 1.9 Comparison of age-adjusted incidence rate (AAR) per 100 000 breast for and lung cancer

			AAR	
		Breast	Trachea, bronchus and lung	
Year studied	Country	(F)	(M)	(F)
1978–1982	USA (Connecticut) White	77.8	64.3	25.3
	Black	61.3	89.8	21.9
1979–1982	UK (Oxford)	61.3	68.8	19.5
1978–1981	Japan (Miyanzi)	25.0	–	–
1989	India: Delhi	28.3	11.9	2.2
	Bombay	26.1	14.6	3.7
	Madras	24.6	11.1	1.7
	Bangalore	22.3	8.6	1.6
	Barshi (rural)	6.8	2.0	0.0

Sources: International Agency for Research on Cancer (1987); NCRP (1989)

endometrium, ovary and gall bladder, excess calorie intake, low dietary fibre and high saturated fat intakes associated with raised BMI are considered as possible risk factors, cancers of the stomach, cervix and oesophagus in India are commonly seen among poor income groups and are inversely related to low BMI. Other factors such as high salt intake, nitrate/nitrites, and intake of sun-dried fish have all been claimed to be related to stomach and oesophageal cancers. Micronutrients such as beta-carotene, vitamin A, riboflavin, folic acid, vitamin C, iron, zinc and selenium which are now claimed to be potent antioxidant agents that act by suppressing carcinogenesis are often deficient in the diets of poor segments of the Asian populations—a deficiency now likely to be further aggravated by soil micronutrient deficiencies induced by intensive agriculture. It is also unfortunate that in the countries of South Asia, despite their rich biodiversity and the availability of vegetables and fruits, the dietary intake of vegetables and fruits is very low. The possible benefits that could accrue from phytochemicals with anti-carcinogenic properties present in these food sources are currently not being exploited.

The role of food contaminants, especially fungal food contaminants such as aflatoxin, in the pathogenesis of liver cancers has attracted some attention because of the presence of aflatoxin contamination of several foods arising from poor storage (Bhat and Miller, 1991). In Thailand, parasitic diseases are also believed to play a possible contributory role in liver cancers. Nitrosamines in chillies and salted tea consumed in Kashmir are believed to increase the risk of oesophageal cancers frequently seen in that State.

Apart from the low intake of saturated fats in Indian diets, it is possible that phyto-oestrogens in plant foods like soya may also play a role in protection against breast cancers. This could perhaps explain the relatively lower incidence of breast cancers in women of South Asian countries. However, we have no clear evidence as yet to support such a hypothesis. The possible role of curcumin, derived from turmeric, a commonly used food item, in protection against certain types of cancer also merits consideration.

Thus it will be seen that some of the aspects of the prevailing dietary profile among poor sections of South and South-East Asian populations could favour the development of certain types of cancer, indicating that the lack of affluence in a majority of these populations does not confer freedom from cancer risks. On the other hand, there are other aspects of the diets which are beneficial.

With rising affluence and with a burgeoning middle class, cancer risks associated with affluence, of the types seen in developed countries, could emerge as important risk factors among Asian populations as well. Indeed, this is already happening. There are indications of rising incidence of cancers of the breast, colon and lung, previously relatively low in comparison to Western countries. Thus, the countries of South and South-East Asia which have not as yet shed their problems of poverty and diseases associated with deprivation, will soon face a double burden, of having to combat cancers arising from nutritional deficiencies and traditional dietary habits among the poor on the one hand, and cancers arising from dietary errors and excesses and unhealthy lifestyles on the other. The decades ahead will thus pose a challenge to Asian countries with respect to containment of control of chronic degenerative diseases and cancer.

Conclusion

The changing profile of diseases in Asia, characterised by a steady decline in the incidence of infectious diseases and a rise in degenerative diseases and cancers, carries highly disturbing far-reaching implications to the health systems of these countries. The emerging chronic diseases are generally far more expensive to treat, require much longer duration of treatment, and yield far less rewarding results than acute communicable diseases. Together with increasing demands for the care of the aged, whose numbers are also gradually increasing, the overall cost of health care in Asian countries will escalate very steeply in the coming decades. This is the price of 'development'. The resources available for health care in most of these countries, however, are currently far too meagre even to meet basic health needs. Policy-makers and planners of these countries in the next few decades will be hard put to make agonising choices with respect to the allocation of meagre resources between the care of the old and chronically ill and the care of the young and acutely ill; between the rural poor and the expanding urban middle class. This cruel dilemma will underscore the need for the institution and vigorous implementation of appropriate preventive measures consisting of the avoidance of dietary errors and excesses, and the promotion of healthier lifestyles. The countries of South and South-East Asia can learn a great deal in this regard from the experience of Europe and North America.

References

Ahuja MMS. Epidemiological studies on diabetes mellitus in India. In: Ahuja MMS, ed. *Epidemiology of Diabetes in Developing Countries*. New Delhi: Interprint, 1979, pp. 29–38

Barker DJP. Fetal origins of coronary heart disease. *British Medical Journal*, 1995; **311**: 171–174

Bhat RY, Miller JD. Mycotoxins and food supply. *Food, Nutrition and Agriculture*, 1991; **1**: 27–31

Bhatnagar D, Durrington PN. Does measurement of apoliproteins add to the clinical diagnosis and management of dyslipidaemias? *Current Opinions in Lipidology*, 1993; **4**: 299–304

Bhatnagar D, Anand IS, Durrington PN *et al*. Coronary risk factors in people from the Indian subcontinent living in West London and their siblings in India. *Lancet*, 1995; **345**: 405–409

Buch MN. Integration of environmental considerations into city planning in intermediate cities. 1991. Unpublished paper presented at ESCAP Conference, Bogor, Indonesia

Chadha SL, Radhakrishnan S, Ramachandran K, Kaul U, Gopinath M. Epidemiological study of coronary heart disease in urban population of Delhi. *Indian Journal of Medical Research*, 1990; **92**; 424–430

Chadha SL, Gopinath N, Shekhawat S. Dietary factors and urban rural incidence of coronary heart disease. *Indian Cardiothoracic Journal*, 1996; **2**

Cremer P, Nagel D, Labrot B *et al*. Lipoprotein (a) as predictor of myocardial infarction in comparison to fibrinogen, LSL cholesterol and other risk factors: results from the prospective Gottingen Risk Incidence and Prevalence Study (GRIPS). *European Journal of Clinical Investigation*, 1994; **24**: 444–453

Doll R, Peto R. *The Causes of Cancer: Qualitative Estimates of Avoidable Risks of Cancer in the United States*. New York: Oxford University Press, 1981

Food and Agriculture Organization (FAO). Micronutrients and the nutrient status of soil: a global study. *FAO Soils Bulletin*, 1982; **48**

Gopalan C. *Nutrition in Developmental Transition in South-East Asia*. Regional Health Paper SEARO/WHO, No 21. New Delhi: CBS, 1992

Gopalan C. 'Micronutrient' Deficiencies—Public Health Implications. *Nutrition Foundation of India Bulletin*, 1994; **15**: 1–6

Gopalan C. Coronary heart diseases in Delhi—the possible role of air pollution (Reviews and Comments). *Nutrition Foundation of India Bulletin*, 1995; **16**: 6–7

Hales CN, Barker DJP. Type 2 (non-insulin dependent) diabetes mellitus: the thrifty phenotype hypothesis. *Diabetologia*, 1992; **35**: 595–601

International Agency for Research on Cancer. *Cancer Incidence in Five Continents. Vol V*. Lyon: IARC, 1987

Jacobson MS. Cholesterol oxides in Indian ghee: possible cause of unexplained high risk of atherosclerosis in Indian immigrant populations. *Lancet*, 1987; **ii**: 656–658

Kanwar JS. Inaugural address at Micronutrient Workshop. Andhra Pradesh Agricultural University, Hyderabad, India, 1990

Kestin M *et al*. Cardiovascular disease risk factors in free living men. Comparison of two prudent diets, one based on lacto-vegetarianism and the other allowing meat. *American Journal of Clinical Nutrition*, 1989; **50**: 280–287

National Cancer Registry Project (NCRP). Biennial Report 1988–89. New Delhi: Indian

Council of Medical Research, 1989

Ramachandran A, Snehalatha C, Dharmaraj D, Viswanathan M. Prevalence of glucose intolerance in Asian Indians—urban–rural difference and significance of upper-body adiposity. *Diabetes Care*, 1992; **15**: 1348–1355

Ramaiya KL, Kodali VRR, Alberti KGMM. Epidemiology of diabetes in Asians of the Indian subcontinent. *International Journal of Diabetes in Developing Countries*, 1990; **11**: 15–35

Ramaiya KL, Swai AB, McLarty DG, Bhopal RS, Alberti KG. Prevalence of diabetes and cardiovascular disease risk factors in Hindu Indian subcommunities in Tanzania. *British Medical Journal*, 1991; **303**: 271–276

SEAMIC Health Statistics 1993. International Medical Foundation of Japan, 1993

Shaukat N. Coronary artery disease in Indo-origin people: possible aetiological mechanisms and preventive measures. *Practical Diabetes International*, 1995; **17**, 273–275

Simopoulos AP. Genetic variation and nutrition. *Nutrition Today*, 1995; **30**: 157–167

United Nations Development Programme (UNDP). *Human Development Report 1993*. New York: Oxford University Press for UNDP, 1993

United Nations Development Programme (UNDP). *Human Development Report 1995*. New York: Oxford University Press, 1995

World Health Organization. Study Group Report on Diabetes Mellitus. Technical Report Series no. 727. Geneva: WHO, 1985

World Health Organization. *The World Health Report 1995: Bridging the gaps*. Geneva: WHO, 1995

World Health Organization. *World Health Statistics (annual)* 1994. Geneva: WHO, 1995

Yajnik CS. Diabetes and insulin resistance syndrome in Indians. *Nutrition Foundation of India Bulletin*, 1995; **16**: 1–5

1.3 Diet-related non-communicable diseases in China

Chen Chunming

Chinese Academy of Preventive Medicine, Beijing, China

China has a population of 1.2 billion, a quarter of whom live in urban centres. With the rapid economic development over the past 18 years, the lives of people have improved, and incomes have increased dramatically. However, the disparities between rich and poor are widening, generating sufficient government concern to cause action to be taken to mitigate the problem. Over 70 million people (7.8% of the rural population) are located in poor areas, and the government has recently launched a national programme on poverty alleviation, aiming for the eradication of poverty by the year 2000. Undernutrition is a significant problem, with the national average for the prevalence of underweight children below five years of age at 17.9% in 1992 (Chang, 1994). Problems of overnutrition are also emerging since the diet and lifestyle of the population have been rapidly changing.

In 1994, mortality due to non-communicable diseases accounted for 66% of the total mortality (76% urban and 64% rural) (Table 1.10). Over 90% of the non-communicable disease mortality was attributed to cancer, cardiovascular diseases, chronic respiratory diseases, digestive and urogenital diseases. Of these, 38% of the mortality was attributed to cardiovascular diseases, 22% to cancer and 28% to chronic obstructive pulmonary diseases (COPD) (MOPH/CAPM, 1996).

Status and trends of chronic diseases in China

Cardiovascular diseases

Disease surveillance data show that cerebrovascular and ischaemic diseases were the principal cause of death both in urban and rural areas (MOPH/CAPM, 1996) (Table 1.11).

Table 1.12 compares data collected in a 1986 survey of the urban population of nine provinces and four urban populations (Beijing and Hebei in the north, and Zhejiang and Guangdong in the south) in 1990.

According to data collected by MONICA-China, in 1987 the incidence of stroke in men in the north ranged from 3.8 to 8.7 per thousand, while it ranged

Table 1.10 Mortality and infant mortality (per thousand)

	1994	1991
Mortality	5.74	6.21
IMR	32.04	33.17

Source: Chinese Ministry of Public Health and Chinese Academy of Preventive Medicine (MOPH/CAPM) (1991; 1994)

Table 1.11 Total mortality from cerebrovascular disease and ischaemic heart disease disaggregated from urban and rural areas for the years 1991 and 1994

	Year	Mortality per thousand population		
		Total	Urban	Rural
Cerebrovascular disease	1994	0.84	0.97	0.80
	1991	0.70	0.88	0.65
Ischaemic heart disease	1994	0.26	0.42	0.22
	1991	0.21	0.35	0.17

Source: Chinese Ministry of Public Health and Chinese Academy of Preventive Medicine (MOPH/CAPM) (1996)

Table 1.12 Prevalence of cardiovascular disease and hypertension in population aged over 20 (per thousand)

	CVD	CHD	HT
1986: 9 cities	7.00	16.01	48.90
1990: Beijing	20.23	80.13	99.96
1990: urban in Hebei Prov.	17.86	42.66	62.96
1990: urban in Zheijang Prov.	7.78	41.57	60.22
1990: urban in Guangdong	13.00	14.47	40.96

Source: Chen and Shao (1994)

from 1.3 to 3.2 in the south. In 1993, the incidence increased to between 4.1 and 11.1 in the north and remained unchanged in the south (MONICA, 1995). It is estimated that there are 1.5 million annual deaths due to stroke alone. Of the 5 million stroke patients, 75% lost the ability to be involved in productive labour while 40% were seriously disabled. The estimated number of hypertensive patients in China is currently about 90 million. These trends are also illustrated in Table 1.13.

Cancer

Mortality due to cancer of the digestive tract accounts for 60% of cancer mortality while 20% is due to respiratory tract cancer. Mortality from digestive cancer in urban areas is about 50% of the total cancer mortality, while it is 66% in rural areas of China. Mortality from respiratory cancer on the other hand is higher in urban areas, accounting for about 30% of the total cancer mortality while contributing only 16% in rural areas. National cancer trends are shown in Table 1.14. There was a marked sex difference evident in the mortality rates from lung, stomach and liver cancer in urban China in 1994, as shown in Table 1.15.

Lung cancer mortality was closely related to smoking. Seventy per cent of adults aged over 15 smoke, and the population pattern of the smoker is shifting towards an increase in the younger age groups, with more young adults starting smoking while more older people are giving it up. It is not unlikely that lung cancer mortality will increase even more rapidly in future decades. It is estimated that lung cancer mortality will be 19.4 per 100 000 in the year 2000, and will reach 40 per 100 000 in 2030 (MOPH/CAPM, 1996).

Table 1.13 The increase in the prevalence (percentage) of hypertension among population aged over 15, comparing data on blood pressure measurements

	1958–1959	1979–1980	1991
National survey	5.1	7.7	11.9
Beijing survey	7.4	13.7	19.7

Source: Chinese National Survey Team (1982, 1993)

Table 1.14 Cancer mortality changes from
1990 to 1994 (national average, per 100 000)

	1994	1990
Lung cancer	16.07	13.84
Stomach cancer	16.57	19.55
Liver cancer	16.63	15.88
Oseophageal cancer	10.53	10.62

Source: Chinese Ministry of Public Health and
Chinese Academy of Preventive Medicine
(MOPH/CAPM) (1996)

Table 1.15 Sex difference in the mortality rates from
lung, stomach and liver cancer in urban China in 1994

	Cancer mortality per 100 000	
	Males	Females
Lung cancer	40.6	16.7
Stomach cancer	21.0	8.7
Liver cancer	27.1	9.4

Source: Chinese Ministry of Public Health and Chinese
Academy of Preventive Medicine (MOPH/CAPM) (1996)

Diabetes mellitus

The prevalence of diabetes mellitus in Beijing in 1989 was 1.2% of the population
aged over 15 years, 0.9% for males and 1.4% for females (Yen *et al*, 1990). A repeat
survey in Beijing in 1994 (Yuan, in press) showed that the prevalence of diabetes
mellitus had increased to 3.4%. Among people aged over 60, 15–20% are
diabetic. The estimated number of diabetic patients in China is 20 million.

Chronic obstructive pulmonary diseases (COPD)

The mortality attributed to COPD in 1994 was 105.6 per 100 000: 63.0 per
100 000 in urban areas and 115.7 per 100 000 in rural areas. Half the mortality is
attributable to chronic bronchitis (MOPH/CAPM, 1996).

Risk factors

Dietary pattern changes

Along with economic development and the increase in income of the people, food
security at household level appears to be solved. In terms of national averages
and household income group comparisons, the caloric needs have been met. The
average protein intake is 64 g *per capita* per day. Between 1990 and 1992, meat

consumption of urban households increased substantially; 75% of the households in the urban area of the sampled provinces or municipalities have increased their meat consumption by at least 20% within the past two years, with one-third of these households increasing by 50–100%. In rural households, a greater increase in meat consumption was seen in the more developed provinces and among richer households. Edible oil consumption has also increased markedly, both in urban and rural households (Chen, in press).

As a result of these dramatic and rapid changes, the diet shows a reduction in the contribution of cereals to the total energy intake and an increase in the energy share of fat (Chen, in press). Before the period 1990–1992, cereal energy contribution was 60–70% in urban households and around 80% in rural households. Since that time, at least 75% of urban households have reduced cereal energy content to below 60%. The reduction of cereal contribution from 80–85% to around 70–75% is a sign of dietary improvement in rural populations. The richer households in Beijing and Guangdong (about 25% of total households) reduced cereal energy content to below 55% in 1992 (Chen, in press). The same study shows that there is a further reduction of cereal energy share along with economic development; half the urban households in Beijing have reduced cereal energy contribution to under 50%, and in Guangdong the richest 25% of households have even reduced it to 39%.

Energy share of fat in the diet has dramatically increased. Seventy-five per cent of the urban households had fat energy over 30% of total energy intake, while in the richest 25% of households, it went up to 35%, and increased even as high as 39% of total energy intake in the richest 10% of households in Guangdong, in 1992. In rural households, the average fat energy share increased from around 13% to 21% during 1990–1992 (Ge, 1996); most of the households had a fat energy intake higher than 15% of total energy intake. It is worth noticing that half the rural households in Beijing Municipality and in Guangdong increased fat intakes to 29–33% of total energy. A study in Beijing (Bei *et al*, in press) reveals that between 1989 and 1995 vegetable oil intakes increased by 13 g/person/day and fat intake of people aged 35–74 increased from 30% to 33%. The effectiveness of nutrition education in reducing oil consumption appeared to be very low from an evaluation in a Non-Communicable Disease Demonstration Area in Beijing (Bei *et al*, in press).

Cholesterol intake in the diet was maintained at 400–500 mg per day. Serum cholesterol in 1989 is shown in Table 1.16. Correlation analysis in this data set showed that serum cholesterol level was positively correlated to blood pressures (data not shown).

Salt intake

Salt intake in China varied geographically, ranging from 13–17 g per person in the north to 11–15 g in the south. A positive correlation between salt intake and

Table 1.16   Serum cholesterol in 1989

| Age group | Serum cholesterol (mg/dl) | |
	Males	Females
35–44	166.2	150.0
45–59	178.7	183.5
60–75	171.7	187.7

Source: Bei J *et al* (in press)

blood pressure was also seen. Community education on salt intake reduction changed people's behaviour. The intervention group reduced salt intake from 12.5 g to 8.8 g between 1989 and 1995 while the average salt intake of the control group remained at 12.4 g throughout this period (Ge, 1996).

Calcium intake

The Chinese diet is usually low in calcium, with intakes around 400–500 mg/day, if little or no dairy product is consumed (Ge, 1996). Milk consumption in China is very low; even in the cities where milk is available, it is mostly consumed by children and the elderly. The national average for milk consumption is only 11 kg *per caput* per year for the urban population.

Alcohol intake

Alcohol intake is increasing along with increases in income, especially among the younger generation. The intake of alcohol was equivalent to 15 g of wine (with 12% alcohol) per day in 1992, 20 g for urban and 13 g for rural population (Ge, 1996). A study of the elderly in Beijing showed that the percentage of people consuming alcohol was 13% in 1989 and reached 16% in 1995 among people aged 35–70. A five-year education campaign helped maintain the percentage of alcohol consumers, 13.2% in 1989 and 13.6% in 1994 in the Demonstration Area in Beijing, while the rate kept rising from 12.9% to 15.9% in the control area during that same period (Bei *et al*, in press).

Smoking

Estimates of smoking among the Chinese during the years 1984 and 1991 based on a random sample survey indicated that 58% of males over the age of 15 smoked. The highest incidence of smoking in males over the age of 15 in 1991 was in Yunnan province (74.1%) while the lowest was in Hainan (50.3%). Among females, the highest smoking rate was in Tianjin Municipality (18.8%) and the lowest was in Guangdong Province (1.2%) (Nui *et al*, in press).

Hypertension

The prevalence of hypertension in middle age is high in China. A survey in the East District of Beijing among the age range 40–45 in 1989 showed a sudden rise from 73.9 to 140.9 per thousand. The prevalence of hypertension is highest at 324.8 per thousand among those aged 65. The prevalence is substantially different between those who are illiterate or have only a primary education (308.3 per thousand) and those with middle school or university education (85.5 per thousand). Salt intake and BMI are positively associated with high blood pressure in Chinese adults (Ge, 1996).

A community management programme for hypertensives showed that behavioural change was an important factor responsible for several beneficial effects: smoking rate reduced to 13.8% during the years 1989 and 1994 in the intervention group, a statistically significant reduction compared to controls who remained at 34.1% during the same period (Bei *et al*, in press). Alcohol consumption also decreased from 5.9% to 1.8% in the intervention group, while increasing by 1.1% in the control group (from 13.6% to 14.7%). Consequently the percentage of individuals with normal blood pressure in the intervention group increased significantly (Bei *et al*, in press).

Body Mass Index

The Body Mass Index (BMI) of adults has been gradually going up in China. The percentage of people with BMI over 25 increased from 7.2% in 1982 to 14.9% in 1992 among urban adults aged 20–45. Among rural populations it was 5.5% and 8.4% respectively (Chen, in press). Among people aged over 20, 31–53% were overweight in the East District of Beijing. There was a significant increase in overweight individuals in the middle age group, namely 36.5% in men and 53.1% in women. BMI has been identified as one of the risk factors for hypertension in that area (Bei *et al*, in press).

Conclusion

In conclusion, during the process of economic development and improvement in the economic status of the people, non-communicable diseases are emerging along with the changes in the risk factors predisposing to chronic disease. This is a matter of great concern from the public health as well as the economic viewpoint, and preventative measures should be taken promptly to avoid the disasters resulting from a dramatic increase of disease burden, especially in developing countries in transition such as China where nutritional deficiencies and problems associated with overnutrition co-exist.

References

Bei J, Yan DY *et al.* Community prevention on non-communicable diseases and control of risk factors: five year evaluation, in press

Chang Y, Zhai F, Li W, Ge K, Jin D, de Oris M. Nutritional status of preschool children in poor rural areas of China. *Bulletin of the World Health Organization*, 1994; **72**: 109

Chen CM. The nutrition status of Chinese people. Proceedings of the 7th Asian Congress of Nutrition. *Biomedical and Environmental Sciences*, 1996; **2**: in press

Chen CM, Shao ZM. *Food, Nutrition and Health Status of Chinese in Seven Provinces*, 1990. Beijing: China Statistical Publishing House, 1994

Chinese Ministry of Public Health. *1986 Survey on Health Services in 9 Provinces/Municipalities.* Beijing: Chinese Ministry of Public Health, 1987

Chinese Ministry of Public Health and Chinese Academy of Preventive Medicine. *1991 Annual Report on Chinese Disease Surveillance.* Beijing: Hua Xia Publishing House, 1993

Chinese Ministry of Public Health and Chinese Academy of Preventive Medicine. *1994 Annual Report on Chinese Disease Surveillance.* Beijing: Hua Xia Publishing House, 1996

Chinese National Survey Team. Report of Nationwide Survey of Hypertension, 1982 (In-house publication)

Chinese National Survey Team. Report of Nationwide Survey on Hypertension, 1993 (In-house publication)

Ge KY. *The Dietary and Nutritional Status of Chinese Population (1992 National Nutrition Survey).* Beijing: CAPM/People's Publishing House, 1996

MONICA Study Group. MONICA Report of China, 1995 (In-house publication)

Nui SR, Wang GH *et al. Report of Survey on Smoking in 1991*, 1996, in press

Yen, DY *et al.* The report of survey on non-communicable diseases in East District of Beijing. *Disease Surveillance*, 1990; **5**: 174–176

Yuan SY *et al.* Prevalence of diabetes in Beijing. *Chinese Journal of Endocrinology and Metabolism*, 1996, in press

1.4 Diet-related non-communicable diseases in the Caribbean and Latin America

Dinesh P. Sinha

Caribbean Food and Nutrition Institute (PAHO/WHO), Kingston, Jamaica, West Indies

Nations at various stages of their socio-economic development experience different patterns of morbidity and mortality. In the early stages of development, countries face the onslaught of nutritional deficiencies and communicable diseases. The victims are mostly children, many of whom die, making life expectancy low. As development proceeds and life expectancy increases, the brunt of diseases and death shifts gradually from children to people in middle and later life, in which the major problems, such as obesity and chronic non-communicable diseases, are mostly lifestyle-related. Omran (1971) described this continuum of changes in the mortality pattern as the 'epidemiological transition', a phenomenon now generally recognised by many as inevitable in the economic development process. As a result of developments in the past 30 years, the countries of the Caribbean and Latin America have experienced the epidemiological transition and massive degrees of obesity and a very high rate of morbidity and mortality due to diabetes, high blood pressure, heart disease, stroke and cancer have replaced undernutrition and infectious diseases as public health problems. This paper presents a status report on mortality due to diet-related non-communicable diseases in the Caribbean and Latin America and relates the changing food pattern in the Caribbean and its relationship to these changing disease patterns.

Changing patterns of mortality

While there is much to be desired in the accuracy of diagnosis and reporting of the causes of deaths, Caribbean and the Latin American countries do have a consistent reporting system for most deaths. Apart from using these data at the national level for various purposes, they are reported to the Pan American Health Organization (PAHO/WHO) every four years. PAHO then produces standardised death rates for all countries using a reference population (PAHO, 1990). Since the number of deaths from various causes in some of the Caribbean countries are very small, the Caribbean Food and Nutrition Institute (CFNI) recently acquired data on the number of deaths from five chronic diseases mentioned above for the years 1986–1991. Using the same reference population as PAHO, it has calculated mean annual age-standardised death rates (Sinha, 1995a). Some of these results are presented below, including a comparison of the rates from the Caribbean and Latin America with those of Canada and the USA.

An examination of the data on the patterns of deaths between the late 1950s or early 1960s and those of the 1990s shows that the main burden of deaths has shifted from young children (0–4 years) to middle-aged (35–64 years) and older (65 years and above) persons (PAHO, 1966; 1990). Thus in Saint Lucia in 1958 and Dominica in 1961 more than half the deaths were in children under five. By 1990, the pattern shifted and more than three-quarters of the deaths were in middle-aged and older persons. In Barbados in 1990, only 3% of deaths were in children under five, 76% of deaths were in people above 65 years of age, a pattern typical of industrialised countries (e.g. the USA). A similar pattern was noticed in Costa Rica, Chile and Cuba.

The causes of deaths have also changed during this period of time. During the mid-1960s in the Caribbean, 14–54% of deaths were due to infectious diseases and nutritional deficiency disorders and 10–45% due to the five major chronic diseases; during the 1980s these figures changed to 2–7% and 25–57% respectively (Figure 1.1) (PAHO, 1966; 1990; Sinha, 1995b). A similar picture again can be noticed in some of the Latin American countries (Figure 1.2).

Comparison of the deaths due to hypertensive disease, diabetes, stroke (cerebrovascular disease) and coronary heart disease (CHD) in the Caribbean with those from Canada and the USA is very revealing. Death rates due to diabetes, hypertension and stroke in the Caribbean far exceeded those of North America, whereas the rates for CHD were higher in North America than in most Caribbean countries. Cancers in which diet has been implicated are also major causes of deaths in the Caribbean. Comparisons of death rates for cancers of breast, prostate, colon, rectum and stomach in the Caribbean have been made with those of Canada and the USA. Breast cancer mortality was almost as high in six Caribbean countries as in North America, while prostate cancer rates were higher in 11 countries. Compared with Canada and the USA, rates for colorectal cancer were low in all Caribbean countries (PAHO, 1996).

Changing nutritional status of the population in the Caribbean

The nutritional status of the Caribbean people has been changing rapidly. Kwashiorkor and marasmus in children, once a common sight, are infrequent, and anaemia appears to be on the decline. Available data from some of the countries indicate that 17–45% of pre-school children were malnourished during the 1960s and early 1970s. By the late 1980s and early 1990s, this picture had dramatically changed (Table 1.17) (Sinha, 1995a).

A large proportion of the population, particularly females, are reported to be obese, as early as in their teenage years. Occasional surveys conducted since the 1970s in different countries reveal that obesity is a highly prevalent condition in the Caribbean. It was evident from these surveys that 7–20% of males and 20–48% of females above 15 years of age were obese (Sinha, 1984).

Changing food situation in the Caribbean and its relationship to chronic disease mortality

The food situation

Agriculture and associated economic activities continue to play a major role in the social life of the Caribbean. Nevertheless, these countries have always depended on outside sources for most of their food needs. In recent years, despite a decline in agricultural production in most countries, food availability has increased as a result of food imports. The increase in food availability is mostly

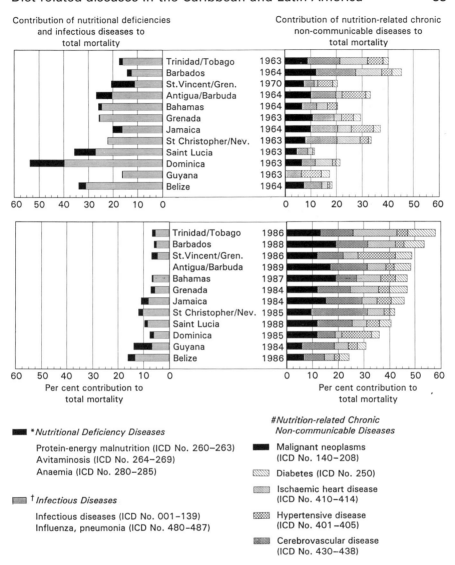

Figure 1.1   Changing mortality patterns in the Caribbean. (Data provided by countries to the Health Situation Analysis Program of the PAHO Health and Development Division and stored in the PAHO Mortality Database, Washington, DC (PAHO, 1996))

from foods from animal sources and fats. This is further compounded by the present low intake of fruits, vegetables, roots and tubers which may be partly responsible for the changing disease pattern.

Most of the data on food availability are from food balance sheets since actual

34 D. P. Sinha

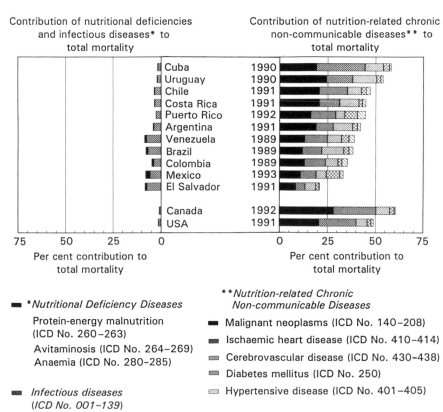

Contribution of nutritional deficiencies and infectious diseases* to total mortality

Contribution of nutrition-related chronic non-communicable diseases** to total mortality

Per cent contribution to total mortality

Per cent contribution to total mortality

■ *Nutritional Deficiency Diseases

Protein-energy malnutrition (ICD No. 260–263)
Avitaminosis (ICD No. 264–269)
Anaemia (ICD No. 280–285)

■ Infectious diseases (ICD No. 001–139)

**Nutrition-related Chronic Non-communicable Diseases

■ Malignant neoplasms (ICD No. 140–208)
■ Ischaemic heart disease (ICD No. 410–414)
▦ Cerebrovascular disease (ICD No. 430–438)
▨ Diabetes mellitus (ICD No. 250)
▨ Hypertensive disease (ICD No. 401–405)

Figure 1.2 Changing mortality patterns in Latin America. (Data provided by countries to the Health Situation Analysis Program of the PAHO Health and Development Division and stored in the PAHO Mortality Database, Washington, DC (PAHO, 1996))

food consumption data on the adult population are limited. In the Caribbean, regular food balance sheets have been available from the 12 independent countries since the 1960s (FAO, 1990). On the basis of the recommended dietary allowance for the Caribbean (CFNI, 1994), which is set at an average of 2250 kcal of energy and 43 g of protein per person per day to meet the population goal, an analysis of the available food data from 1961–1963 to 1988–1990 showed a definite increase in the total energy available per person per day. Protein availability was nearly sufficient in all countries in the early 1960s and further increased in all countries in the late 1980s, to levels of 30–130% above the population goal. Thus calorie and protein availability has improved significantly in the past 25 years and enough calories and protein are presently available to meet the requirements of the total population. Most of the increase in calorie availability is due to an increase in total fat consumption, largely caused by an

Table 1.17 Levels of malnutrition (weight-for-age <80% of standard) in pre-school children in the countries of the Caribbean (late 1980s and early 1990s)

Negligible levels of malnutrition (<5%)	Minor levels of malnutrition (5–10%)	Moderate levels of malnutrition (>10%)
Antigua and Barbuda	Belize	Guyana
Bahamas	Grenada	
Barbados	Jamaica	
British Virgin Islands	St Christopher-Nevis	
Cayman Islands	Saint Lucia	
Dominica	Trinidad and Tobago	
Montserrat		
St Vincent and the Grenadines		
Turks and Caicos Islands		

increase in foods from animal sources, mostly meats, milk and milk products. In fact, meat (beef, pork, poultry) is the largest contributor of fat, followed by milk and milk products (butter), and separated fat (lard and vegetable oil) comes next. The contribution of seafoods is very small (Figure 1.3).

Among the complex carbohydrate sources, the amount of cereals has increased in six Eastern Caribbean countries. Almost all countries have more than sufficient cereals available for consumption. Requirements for roots, tubers,

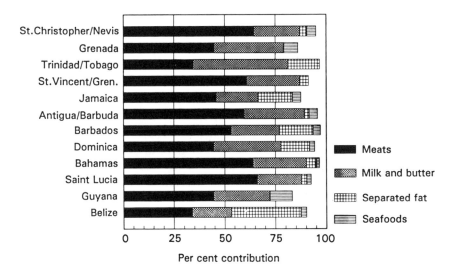

Source: FAO (1990)

Figure 1.3 Contribution of fat to the diet in the Caribbean (FAO, 1990)

legumes, fruits and vegetables, which most Caribbean countries can produce in sufficient quantities, are not, however, met by any of the countries, and most countries show gross deficiencies in these sources of food. Sugar consumption in the Caribbean is very high, despite the fact that, unlike in the past, not all countries in the Caribbean currently produce sugar.

It is therefore evident that in the countries of the Caribbean, on a population basis, there is no deficit in calories and protein. Availability of animal foods, fats and oils, has been increasing consistently. Sugar consumption is high but there is a gross deficiency of complex carbohydrate foods and fruits, vegetables, roots, tubers and legumes. This trend is typically the one against which the experience of the past 30 years of research in nutrition and health warns us.

Evidence for the relationship between diet and health in the Caribbean

It is evident that in the Caribbean, food availability, and thus the food consumption patterns, has rapidly changed. Indeed, these changes are conducive to an increase in chronic non-communicable disease. Is there any support for the assumption that changing dietary patterns may have been responsible for the changing disease patterns? Ecological studies show that this may be so.

Allowing for a time lag of 5–7 years between dietary change and chronic disease prevalence, an analysis of these two data sets—food consumption patterns and disease prevalence—shows that the countries with higher *per caput* calorie availability also have significantly higher mortality due to diabetes mellitus. Similarly, countries with higher *per caput* fat availability also have higher mortality due to CHD, while death rates due to CHD are inversely related to *per caput* availability of fruits and vegetables and roots and tubers. Cancers of several sites have also been found to be significantly related to the availability of fat and dietary fibre (Sinha, 1995a). Thus the countries which have higher *per caput* fat availability also have higher mortality due to prostate, breast and colorectal cancers. While no relationships have been shown between colorectal cancer and total carbohydrate foods, it is inversely related to *per caput* availability of cereals, roots and tubers. Another interesting finding is the relationship between types of fat and mortality due to cervical cancer. While the variation in total fat availability is not related to cervical cancer mortality, higher availability of fat from plant sources (oils) is directly related and fat from animal sources is inversely related to cervical cancer mortality.

References

CFNI. *Recommended Dietary Allowances for the Caribbean*. Kingston, Jamaica: Caribbean Food and Nutrition Institute Press, 1994

Food and Agriculture Organization of the United Nations (FAO). *Food Balance Sheets 1986–88*. Rome: FAO, 1990

Omran AR. The epidemiological transition—a theory of epidemiology of population change. *Milbank Memorial Fund Quarterly*, 1971; **4**: 509–515

PAHO. *Health Conditions in the Americas, 1961–64*. Scientific Publication No 138. Washington, DC: Pan American Health Organization, 1966

PAHO. *Health Conditions in the Americas*, 1990 Edition, Vol 1. Scientific Publication No 524. Washington, DC: Pan American Health Organization, 1990

Sinha DP. Obesity and related diseases in the Caribbean. *Cajanus*, 1984; **17**: 79–106

Sinha DP. Changing patterns of food, nutrition and health in the Caribbean. *Nutrition Research* 1995a; **15**: 899–938

Sinha, DP. *Food, Nutrition and Health in the Caribbean—A Time for Re-examination*. Kingston, Jamaica: Caribbean Food and Nutrition Institute Press, 1995b

1.5 Diet-related non-communicable diseases in the Middle East countries

Abdulrahman O. Musaiger

United Arab Emirates University, Al Ain, United Arab Emirates

Most of the Middle East countries have faced profound demographic, socio-economic and behavioural transformation during the past three decades. These changes in diet and lifestyle have led to great changes in the health and nutritional status of the population. Infectious diseases and undernutrition have gradually disappeared, and chronic non-communicable diseases, such as heart disease, diabetes mellitus and cancer, are becoming more prevalent. However, in a region as vast and varied as the Middle East, stretching from Libya to Iran, with countries that range from the poorest to the richest in the world, the study of chronic non-communicable diseases is difficult. Therefore, we divided these countries into three categories, based on two relevant indicators: *per capita* GNP and Daily Energy Supply (DES), derived from FAO Food Balance Sheets (FAO, 1990):

1. High-income countries with *per capita* GNP above US$6000 and DES above 3000 kcal/*caput*. This group includes petroleum-exporting countries: Libya, Saudi Arabia, Kuwait, United Arab Emirates (UAE), Qatar, Bahrain and Oman.
2. Intermediate-income countries with *per capita* GNP between US$600 and $3000, and DES between 2700 and 3300 kcal/*caput*. This group includes Cyprus, Egypt, Iraq, Iran, Jordan, Lebanon, Syria, Tunisia and Turkey.

3. Low-income countries with *per capita* GNP below US$500 and DES between 2000 and 2300 kcal/*caput*. This group includes Djibouti, Somalia, Sudan and Yemen.

Changes in food consumption patterns

In general, the food situation in the Middle East has markedly improved during the three decades from 1960 to 1990. However, the change in food habits is not the same in the three groups of countries. In the *high-income countries*, the traditional diet, which consisted of dates, milk, fresh vegetables and fruits, whole wheat bread and fish, has changed to a more Westernised diet, with an excess intake of energy-dense foods rich in fat and free sugars and deficient in complex carbohydrates (Musaiger, 1994), with the daily energy intake exceeding 3000 kcal/*caput*. Sugar consumption is rising despite being already very high (30–40 kg/*caput*/annum), its contribution to the total energy intake ranging between 10 and 15%. The same trend may be seen for fat consumption, both vegetable and animal, which is now estimated at around 30 kg/*caput*/annum, contributing over 30% to the total energy intake (FAO, 1990).

The average *per caput* calorie supply in the *intermediate-income* countries is between 2700 and 3000 kcal. Cereals contribute more than half the calorie supply. Sugar consumption has also risen considerably to reach an average level of 30–40 kg/*caput*/annum. Similarly, fat consumption has increased in several countries and it contributes 20–25% of the DES. The change in habitual dietary intakes in these countries is mainly due to the shift to middle and upper social classes in the two decades (1970–1990) following the economic boom and the development of industry and services. Most of the people now live in large cities which are gradually adopting the eating habits and lifestyles of the wealthier classes elsewhere (FAO, 1990).

The *low-income* countries have the same food consumption characteristics as many poor countries in the world. The daily caloric supply is insufficient (2000–2300 kcal) and cereals contribute 60–80% of total calorie intake (Table 1.18). It is worth mentioning, however, that in the large cities of these low-income countries, the higher social classes have similar dietary intakes to their counterparts in the intermediate- and high-income countries.

Diet-related chronic non-communicable diseases

Trends in morbidity and mortality have changed dramatically in the high-income countries (especially in the Arab Gulf countries) and in some parts of the intermediate-income countries. In the low-income countries, chronic non-communicable diseases are not common health problems, and there are no reliable reports of their prevalence in the community.

Table 1.18 Contribution (percentage) of nutrients to Daily Energy Supply (DES) in the Middle East countries

	Low-income countries	Intermediate-income countries	High-income countries
Carbohydrates	55–75	60–70	59–60
Fats	15–20	20–25	29–30
Proteins	10–12	10–11	10–12
Complex carbohydrates	60–70	50–60	45–50
Sugar	3–12	9–12	10–15
Animal fat	4–7	4–10	11–15
Cereals	60–80	45–65	35–40

Source: FAO (1990)

Chronic non-communicable diseases such as cardiovascular disease, cancer, hypertension and diabetes mellitus have become the major health problems in high-income countries, and in urban areas in intermediate-income countries. Improved standards of living and health services have contributed to a longer life expectancy in these countries. The average life expectancy has reached 61–69 years and 70–76 years in intermediate- and high-income countries respectively, compared with 41–51 years in low-income countries. Deaths due to heart disease represent 30–37% of total deaths in high-income countries, while those due to cancer reached 10–16%. The prevalence of diabetes mellitus among adult populations is very similar to that reported in developed countries at between 10 and 14%.

The increase in *per capita* income has led to a greater availability of cars, televisions and labour-saving household appliances, resulting in the lifestyle of the people in these countries becoming more sedentary, and consequently the physical activity level of the population has significantly diminished. In addition, dietary intake estimates indicate a high intake of energy-rich foods, largely the result of increased fat intakes. The prevalence of obesity in both intermediate- and high-income countries, especially among women, has reached alarming levels. About 30–70% of women in these countries are overweight and obese (BMI > 25), while the prevalence among men was 14–50% (Table 1.19). Epidemiological studies have indicated that obesity is a major risk factor for several chronic diseases (Simopoulos, 1985).

Smoking has increased dramatically in all these countries, especially among young people, and alcohol consumption has also increased in some countries. The fast food industry is booming, and has become the favoured food consumed outside the home for the whole family, particularly among adolescents and young adults. Studies in the region indicate that a substantial proportion of the population has cholesterol levels above that considered to be the upper permissible limit (Alwan, 1993; Al-Nuaim *et al*, 1995).

Table 1.19   Some health indicators in Middle East countries

Health indicators	Low-income countries	Intermediate-income countries	High-income countries
Low birthweight (%)	16–20	13–16	6–8
Infant Mortality Rate (per 1000)	>100	30–80	<25
Life expectancy (years)	41–51	61–69	70–76
Death, heart disease (%)	–	16–31	30–37
Death, cancer (%)	–	2–8	10–16
Adult obesity (BMI >25)			
Males (%)	–	14–20	30–50
Females (%)	–	30–60	50–70
Adult diabetes (%)	–	4–8	10–14

Sources: FAO (1990); Alwan (1993); Musaiger (1994)

Conclusion

With the increase in prevalence of chronic non-communicable diseases as well as the rise in risk factors for these chronic diseases in most intermediate- and high-income Middle East countries, there is little doubt that non-communicable diseases in this part of the world will become a major public health problem. An action plan to prevent and control these diseases is urgently needed. Studies on the causes and magnitude of non-communicable diseases are essential for any intervention programmes. It is important that national governments and policy-makers in these regions initiate nutritional and health education programmes to reverse or contain this dangerous trend. It is recommended that international organisations such as WHO and FAO support research and intervention programmes to overcome these diseases in the countries of the Middle East.

References

Al-Nuaim A, Al-Rubean K, Al-Mazrou Y, Khoja T, Al-Attas O, Al-Daghari N. *National Chronic Metabolic Diseases Survey.* Riyadh: Ministry of Health and King Saud University, 1995

Alwan AAS. Diseases of modern lifestyles: the need for action. *Health Services Journal of the Eastern Mediterranean Region*, 1993; **7**: 24–34

Food and Agricultural Organization (FAO). *A Balanced Diet—A Way to Good Nutrition.* FAO Document NERC/90/4. Rome: FAO, 1990

Musaiger AO. Diet-related chronic diseases in the Arab Gulf countries: the need for action. *Ecology of Food and Nutrition*, 1994; **32**: 91–94

Simopoulos A. The health implications of overweight and obesity. *World Review of Nutrition and Dietetics*, 1985; **43**: 33–40

2
Prenatal influences on disease in later life

David J. P. Barker

Medical Research Council Environmental Epidemiology Unit, University of Southampton, UK

Recent research has shown that babies who are small at birth and during infancy will be at increased risk of developing coronary heart disease and the related disorders, stroke, diabetes and hypertension, during adult life (Osmond *et al*, 1993; Barker, 1995). That a person's destiny and lifespan may be determined before birth is well known. Genetically determined diseases such as Huntington's chorea illustrate how a long period of normal development and adult life can be prematurely brought to an end by the action of inherited defects. We are now seeing that undernutrition *in utero* permanently changes the body's structure and function in ways that 'programme' the appearance of disease in later life.

The main focus for research into the causes of coronary heart disease (CHD) has been the lifestyle of adults. Inappropriate behaviours, such as cigarette smoking and becoming obese, have been shown to hasten destructive processes in the body. Differences in lifestyle, however, fail to explain much about the geography of the disease, its time trends, or why one person gets the disease and another does not. In the search for a new model for the disease an important clue, suggesting that CHD might originate *in utero*, came from studies of death rates among newborn babies in the early years of the century (Barker and Osmond, 1986; 1987). It was found that, across England and Wales, areas that have high death rates from CHD had high death rates among newborn babies in the early years of the century. At that time the usual cause of death among newborn babies was small size.

Rose (1964) had previously reported that siblings of patients with CHD had stillbirth and infant mortality rates that were twice as high as those of controls. He concluded that 'ischaemic heart disease tends to occur in people who come from a constitutionally weaker stock', a conclusion foreshadowing what is known today. Later studies in Norway and Britain (Forsdahl, 1977; Barker and Osmond,

Diet, Nutrition and Chronic Disease: Lessons from Contrasting Worlds.
Edited by P. S. Shetty and K. McPherson © 1997 John Wiley & Sons, Ltd.

1986; 1987) had revealed a geographical relationship between cardiovascular mortality and past infant mortality. While this was initially attributed to events in childhood or adolescence that predispose individuals to CHD (Forsdahl, 1977), studies in Britain, where data on infant mortality were more detailed, clearly pointed to the foetal life as a critical window of early development (Barker and Osmond, 1986; 1987). A focus on intrauterine life, and hence on the mother rather than the child, was a new point of departure for cardiovascular research.

Foetal growth

The body does not increase greatly in size during embryonic life but in the foetal period, from nine weeks after conception, there begins the phase of rapid growth and functional maturation which continues until after birth. The main feature of growth is, of course, cell division. Different tissues of the body grow during periods of rapid cell division, so called critical periods (Widdowson and McCance, 1975). The timing of these 'critical' periods differs for different tissues. The kidney, for example, has a critical period of development in the weeks immediately before birth (Hinchcliffe et al, 1992). Growth depends on nutrients and oxygen. The foetus' main adaptation to lack of these is to slow its rate of cell division, especially in those tissues which are in their 'critical' periods of growth at the time. Cell division slows either as a direct effect of undernutrition on the cell or in response to altered concentrations of growth factors or hormones, of which insulin and growth hormone are particularly important. Even brief periods of undernutrition may permanently reduce the numbers of cells in particular organs (Winick and Noble, 1966; Winick et al, 1968; Widdowson et al, 1972). This is one of the mechanisms by which undernutrition may permanently change or 'programme' the body. Other lasting 'memories' of undernutrition include change in the distribution of cell types, in hormonal feedback, in metabolic activity and in organ structure. The diversity of size and form of babies born after normal pregnancies is remarkable. From studies of birthweight of relatives, Penrose (1954) and others (Morton, 1955; McCance and Widdowson, 1974) have concluded that variation in size at birth is essentially determined by the intrauterine environment rather than the foetal genome.

Table 2.1 shows one of many experiments on animals which have shown that undernutrition of a foetus is followed by persisting long-term effects on physiology and metabolism (Langley and Jackson, 1994). In this experiment, rats born to mothers who had low protein intakes during pregnancy had persistently raised blood pressure. Similar experiments have demonstrated persisting changes in lipid metabolism, carbohydrate metabolism, in insulin response to glucose, and in a range of metabolic, endocrine and immune parameters (Barraclough, 1961; Hahn, 1984; Lucas, 1991; Mott et al, 1991; Smart, 1991). It seems easy to programme the structure and function of animals and there seems no reason why the human body is not equally readily programmed.

Table 2.1 Effects of foetal exposure to maternal low-protein diets on systolic blood pressure in adult rats

Dietary protein (wt %)	n	Mean (SD) systolic blood pressure 9 weeks after birth (mmHg)
18	15	137 ($\pm$4)
12	13	152 ($\pm$3)
9	13	153 ($\pm$3)
6	11	159 ($\pm$4)

Source: Langley and Jackson, 1994

Small size at birth and CHD

It became possible to explore the links between growth *in utero* and later CHD after a search of the archives in Britain revealed three collections of birth records of men and women born 50 years and more ago—in Hertfordshire, Preston and Sheffield. From 1911 onwards, when women in Hertfordshire had their babies they were attended by a midwife (Barker *et al*, 1989; Osmond *et al*, 1993). The local health visitor went to the baby's home throughout infancy and the baby was weighed when it was one year old. Sixteen thousand men and women born in the county from 1911 to 1930 have now been traced. Death rates from CHD fell between those who were small and those who were large at birth (Table 2.2). A study in Sheffield showed that the small babies with high coronary death rates were small in relation to the duration of gestation rather than small because they were prematurely born (Barker *et al*, 1993d).

These findings pose the question of the nature of the processes which link reduced early growth with adult disease. From examining samples of men and women who still live in Hertfordshire, and Sheffield, and in Preston, we now know that babies who were small have, as adults, raised blood pressure, raised

Table 2.2 Standardised mortality ratios from coronary heart disease among 15 726 men and women according to birthweight

Birthweight (pounds (kg))	Standardised mortality ratio	No. of deaths
< 5.5 (2.50)	100	57
5.5–6.5 (2.50–2.95)	81	137
6.5–7.5 (2.95–3.41)	80	298
7.5–8.5 (3.41–3.86)	74	289
8.5–9.5 (3.86–4.31)	55	103
> 9.5 (4.31)	65	47
Total	74	941

Source: Barker *et al*, 1989

serum cholesterol and plasma fibrinogen concentrations and impaired glucose tolerance (Barker *et al*, 1993a)—the main risk factors for CHD. Table 2.3 shows the mean systolic pressures of men and women aged 64–71 years (Law *et al*, 1993). Systolic pressure fell progressively between those who were small at birth and those who were large. The relation between birthweight and blood pressure has now been demonstrated in 21 studies of men, women and children, and there is a secure base for saying that impaired foetal growth is strongly linked to blood pressure at all ages except during adolescence, when the tracking of blood pressure levels which begins in early childhood is perturbed by the adolescent growth spurt (Barker, 1995). Differences in blood pressure associated with birthweight are small in childhood but are magnified throughout life. This suggests that there may be 'amplification' as well as 'initiation processes' (Folkow, 1982; Law *et al*, 1993).

Among the possible mechanisms linking reduced foetal growth and raised blood pressure are persisting changes in vascular structure (Berry *et al*, 1976; Martyn *et al*, 1995a). Reduced blood flow in foetal arteries is known to be associated with persisting loss of elasticity, which in itself may raise blood pressure. Another possible mechanism is exposure to excess glucocorticoids. In animals, modest glucocorticoid excess retards intrauterine growth and programmes raised blood pressure (Benediktsson *et al*, 1993; Edwards *et al*, 1993). An excess of glucocorticoids may occur either from foeto-placental stress and consequent increased foetal glucocorticoid secretion, or from deficiency in the normal placental enzyme barrier which protects the foetus from its mother's glucocorticoids.

Table 2.4 shows the prevalence of non-insulin-dependent diabetes (NIDDM) and impaired glucose tolerance according to birthweight in a group of men in Hertfordshire (Hales *et al*, 1991). The prevalence falls sharply between men who were small at birth and men who were large. There are similar findings in women. This association between birthweight and NIDDM has been replicated by other

Table 2.3 Mean systolic pressure in men and women aged 64–71 years according to birthweight

	Mean systolic pressure	
Birthweight (pounds (kg))	Men (mmHg) (*n*))	Women (mmHg (*n*))
<5.5 (2.50)	171 (18)	169 (9)
5.5–6.5 (2.50–2.95)	168 (53)	165 (33)
6.5–7.5 (2.95–3.41)	168 (144)	160 (68)
7.5–8.5 (3.41–3.86)	165 (111)	163 (48)
>8.5 (3.86)	163 (92)	155 (26)
Total	166 (418)	161 (184)
Standard deviation	24	26

Source: Law *et al*, 1993

Table 2.4 Prevalence of non-insulin-dependent diabetes and impaired glucose tolerance in men aged 59–70 years

Birthweight (pounds (kg))	Number of men	% with impaired glucose tolerance or diabetes	Odds ratio adjusted for body mass index (95% confidence interval)
<5.5 (2.50)	20	40	6.6 (1.5–28)
5.5–6.5 (2.50–2.95)	47	34	4.8 (1.3–17)
6.5–7.5 (2.95–3.41)	104	31	4.6 (1.4–16)
7.5–8.5 (3.41–3.86)	117	22	2.6 (0.8–8.9)
8.5–9.5 (3.86–4.31)	54	13	1.4 (0.3–5.6)
>9.5 (4.31)	28	14	1.0
Total	370	25	

Source: Hales *et al*, 1991

studies in Britain (Phipps *et al*, 1993; McCance *et al*, 1994), in studies in the United States (Valdez *et al*, 1994) and in Sweden (McKeigue *et al*, 1994).

Adult lifestyle and CHD

One response to these and similar findings has been to attribute them to confounding variables, arguing that people exposed to an adverse environment *in utero* are exposed to an adverse environment in adult life, and that it is this later environment that produces the effects attributed to programming. This suggestion can be examined directly, and the associations between birth measurements and coronary risk factors are found to be unchanged after even the most potent adult determinants of risk are allowed for (Barker, 1995). For example, associations between birth size and plasma fibrinogen concentrations are unchanged if smoking is allowed for. Adult lifestyle does, however, add to the effects of intrauterine life. Thus the highest prevalences of impaired glucose tolerance and diabetes, for example, are seen in people who were small at birth and who became obese as adults (Hales *et al*, 1991).

There remains the possibility of unknown confounding variables. One way of examining this is to use social class as an indicator of a range of socio-economic influences, known and unknown. Associations between size at birth and cardiovascular risk factors are found in each social group, whether this is defined at birth or in adult life. Doubt has been cast on the usefulness of data on social class at birth in Hertfordshire because low social class was not associated with low birthweight (Paneth and Susser, 1995). There is, however, no evidence that the differences in birthweight found in different social classes in industrial Britain existed in affluent rural counties like Hertfordshire 70 years ago. Furthermore, the usefulness of the information about social class at birth in Hertfordshire is shown by its associations with different infant feeding practices (Fall *et al*, 1992). Another way of addressing the issue of unknown confounding variables is to test the associations with size at birth in different populations around the world. Studies in several countries have shown that children who were small at birth have raised blood pressure and evidence of impaired response to an oral glucose challenge (Law et al, 1993; 1994; Yajnik et al, 1995). These findings are further evidence that the associations in adults do not reflect unknown confounding variables linked to lifestyle. Since many of the studies were done in countries where child mortality is low, they also argue against suggestions that associations with birth size reflect bias due to differential survival and selective migration (McCance et al, 1994; Paneth and Susser, 1995).

The thin baby and Syndrome X

In Table 2.5 the men shown in Table 2.4 are arranged according to their weight at birth and their current Body Mass Index (BMI). The lowest two-hour plasma glucose concentrations are seen among men who are large at birth and have remained thin. The highest concentrations are among men who are small at birth and have become fat as adults (Hales and Barker, 1992).

Around the world, communities with high prevalences of NIDDM conform to the pattern shown here. They are peoples such as the Ethiopian Jews air-lifted to Israel or the Indians who migrate to this country, whose foetal nutrition was poor but who subsequently became affluent and obese in their adult life. We know something of why people who are small at birth are unable to withstand the stress of becoming obese as adults. There is evidence that they have a reduced number of pancreatic β-cells and hence a reduced capacity to make insulin. These findings, however, are inconclusive. There is stronger evidence that small babies become insulin-resistant (Phillips et al, 1994).

The occurrence of insulin-resistance in adults is characterised in a syndrome, in which diabetes, hypertension and raised plasma triglyceride concentrations coincide in the same patient (Reaven, 1988). The syndrome is associated with increased susceptibility to CHD. Allowing for current BMI, the relative risk of having the insulin-resistance syndrome among people who were 6.5 pounds (2.95 kg) or less at birth is around 10 times higher than among people who were more than 9.5 pounds (4.31 kg) (Barker et al, 1993b). This is a large risk. For comparison, the

Table 2.5   Plasma glucose concentrations in men two hours after 75 g glucose by mouth

	Current body mass index (kg/m^2)			
Birthweight (pounds (kg))	<25.4	25.4–28.0	>28.0	All
<7 (3.12)	6.1	6.9	7.9	6.9
7–8.25 (3.12–3.75)	6.5	6.4	7.5	6.7
>8.25 (3.75)	5.8	6.5	6.6	6.3
All	6.2	6.5	7.2	6.6

Source: Hales et al, 1991

risk of CHD among smokers compared with non-smokers is around 2.

The insulin-resistance syndrome is associated not only with low birthweight but more specifically with thinness at birth, as measured by a low ponderal index (birthweight/length) (Barker and Osmond, 1986; Barker et al, 1993b). Insulin tolerance tests on men and women aged 50 confirm that those who were thin at birth are less sensitive to insulin (Phillips et al, 1994). Babies who are thin at birth lack muscle as well as fat. Muscle is the main peripheral site of insulin action. It is thought that at some point in mid-gestation babies who are born thin become undernourished and unable to sustain their growth. In response their muscles become resistant to insulin. Growth of muscle was therefore sacrificed but the brain, which does not require insulin to metabolise glucose, was spared.

The short baby and abnormal lipid metabolism and blood coagulation

Another kind of baby at increased risk of CHD is short at birth in relation to the size of its head (Barker et al, 1993a; 1993c; Barker, 1995). Like the thin baby, the birthweight of the short baby is usually within the normal range. Its shortness is thought to be a consequence of undernutrition in late gestation. The foetus utilises an adaptive response present in mammals to divert oxygenated blood away from the trunk to sustain the brain. The liver is one of the organs whose growth is prejudiced by this. The liver has a central role in the synthesis and excretion of cholesterol and in the control of blood coagulation. Disturbance of cholesterol metabolism and blood clotting are both important features of CHD.

Abdominal circumference at birth, which reflects the size of the liver, is remarkably predictive of serum cholesterol, blood clotting and death from CHD in adult life. Table 2.6 shows how men and women in middle life who had small abdominal circumferences at birth have raised concentrations of cholesterol, in particular low-density lipoprotein cholesterol (Barker et al, 1993c). The difference in concentrations between people who had small abdominal circumferences at birth and those who had large circumferences is equivalent to around 30%

Table 2.6 Mean serum lipid concentrations according to abdominal circumference at birth in men and women aged 50–53 years

Abdominal circumference (inches (cm))	No. of people	Total cholesterol (mmol/l)	Low-density lipoprotein cholesterol (mmol/l)
<11.5 (29.2)	53	6.7	4.5
11.5–12.0 (29.2–30.5)	43	6.9	4.6
12.0–12.5 (30.5–31.8)	31	6.8	4.4
12.5–13.0 (31.8–33.0)	45	6.2	4.0
>13.0 (33.0)	45	6.1	4.0
Total	217	6.5	4.3

Source: Barker et al, 1993c

difference in risk of CHD. Findings for plasma fibrinogen concentrations, a measure of coagulability, are similarly strong (Martyn *et al*, 1995b).

In keeping with these associations, a small abdominal circumference at birth is also associated with raised death rates from CHD (Barker *et al*, 1995). This, however, is only seen in babies of below average weight. In large babies the trend is reversed, so that it is the large baby with the large abdominal circumference who is at increased risk. This kind of baby is known to result from a pregnancy in which the mother develops diabetes. The foetus is exposed to abnormally high concentrations of glucose and is therefore, in a sense, overnourished. In these babies the abdomen enlarges rapidly in late gestation. It seems that accelerated as well as reduced liver growth in late gestation is linked to later CHD.

Experiments in rats have shown how undernutrition may permanently alter the way the liver metabolises glucose (Desai *et al*, 1994). Phospho-enol-pyruvate-carboxy-kinase is largely made in the peri-portal area of the liver and is part of the process by which glucose is synthesised. Glucokinase is made in the peri-venous cells and participates in the breakdown of glucose. A low-protein maternal diet during gestation is followed by a permanent change in the balance of the two enzymes in favour of synthesis, even if followed by normal protein intake after birth, while a low-protein diet after birth has no such effect. An interpretation of these findings is that undernutrition programmes the zonal structure of the liver, enhancing the development of the peri-portal cells in relation to the peri-venous cells.

The rate of cell division in the foetus falls in late gestation and growth slows down (Tanner, 1989). After birth, growth mainly consists of the development and enlargement of existing cells rather than addition of new ones. The growth of babies who were short at birth, and had reduced abdominal circumferences, tends to slow markedly after birth (Villar *et al*, 1984). In men, failure of infant growth is highly predictive of CHD (Barker *et al*, 1989; Osmond *et al*, 1993). Figure 2.1 shows that, among the Hertfordshire men, those who were small at one year were three times as likely to develop or die of CHD as those who were large. These associations between CHD and weight at one year do not depend on the way in which the infant was fed subsequent to birth. Low weight gain during infancy is associated with enlargement of the left ventricle in adult life, now known to predict CHD independently of raised blood pressure (Vijayakumar *et al*, 1995). One explanation for this association is that, in the short baby, the structure of the heart is permanently changed by adaptive responses occurring before birth. Redistribution of blood flow in favour of the brain is associated with an increase in left ventricular blood flow and also a possible increase in peripheral resistance.

The small baby and raised blood pressure

The thin and short babies are two forms of disproportionate babies, whose growth was restricted at different stages of gestation and in whom different tissues, muscle and liver, were sacrificed to sustain the brain. Perhaps the origins

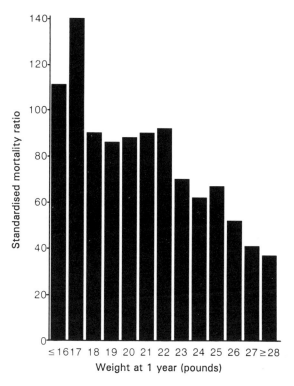

Figure 2.1 Standardised mortality ratios for coronary heart disease in 8175 men according to their weight at one year of age (Barker *et al*, 1989)

of CHD partly lie in the disproportionate size of the human brain, in comparison with that of other mammals. Adaptive responses that protect the brain do so at costs to other tissues. In the Third World many babies are born proportionately small rather than disproportionate. They are thought to have established a slow trajectory of growth in early gestation which they are able to sustain in late gestation and thereby avoid becoming disproportionate. A slow growth trajectory is a major adaptation to undernutrition because it reduces the demand for nutrients in foetal life (McCance and Widdowson, 1974). As far as we know, the proportionately small baby does not develop CHD (Barker, 1995). It does, however, develop raised blood pressure. Persisting elevation of blood pressure is associated with interference with growth at any stage of gestation and is seen in small, thin or short babies.

The placenta

In the ewe, undernutrition in early pregnancy will lead to placental enlargements, thought to be an adaptation to enable extraction of more nutrients for the foetus

Table 2.7   Mean systolic blood pressure (mmHg) of men and women aged 46–54 years, born after 38 completed weeks of gestation, according to placental weight and birthweight

| Birthweight (pounds (kg)) | Placental weight (pounds (kg)) | | | | |
	< 1.0 (0.45)	1.0–1.25 (0.45–0.57)	1.25–1.5 (0.57–0.68)	> 1.5 (0.68)	All
<6.5 (2.95)	149 (24)	152 (46)	151 (18)	167 (6)	152 (94)
6.5–7.5 (2.95–3.41)	139 (16)	148 (63)	146 (35)	159 (23)	148 (137)
>7.5 (3.41)	131 (3)	143 (23)	148 (30)	153 (40)	149 (96)
All	144 (43)	148 (132)	148 (83)	156 (69)	149 (327)

Figures in parentheses within the main body of the table are numbers of subjects
Source; Barker *et al*, 1990

(McCrabb *et al*, 1992). This will only occur, however, if the ewe is well nourished before mating—one of many pointers to the importance to the foetus of the mother's nutritional state before conception (Hales *et al*, 1991). There is evidence that placental enlargement may also be an adaptive response in humans. Mothers who are anaemic, who exercise heavily, or who live at higher altitudes have babies with large placentas (Godfrey *et al*, 1991; Clapp and Rizk, 1992; Wheeler *et al*, 1994). Our observations suggest, however, that expansion of the placenta may be an adaptation that exacts a long-term price. The blood pressures of a group of men and women in Preston were measured and are shown in Table 2.7 by their birthweights and placental weight (Barker *et al*, 1990). Systolic pressure tended to fall with increasing birthweight. At any birthweight, however, systolic pressure tended to rise as placental weight increased so that the highest pressures were in people who in foetal life allocated more resources to placental development.

Other studies have shown that disproportionate placental enlargement is followed in adult life not only by elevated blood pressure, but by impaired glucose tolerance, disordered blood coagulation and death from CHD (Barker *et al*, 1993d; Phipps *et al*, 1993; Barker, 1995). Placental enlargement therefore seems a general marker of foetal undernutrition and its consequences, rather than a specific marker of later hypertension.

Factors in childhood and adolescence

Although the potential importance of living conditions in childhood and adolescence has been emphasised by some authors, we do not yet know whether socio-economic influences that affect nutrition and infection in childhood (and thereby influence postnatal growth) can modify the effects of suboptimal growth *in utero*. Because associations between birth measurements and CHD are found in childhood it should be possible to carry out short-term follow-up studies linking measures of foetal growth and growth through childhood to the emergence of risk factors.

Inter-generational effects

During the winter of 1944 there was widespread famine in western Holland. The famine, however, ended abruptly after seven months when Holland was liberated. A group of babies conceived during the famine was born after liberation. They had low birthweights, but attained normal height as adults; when these girls had babies, in their turn, they were small (Lumey, 1992). It seems that their foetal experience had permanently constrained their ability to deliver nutrients to their own foetuses. There is other evidence suggesting that a constraint on nutrient delivery to the foetus is established during the mother's foetal life. The nature of this constraint is unknown but it could be through changes in the structure of the mother's ovaries or uterus, which are laid down in foetal life.

Conclusion

This brief review of what is known in animals and humans allows a number of conclusions.

- Restriction of nutrients *in utero* permanently changes, or programmes, the physiology and structure of the body.
- Experiments on animals have established that undernutrition at different times in early life has different effects. In late gestation, undernutrition leads to disproportionate growth, as in the thin or short human baby, while in early gestation it leads to proportionate loss of body size. Disproportionate growth rather than small size may hold a key to the origins of CHD.
- The rapidly growing baby is more vulnerable to undernutrition.
- Foetal undernutrition, which programmes the body, itself results from inadequate maternal intake of food before and during pregnancy, inadequate transport of nutrients, or of transfer through the placenta.

New model of CHD

A new paradigm to predict the causation of CHD is emerging (Barker, 1994). Under the old model an inappropriate lifestyle, including cigarette smoking and lack of exercise, leads to accelerated destruction of the body in middle and late life, including the more rapid development of atheroma, raised blood pressure, and the development of insulin resistance. Under the new model CHD results not primarily from external forces but from the body's self-organisation, homeostatic settings of enzyme activity, cell receptors, and hormonal feedback, which are established in response to undernutrition *in utero* and lead eventually to premature death.

References

Barker DJP. *Mothers, Babies, and Disease in Later Life*. London: British Medical Journal Publishing Group, 1994

Barker DJP. Fetal origins of coronary heart disease. *British Medical Journal*, 1995; **311**: 171–174

Barker DJP, Osmond C. Death rates from stroke in England and Wales predicted from past maternal mortality. *British Medical Journal*, 1987; **295**: 83–86

Barker DJP, Osmond C. Infant mortality, childhood nutrition, and ischaemic heart disease in England and Wales. *Lancet*, 1986; **i**: 1077–1081

Barker DJP, Winter PD, Osmond C, Margetts B, Simmonds SJ. Weight in infancy and death from ischaemic heart disease. *Lancet*, 1989; **ii**: 577–580

Barker DJP, Bull AR, Osmond C, Simmonds SJ. Fetal and placental size and risk of hypertension in adult life. *British Medical Journal*, 1990; **301**: 259–262

Barker DJP, Gluckman PD, Godfrey KM, Harding JE, Owens JA, Robinson JS. Fetal nutrition and cardiovascular disease in adult life. *Lancet*, 1993a; **341**: 938–941

Barker DJP, Hales CN, Fall CHD, Osmond C, Phipps K, Clark PMS. Type 2 (non-insulin dependent) diabetes mellitus, hypertension and hyperlipidaemia (syndrome X): relation to reduced fetal growth. *Diabetologia*, 1993b; **36**: 62–67

Barker DJP, Martyn CN, Osmond C, Hales CN, Fall CHD. Growth *in utero* and serum cholesterol concentrations in adult life. *British Medical Journal*, 1993c; **307**: 1524–1527

Barker DJP, Osmond C, Simmonds SJ, Wield GA. The relation of small head circumference and thinness at birth to cardiovascular disease in adult life. *British Medical Journal*, 1993d; **306**: 422–426

Barker DJP, Martyn CN, Osmond C, Wield GA. Abnormal liver growth in utero and death from coronary heart disease. *British Medical Journal*, 1995; **310**: 703–704

Barraclough CA. The production of anovulatory, sterile rats by single injections of testosterone propionate. *Endocrinology*, 1961; **68**: 62–67

Benediktsson R, Lindsay RS, Noble J, Seckl JR, Edwards CR. Glucocorticoid exposure *in utero*: new model for adult hypertension. *Lancet*, 1993; **341**: 339–341

Berry CL, Gosling RG, Laogun AA, Bryan E. Anomalous iliac compliance in children with a single umbilical artery. *British Heart Journal*, 1976; **38**: 510–515

Clapp JF III, Rizk KH. Effect of recreational exercise on midtrimester placental growth. *American Journal of Obstetrics and Gynecology*, 1992; **167**: 1518–1521

Desai M, Crowther N, Lucas A, Hales CN. Programming of hepatic metabolism by low protein diet during early life. *Diabetic Medicine*, 1994; **11**: 537

Edwards CRW, Benediktsson R, Lindsay RS, Seckl JR. Dysfunction of placental glucocorticoid barrier: link between fetal environment and adult hypertension? *Lancet*, 1993; **341**: 355–357

Fall CHD, Barker DJP, Osmond C, Winter PD, Clark PMS, Hales CN. Relation of infant feeding to adult serum cholesterol concentration and death from ischaemic heart disease. *British Medical Journal*, 1992; **304**: 801–815

Folkow B. Physiological aspects of primary hypertension. *Physiological Reviews*, 1982; **62**: 347– 504

Forsdahl A. Are poor living conditions in childhood and adolescence an important risk factor for arteriosclerotic heart disease? *British Journal of Preventive and Social Medicine*, 1977; **31**: 91–95

Godfrey KM, Redman CWG, Barker DJP, Osmond C. The effect of maternal anaemia and iron deficiency on the ratio of fetal weight to placental weight. *British Journal of Obstetrics and Gynaecology*, 1991; **98**: 886–891

Hahn P. Effect of litter size on plasma cholesterol and insulin and some liver and adipose tissue enzymes in adult rodents. *Journal of Nutrition*, 1984; **114**: 1231–1234

Hales CN, Barker DJP. Type 2 (non-insulin dependent) diabetes mellitus: the thrifty phenotype hypothesis. *Diabetologia*, 1992; **35**: 595–601

Hales CN, Barker DJP, Clark PMS *et al*. Fetal and infant growth and impaired glucose tolerance at age 64. *British Medical Journal*, 1991; **303**: 1019–1022

Hinchcliffe SA, Lynch MRJ, Sargent PH, Howard CV, Van Velzen D. The effect of intrauterine growth retardation on the development of renal nephrons. *British Journal of Obstetrics and Gynaecology*, 1992; **99**: 296–301

Langley SC, Jackson AA. Increased systolic blood pressure in adult rats induced by fetal exposure to maternal low protein diets. *Clinical Science*, 1994; **86**: 217–222

Law CM, de Swiet M, Osmond C *et al*. Initiation of hypertension *in utero* and its amplification throughout life. *British Medical Journal*, 1993; **306**: 24–27

Law CM, Gordon GS, Shiell AW, Barker DJP, Hales CN. Thinness at birth and glucose tolerance in seven-year-old children. *Diabetic Medicine*, 1994; **12**: 24–29

Lucas A. Programming by early nutrition in man. In: Bock GR, Whelan J, eds. *The Childhood Environment and Adult Disease*. Chichester: John Wiley and Sons, 1991: 38–55

Lumey LH. Decreased birthweights in infants after maternal in utero exposure to the Dutch famine of 1944–45. *Paediatric and Perinatal Epidemiology*, 1992; **6**: 240–253

Martyn CN, Barker DJP, Jespersen S, Greenwald S, Osmond C, Berry CL. Growth *in utero*, adult blood pressure and arterial compliance. *British Heart Journal*, 1995a; **73**: 116–121

Martyn CN, Meade TW, Stirling Y, Barker DJP. Plasma concentrations of fibrinogen and factor VII in adult life and their relation to intra-uterine growth. *British Journal of Haematology*, 1995b; **89**: 142–146

McCance RA, Widdowson EM. The determinants of growth and form. *Proceedings of the Royal Society of London: Biological Sciences*, 1974; **185**: 1–17

McCance DR, Pettitt DJ, Hanson RL, Jacobsson LTM, Knowle WC, Bennett PH. Birthweight and non-insulin dependent diabetes: 'thrifty genotype', 'thrifty phenotype', or 'surviving small baby genotype'. *British Medical Journal*, 1994; **308**: 942–945

McCrabb GJ, Egan AR, Hosking BJ. Maternal undernutrition during mid-pregnancy in sheep: variable effects on placental growth. *Journal of Agricultural Science*, 1992; **118**: 127–132

McKeigue PM, Leon DA, Berglund L, Mohren R, Lithell HO. Relationship of birthweight and ponderal index to non-insulin dependent diabetes and insulin response to glucose challenge in men aged 50–60 years. *Diabetic Medicine*, 1994; **11**: suppl 17

Morton NE. The inheritance of human birthweight. *Annals of Human Genetics*, 1955; **20**: 123–134

Mott GE, Lewis DS, McGill HC. Programming of cholesterol metabolism by breast or formula feeding. In: Bock GR, Whelan J, eds. *The Childhood Environment and Adult Disease*. Chichester: John Wiley and Sons, 1991: 56–76

Osmond C, Barker DJP, Winter PD, Fall CHD, Simmonds SJ. Early growth and death from cardiovascular disease in women. *British Medical Journal*, 1993; **307**: 1519–1524

Paneth N, Susser M. Early origin of coronary heart disease (the 'Barker hypothesis'). *British Medical Journal*, 1995; **310**: 411–412

Penrose LS. Some recent trends in human genetics. *Caryologia*, 1954; **6** (suppl): 521–529

Phillips DIW, Barker DJP, Hales CN, Hirst S, Osmond C. Thinness at birth and insulin resistance in adult life. *Diabetologia*, 1994; **37**: 150–154

Phipps K, Barker DJP, Hales CN, Fall CHD, Osmond C, Clark PMS. Fetal growth and impaired glucose tolerance in men and women. *Diabetologia*, 1993; **36**: 225–228

Reaven GM. Banting Lecture 1988. Role of insulin resistance in human disease. *Diabetes*, 1988; **37**: 1595–1607

Rose G. Familial patterns in ischaemic heart disease. *British Journal of Preventive and Social Medicine*, 1964; **18**: 75–80

Smart JL. Critical periods in brain development. In: Bock GR, Whelan J, eds. *The Childhood Environment and Adult Disease.* Chichester: John Wiley and Sons, 1991: 109–128

Tanner JM. *Foetus into Man: Physical Growth from Conception to Maturity.* Second Edition. Ware: Castlemead Publications, 1989

Valdez R, Athens MA, Thompson GH, Bradshaw BS, Stern MP. Birthweight and adult health outcomes in a biethnic population in the USA. *Diabetologia*, 1994; **37**: 624–631

Vijayakumar M, Fall CHD, Osmond C, Barker DJP. Birthweight, weight at one year and left ventricular mass in adult life. *British Heart Journal*, 1995; **73**: 363–367

Villar J, Smeriglio V, Martorell R, Brown CH, Klein RE. Heterogenous growth and mental development of intrauterine growth-retarded infants during the first 3 years of life. *Paediatrics*, 1984; **74**: 783–791

Wheeler T, Sollero C, Alderman S, Landen J, Anthony F, Osmond C. Relation between maternal haemoglobin and placental hormone concentrations in early pregnancy. *Lancet*, 1994; **343**: 511–513

Widdowson EM, McCance RA. A review: new thoughts on growth. *Paediatric Research*, 1975; **9**: 154–156

Widdowson EM, Crabb DE, Milner RDG. Cellular development of some human organs before birth. *Archives of Disease in Childhood*, 1972; **47**: 652–655

Winick M, Noble A. Cellular response in rats during malnutrition at various stages. *Journal of Nutrition*, 1966; **89**: 300–306

Winick M, Fish I, Rosso P. Cellular recovery in rat tissues after a brief period of neonatal malnutrition. *Journal of Nutrition*, 1968; **95**: 623–626

Yajnik CS, Fall CHD, Vaidya U *et al.* Fetal growth and glucose and insulin metabolism in four-year-old Indian children. *Diabetic Medicine*, 1995; **12**: 330–336

Discussion

David A. Leon

Epidemiology Unit, London School of Hygiene & Tropical Medicine, UK

When first articulated in its modern guise by Barker, the 'foetal origins' hypothesis was received with an element of scepticism among people working in public health and epidemiology. In retrospect this is not surprising. The focus of work on non-communicable diseases in recent decades has been on the role of factors operating in adult life. The proposition that there may be important influences on risk that are determined in *infancy*, or even earlier, was regarded by some as an unwelcome diversion, one that could even undermine efforts to persuade people to modify their adult lifestyles. It is apparent, however, that the notion of early origins of adult disease is being given increasing weight in the light of rapidly accumulating evidence that events and processes in foetal life are directly related to adult physiology and disease risk.

There are many issues raised in Barker's paper that deserve attention. Rather than taking up detailed questions of mechanism, however, this paper considers some broader issues. These are (i) the concept of 'programming', (ii) the relationship of foetal influences to risk factors operating at other points in the life-course, and (iii) the nature and determinants of foetal growth *per se*.

Programming

Over the past few decades, aetiological research in cancer and cardiovascular disease has been preoccupied with exposures (whether internal or external) that have an adverse effect on risk. These range from carcinogenic exposures in the workplace to exposure to adverse levels or types of dietary fat intake. More recently, attention has been given to exposures that appear to be protective, such as consumption patterns of fresh fruit and vegetables that appear to act in part by eliminating or minimising the effect of adverse exposures (e.g. dietary antioxidants). The concept of modulation of disease risk through permanent changes in the body's structure and function ('programming') is a less familiar idea in the epidemiological literature, although interesting examples may be found. For instance, the protective effect of a young age at first birth on subsequent breast cancer risk described first by MacMahon *et al* (1970) may be viewed as an example of programming in early adult life. This protective effect is thought to arise because first pregnancy appears either to lead to a permanent reduction in the number of breast tissue stem-cells, from which many tumours are thought to arise, or reduces the sensitivity of these cells to carcinogenic insults (Moolgavkar *et al*, 1980; Pike *et al*, 1993). This is in contrast to the non-programming mechanism that is thought to underlie the recently observed association between various birthweight and perinatal complications and risk of breast cancer in a woman's offspring (Ekbom *et al*, 1992; Sanderson *et al*, 1996). These factors may, instead, modulate foetal exposure to the direct carcinogenic influence of maternal oestrogens (Trichopoulos, 1990).

Early programming of risk of developing adult obesity was suggested by Ravelli and colleagues (Ravelli *et al*, 1976), who found that male offspring of women exposed to the Dutch famine of 1944–1945 while in the their last trimester of gestation had reduced rates of obesity in young adult life. They speculated that this was consistent with nutritional deprivation in pregnancy affecting a critical period of development of adipose-tissue cellularity. Studies of Pima Indians in the early 1980s have suggested an important role for the prenatal environment in determining risks of obesity (Pettitt *et al*, 1983) as well as of non-insulin-dependent diabetes mellitus (Pettitt *et al*, 1988).

Based on their work on gestational diabetes, Frienkel and Metzger (1979)

... nced the concept of *fuel-mediated teratogenesis*. They proposed that some cell types such as brain cells, fat cells, muscle cells and pancreatic β-cells have relatively 'terminal structures' and limited replicative capacity. They went on to suggest that:

> the total endowment and functions of these cells in the offspring may be influenced by intrauterine and perinatal events ... Thus, the period of intrauterine development presents an interval in which nurture, as exemplified by the character of maternal fuels, may influence nature, as represented by the intrinsic genetic endowment of the fetus.

'In utero'–adult interactions

Regardless of the extent to which early influences may determine susceptibility to later disease, there can be no question that influences acting at other points in the life-course are important. One of the tasks before us is to integrate the new insights into the role of foetal factors with the substantial body of knowledge about adult risk factors. Empirical human evidence showing how the early and late factors mesh together to determine disease risk is not extensive. Barker's own studies (Hales *et al*, 1991) suggest that among those who are small at birth it is those who are subsequently obese who have the highest prevalence of impaired glucose tolerance (see Table 2.5). Barker himself comments that 'people who are small at birth are unable to withstand the stress of becoming obese as adults' (page 46).

The role of adult adiposity in unmasking the association between impaired foetal growth and later physiological function is supported by recent data from Sweden (Leon *et al*, 1996; Lithell *et al*, 1996). These suggest that among men in the bottom third of the distribution of adult Body Mass Index (BMI) there is no association of size at birth with blood pressure or insulin-mediated glucose uptake. This type of interaction is remarkably similar to a striking 'gene–environment' interaction recently reported by Clausen and others (Clausen *et al*, 1995), who showed that polymorphisms at the IRS-1 locus were only associated with insulin resistance in adults among men who had relatively high BMIs.

The parallel with gene–environment interaction may be more than superficial. It may be fruitful to hypothesise that *in utero* circumstances as well as genotype impart a susceptibility to later disease that is only revealed in certain environments or adult circumstances. By framing the problem in this way, we may avoid the sterile argument about the relative importance of early or late influences on adult risk, and see that even if *in utero* effects are irreversible, this is not equivalent to saying that a person's fate is sealed at birth.

Understanding foetal growth

The current epidemiological evidence linking impaired foetal growth with the risk of later disease uses crude measures of *in utero* development. Birthweight, birth length, and placental weight or various ratios of one to the other are among the most common indices that have been employed. There is, however, a need to use more sophisticated ways of characterising foetal growth, such as taking account of gestational age. In this area, however, we can go beyond measures based on size at birth alone. We have recently argued that using attained adult height as an index of genetic growth potential, those people who are tall as adults but were relatively small at birth failed to attain their growth potential *in utero*. It is this subgroup that appears to have particularly raised blood pressure in our Swedish studies (Leon *et al*, 1996).

Foetal growth is determined by a range of different factors. These include foetal genotype, fixed maternal characteristics such as frame size and genotype, and factors that can vary from one pregnancy to the next including pre-pregnancy weight, smoking, and so on. Estimates of the contribution of each of these factors to the variance in birthweight involve a number of questionable assumptions. However, Robson (1978) suggests that over a third of the variance may be explained by a combination of fixed maternal factors plus foetal genotype. Studies aimed at examining the degree to which these different sources of variation in foetal growth are associated with disease susceptibility in later life are a priority. Within this broader framework, it is worth noting that maternal diet in pregnancy may be of less importance than is sometimes implied: trials in pregnancy have demonstrated that dietary supplementation results in minimal changes in size at birth and may even be harmful (Kramer, 1993). Maternal pre-pregnancy nutritional status may be a considerably more important factor, although whether this influences later disease risk in the offspring as well as foetal growth is yet to be established.

Finally, it is important not to overlook the possibility that at least some of the associations between size at birth and later disease risk may be due to a common genetic factor. For instance, it is plausible that the association between size at birth and non-insulin-dependent diabetes may be due to a common genetic pathway: a genetic defect in insulin action may affect foetal growth as well as predispose to diabetes. A study that explicitly attempts to differentiate between the effects of genotype from *in utero* programming on later disease risk has yet to be undertaken. It may be that both mechanisms are in operation.

References

Clausen JO, Hansen T, Bjorbaek C *et al*. Insulin resistance: interactions between obesity and a common variant of insulin receptor substrate-1. *Lancet*, 1995; **346**: 397–402

Ekbom A, Trichopoulos D, Adami HO, Hsieh CC, Lan SJ. Evidence of prenatal influences on breast cancer risk. *Lancet*, 1992; **340**: 1015–1018

Freinkel N, Metzger BE. Pregnancy as a tissue culture experience: the critical implications of maternal metabolism for fetal development. In: *Pregnancy Metabolism, Diabetes and the Fetus (Ciba Foundation Symposium No. 63)*. Amsterdam: *Excerpta Medica*, 1979: 3–23

Hales CN, Barker DJP, Clark PMS *et al*. Fetal and infant growth and impaired glucose tolerance at age 64. *British Medical Journal*, 1991; **303**: 1019–1022

Kramer MS. Effects of energy and protein intakes on pregnancy outcome: an overview of the research evidence from controlled clinical trials. *American Journal of Clinical Nutrition*, 1993; **58**: 627–635

Leon DA, Koupilova I, Lithell HO *et al.* Failure to realise growth potential *in utero* and adult obesity in relation to blood pressure in 50 year old Swedish men. *British Medical Journal*, 1996; **312**: 401–406

Lithell HO, McKeigue PM, Berglund L, Mohsen R, Lithell U, Leon DA. Relation of size at birth to non-insulin-dependent diabetes and insulin response to glucose challenge in men aged 50–60 years. *British Medical Journal*, 1996; **312**: 406–410

MacMahon B, Cole P, Lin TM *et al.* Age at first birth and breast cancer risk. *Bulletin of the World Health Organization*, 1970; **43**: 209–221

Moolgavkar SH, Day NE, Stevens RG. Two-stage model for carcinogenesis: epidemiology of breast cancer in females. *Journal of the National Cancer Institute*, 1980; **65**: 559–569

Pettitt DJ, Baird HR, Aleck KA, Bennett PH, Knowler WC. Excessive obesity in offspring of Pima Indian women with diabetes during pregnancy. *New England Journal of Medicine*, 1983; **308**: 242–245

Pettitt DJ, Aleck KA, Baird HR, Carraher MJ, Bennett PH, Knowler WC. Congenital susceptibility to NIDDM: role of intrauterine environment. *Diabetes*, 1988; **37**: 622–628

Pike MC, Spicer DV, Dahmoush L, Press MF. Estrogens, progesterones, normal breast cell proliferation, and breast cancer risk. *Epidemiologic Reviews*, 1993; **15**: 17–35

Ravelli GP, Stein ZA, Susser MW. Obesity in young men after famine exposure *in utero* and early infancy. *New England Journal of Medicine*, 1976; **295**: 349–353

Robson EB. The genetics of birth weight. In: Falkner F, Tanner JM, eds. *Human Growth. Vol. 1: Principles and Prenatal Growth.* London: Baillière Tindall, 1978: 285–297

Sanderson M, Williams MA, Malone KE *et al.* Perinatal factors and the risk of breast cancer. *Epidemiology*, 1996; **7**: 34–37

Trichopoulos D. Hypothesis: does breast cancer originate *in utero*? *Lancet*, 1990; **335**: 939–940

3
Cardiovascular disease and diabetes in migrants—interactions between nutritional changes and genetic background

Paul M. McKeigue

Epidemiology Unit, London School of Hygiene & Tropical Medicine, UK

Early studies of migrant groups such as Japanese-Americans helped to establish that many of the international variations in rates of cardiovascular disease and cancer were attributable to differences in diet and other environmental influences, rather than to genetic variation. More recent studies of migrants of African and South Asian descent have suggested a more complex picture in which changes in nutritional status interact with genetic background. Mortality from coronary heart disease (CHD) is higher in South Asian migrants than in other ethnic groups living in the same countries, not only in the United Kingdom where migration from South Asia has occurred relatively recently, but also in countries where migration occurred many generations ago. The high rates of CHD in South Asian people are accompanied by high prevalence of non-insulin-dependent diabetes mellitus (NIDDM). It is now clear that this high prevalence of diabetes is only one manifestation of a pattern of metabolic disturbances related to central obesity and insulin resistance. This syndrome includes raised plasma very-low-density lipoprotein triglyceride and low plasma high-density (HDL) lipoprotein cholesterol. South Asian migrants have a marked tendency to central obesity, even when not overweight by conventional criteria: in this respect South Asians differ from Native American, Pacific and Aboriginal Australian populations

Diet, Nutrition and Chronic Disease: Lessons from Contrasting Worlds.
Edited by P. S. Shetty and K. McPherson © 1997 John Wiley & Sons, Ltd.

where high prevalence of NIDDM occurs in association with generalised obesity. The high rates of CHD in South Asians are most easily explained by the metabolic disturbances associated with this central obesity/insulin resistance syndrome, although the mechanism by which these disturbances lead to atherosclerosis is not clear.

In people of black African descent settled in Europe and the Americas, average blood pressures are consistently higher than in people of European descent, and mortality from strokes and other sequelae of hypertension are also high. The reasons for this susceptibility of black African populations to hypertension are not understood. Hypertension in black populations is strongly associated with glucose intolerance, and obesity is a common factor in both disturbances. Despite the high prevalence of diabetes and hypertension in Afro-Caribbean and African migrants to the UK, mortality from CHD in these groups is much lower than in the general population of the UK. In comparison with Europeans, Afro-Caribbean and African-American men tend to have a more favourable pattern of plasma lipids: lower plasma triglyceride and higher plasma HDL cholesterol. This relative absence of the lipid disturbances that usually accompany obesity and glucose intolerance may account for the relative immunity of Afro-Caribbean and African men to CHD.

The patterns of cardiovascular disease in South Asian and African people settled in Europe and the Americas appear to reflect different patterns of susceptibility to the metabolic complications of obesity. In South Asians high rates of CHD and diabetes occur in association with central obesity, plasma lipid disturbances and insulin resistance. In migrants of black African descent high rates of hypertension, stroke and diabetes occur, but rates of CHD remain much lower than in Europeans. It is likely that the patterns of cardiovascular disease and diabetes now emerging in urban populations in South Asia and West Africa will be similar to those already observed in migrants from these countries.

Cardiovascular disease and cancer mortality in Japanese migrants to the United States

Studies in which Japanese migrants to the USA were compared with Japanese living in Japan and with US whites have made a key contribution to our understanding of the aetiology of cardiovascular disease and several cancers (Haenszel and Kurihara, 1968; Worth et al, 1975). Breast cancer incidence rates, for instance, are four to seven times higher in the USA than in China or Japan. When Chinese or Japanese women migrate to the USA, breast cancer risk rises over several generations to approach the levels among US whites (Ziegler et al, 1993). For colorectal cancer, the risk in Asian migrants rises towards that in US whites within a single generation, suggesting that environmental influences in adult life determine disease risk. The Ni-Hon-San study, comparing Japanese men in Japan, Hawaii and California, demonstrated that mortality from CHD in

Japanese migrants to the USA was about twice as high as in Japan, although still much lower than in US whites (Worth *et al*, 1975). These migrant studies demonstrated that the differences between Japan and the USA in rates of CHD, colon cancer and breast cancer were unlikely to be genetically determined. Dietary changes, especially increased fat intake, were implicated as the key factors in the increased risk associated with migration to the USA.

Mortality of migrants to England

Large-scale migration to England from outside Europe is a more recent phenomenon, although migration from Ireland and Scotland has occurred freely for several generations. Large-scale migration to England from the Caribbean began in the 1950s. Migration from South Asia (India, Pakistan, Bangladesh and Sri Lanka) did not occur on a large scale until around 1960, and reached a peak just before immigration restrictions were imposed in 1966. Two main groups have migrated from Africa: people of South Asian descent, who have migrated from Kenya, Uganda and other countries in East Africa; and migrants of black African descent who have come mainly from Nigeria and Ghana. At the census in 1991, about 200 000 people identified their ethnic group as Black African.

From 1970 onwards, country of birth was recorded on death certificates in England and Wales, making it possible to calculate mortality rates by country of birth using population denominators from the national census. We have analysed mortality data for the years around the most recent census in 1991, and the results are shown in Table 3.1. To ensure consistency between recording of country of birth on death certificates and census, it is necessary to group the countries of South Asia together, and to group northern and southern Ireland together. About 15% of the group defined as 'West/Southern African' are people of European descent born in what is now Zimbabwe; in published census tables these individuals are grouped together with West Africans.

Table 3.1 Standardised mortality ratios (SMRs) for ischaemic heart disease and stroke in England and Wales in 1989–1992 by country of birth, ages 20–69 years

| | Ischaemic heart disease | | | | Stroke | | | |
| | SMR | | Deaths | | SMR | | Deaths | |
Country of birth	M	F	M	F	M	F	M	F
Scotland	120	130	3066	1099	125	125	554	416
Ireland	124	120	3995	1398	138	123	758	553
South Asia	146	151	3348	882	155	141	594	344
Caribbean	46	71	592	236	168	157	360	212
West/Southern Africa	16	81	56	62	26	67	271	181

England and Wales in 1991 = 100

The highest mortality rates from ischaemic heart disease (IHD) are in men and women born in South Asia, whose rates are about 50% higher than the national average. This contrasts with the remarkably low rates of IHD in Caribbean-born and African-born migrants. Stroke mortality shows a different picture: although mortality is high in South Asian-born men and women, the highest rates are in Caribbean- and African-born migrants. Stroke mortality in Caribbean-born men and women has fallen more rapidly than in the general population since 1970. Thus the relative risk of death from stroke in Caribbean-born women compared with the national average has fallen from about 2.3 to about 1.6. More adequate control of hypertension in Caribbean-born people may account for this. The highest mortality rates from stroke are now in African immigrants. This suggests that stroke mortality is also high in the countries (Nigeria and Ghana) from which most African immigrants originate, at least in the social strata from which migration occurred.

Epidemiology of CHD and NIDDM in South Asians

Coronary heart disease

The high mortality from CHD in South Asian migrants to the UK is part of a general pattern in Indians and Pakistanis overseas. From the 1950s onwards, reports began to appear of unusually high rates of CHD in South Asians overseas compared with other groups in the same countries (Danaraj *et al*, 1959; Adelstein, 1963; Sorokin, 1975; Tuomilehto *et al*, 1984). In comparison with high-risk populations such as Europeans in South Africa or the UK, the relative risk for CHD mortality associated with South Asian origin is about 1.4 (Steinberg *et al*, 1988; OPCS, 1990), and in comparison with relatively low-risk groups such as Chinese in Singapore (Hughes *et al*, 1990a) or Africans in Trinidad (Miller *et al*, 1989) the relative risk is about 3. In England and Wales, high coronary mortality is common to Hindus originating from Gujarat in western India, to Sikhs originating from Punjab in northern India, and to Muslims from Pakistan and Bangladesh (Balarajan *et al*, 1984; McKeigue and Marmot, 1988). Reliable population-based coronary mortality data from South Asia are not available, but in two northern Indian cities the prevalence of Minnesota-coded major Q waves on electrocardiograms has been reported to be at least as high as in European populations (Sarvotham and Berry, 1968; Chadha *et al*, 1990). In contrast, very low prevalence rates have been recorded in rural India (Dewan *et al*, 1974; Jajoo *et al*, 1988).

The consistency of the high CHD risk in urban South Asian populations around the world, affecting both sexes and with early onset in men, suggests a common underlying cause. Surveys comparing risk factors in South Asians with other groups have shown that the high CHD rates are not explained by differences in smoking, hypertension, plasma cholesterol, or haemostatic activity

(McKeigue *et al*, 1988; Miller *et al*, 1988). The persistence of excess CHD risk in overseas South Asian populations, even where migration from India occurred more than a century before, suggests that genetic factors may be important in determining susceptibility to the disease.

Diabetes mellitus (NIDDM) in South Asians

One clue to possible explanations for the high rates of CHD in people of South Asian (Indian, Pakistani and Bangladeshi) descent living in urban societies is that prevalence of NIDDM is far higher in urban South Asians than in Europeans. Table 3.2 summarises the results of surveys that have used glucose tolerance tests and WHO criteria to study South Asian populations. The prevalence of 19% in our own survey in the UK (McKeigue *et al*, 1991) is remarkably consistent with surveys in other overseas South Asian populations (Zimmet *et al*, 1983; Omar *et al*, 1985; Miller *et al*, 1989; Dowse *et al*, 1990; Hughes *et al*, 1990b) and in urban India (Ramachandran *et al*, 1988; 1992) as compared to the 4% prevalence in men and women of European descent in the UK (McKeigue *et al*, 1991). In a recent survey of a rural Indian population (Ramachandran *et al*, 1992) prevalence was 3% in the age group 40–64 years, similar to that in Europeans in the UK. Most South Asian patients with coronary disease are not diabetic (Hughes *et al*, 1989), and glucose intolerance alone cannot explain more than a small proportion of the excess coronary risk in South Asian people (Miller *et al*, 1989).

Insulin resistance and central obesity in South Asians

In a study comparing Bangladeshi migrants to east London with native Europeans, we identified a pattern of intercorrelated metabolic disturbances in

Table 3.2 Prevalence of non-insulin-dependent diabetes in South Asians

Year	Place	Age	Prevalence (%)	Reference
Prevalence in South Asians overseas				
1977	Trinidad	35–69	21	Miller *et al*, 1989
1983	Fiji	35–64	25	Zimmet *et al*, 1983
1985	South Africa	30–	22	Omar *et al*, 1985
1990	Singapore	40–69	25	Hughes *et al*, 1990b
1990	Mauritius	35–64	20	Dowse *et al*, 1990
1991	England	40–69	19	McKeigue *et al*, 1991
Prevalence in India				
1985	Urban Karnataka	45–64	29	Ramachandran *et al*, 1988
1992	Urban Madras	45–64	18	Ramachandran *et al*, 1992
1992	Rural Tamil Nadu	45–64	3	Ramachandran *et al*, 1992
Prevalence in Europeans, for comparison				
1991	London	40–69	4	McKeigue *et al*, 1991

Bangladeshi men and women: high prevalence of NIDDM, high levels of insulin and triglyceride after a glucose load, and low HDL cholesterol (McKeigue *et al*, 1988). This pattern corresponds to the insulin resistance syndrome described by others (Reaven, 1988; DeFronzo and Ferrannini, 1991). The occurrence of this syndrome in South Asians was confirmed in a larger study of Indian and Pakistani subjects in west London: the Southall Study. South Asian men and women have a more central distribution of body fat than Europeans, with thicker trunk skinfolds and markedly higher mean waist–hip ratios (WHR) for a given level of Body Mass Index (BMI). This ethnic difference in WHR is equivalent to about two-thirds of one standard deviation in men and about one standard deviation in women (McKeigue *et al*, 1991). In both South Asians and Europeans, we found that glucose intolerance and two-hour insulin were more strongly associated with WHR than with BMI (McKeigue *et al*, 1992), although the ethnic differences in diabetes prevalence and insulin levels were not fully accounted for by the WHR (McKeigue *et al*, 1991). Average BMI and insulin levels are much lower in rural Indians than in urban Indian populations (Snehalatha *et al*, 1994); this is consistent with the urban–rural differences in prevalence of diabetes and CHD that have been described (Sarvotham and Berry, 1968; Dewan *et al*, 1974; Ramachandran *et al*, 1992). A recent study comparing Punjabi migrants to England with their siblings living in rural Punjab showed that the migrants had higher BMI, higher serum insulin, and lower HDL cholesterol than their siblings in India (Bhatnagar *et al*, 1995).

The tendency for South Asians to accumulate intra-abdominal fat without necessarily developing generalised obesity contrasts with other populations at high risk of diabetes, such as Pima Americans (Knowler *et al*, 1981) and Nauruans (Zimmet *et al*, 1977), in whom average BMIs are considerably higher than in populations of European origin. The occurrence of metabolic disturbances associated with insulin resistance in people of South Asian descent in widely different environments, even several generations after migration, suggests that some genetic predisposition to develop insulin resistance exists in this group. The ability to store fat in intra-abdominal depots and to rely on lipid rather than glucose as fuel for muscle may have been an advantage in times of unreliable food supply.

Relationship of lipid disturbances to central obesity

In the Southall Study, WHR was correlated more strongly with plasma triglyceride than with any other metabolic variable. A clue to the possible mechanism of this association may lie in the response of plasma triglyceride levels to glucose challenge. Between fasting and 2 h after a glucose load, the average change in plasma triglyceride was –1% in South Asian men and –6% in European men (McKeigue *et al*, 1991). In both ethnic groups the change in plasma triglyceride levels was directly correlated with WHR; men with central obesity have high fasting triglyceride levels which fall less in response to a glucose load. The most likely mechanism of this effect is that the rise in insulin levels suppresses lipolysis of fat to non-esterified fatty acids (NEFA), which are the main substrate for hepatic triglyceride synthesis. We found that the 2 h plasma NEFA level was correlated with both WHR and plasma triglyceride levels. This association is consistent with the results of two studies which have shown that the rate of decline of NEFA in response to insulin infusion is closely related to elevation of very-low-density lipoprotein (VLDL) triglyceride levels (Yki-Jarvinen and Taskinen, 1988) and to central obesity (Coon et al, 1992). It is likely that the relationship between central obesity and triglyceride levels is mediated through effects on the supply of NEFA to the liver. Raised triglyceride levels in turn may lower plasma HDL cholesterol and cause changes in the composition and size of particles in the LDL fraction (Austin et al, 1990).

Relationship of central obesity to CHD in South Asians

Baseline data from the Southall Study show strong cross-sectional associations of electrocardiographic Q waves in South Asian men with glucose intolerance, elevated insulin and triglyceride levels (McKeigue et al, 1993). Confirmation that this accounts for the high CHD risk will depend on prospective studies. We can test hypotheses about the mechanism of increased CHD risk by studying the distribution of risk factors in different South Asian groups. If the hypothesis that the insulin resistance syndrome underlies the high CHD risk in South Asians is correct, then the disturbances which cause CHD must be consistently present in all the groups originating from South Asia who share the high CHD risk. Although systolic and diastolic blood pressures are correlated with insulin levels in South Asians as in other populations, it is only in Sikhs and Hindus of Punjabi origin that average blood pressures are higher than in Europeans (McKeigue et al, 1991). Average HDL cholesterol is lower in Hindu and Muslim South Asian men than in the native British population, but in Sikh men average HDL cholesterol is no lower than in native British men. It follows that the increased CHD risk in South Asians cannot be mediated mainly through blood pressure or HDL cholesterol. Common to all South Asian populations at high risk of CHD are central obesity, hyperinsulinaemia, high diabetes prevalence and raised triglyceride levels after a glucose load (McKeigue and Marmot, 1988; McKeigue et al, 1991). Factors that are not common to all South Asian populations at risk are: high blood pressure (not Muslims), low HDL cholesterol (not Sikhs) and high fasting triglycerides (not Gujarati Hindus). The increased CHD risk may thus be mediated through some disturbance of lipoprotein metabolism related to increased synthesis of VLDL triglyceride.

Epidemiology of hypertension, NIDDM and CHD in Africans and Afro-Caribbeans

Numerous studies in the USA and the UK have demonstrated that hypertension is commoner and average blood pressures are higher in people of black African descent. The high mortality from stroke and hypertensive end-organ damage in African and Afro-Caribbean migrants to England is similar to that recorded in the African-American population of the USA. When groups of similar socio-economic status are compared in the UK, mortality from CHD is consistently lower in men of black African descent than in those of European descent. It is less clear whether African-Americans share any of this apparent immunity to CHD. Thus in the Charleston Heart Study, the relative risk of death from CHD in black compared with white men was 0.56 in those of low socio-economic status and 0.69 in those of high socio-economic status (Keil *et al*, 1992). Prevalence of NIDDM in people of West African descent in urban societies is almost as high as in South Asians. Table 3.3 summarises surveys which have compared prevalence of NIDDM in Afro-Caribbeans or African-Americans with Europeans: the ratio of diabetes prevalence in people of African descent to that in Europeans was 1.8 in the USA (Harris *et al*, 1987), 2 in Trinidad (Beckles *et al*, 1986) and around 3 in the UK (McKeigue *et al*, 1991; Chaturvedi *et al*, 1993). This dissociation between high prevalence of diabetes and hypertension and relatively low CHD mortality rates in Afro-Caribbean and African-American people has never been explained.

Insulin, lipids and body fat pattern in Afro-Caribbeans

In the Southall Study prevalence of NIDDM in Afro-Caribbean men was almost as high as in South Asian men, but serum insulin levels were similar in Afro-Caribbean and European men (McKeigue *et al*, 1991). Afro-Caribbean men have lower plasma triglyceride and higher HDL cholesterol than European men: in these respects Afro-Caribbean men resemble European women. At 2 h after a glucose load, plasma triglyceride levels are nearly 30% lower in Afro-Caribbean than in European men. These differences in triglyceride and HDL cholesterol levels have been consistently found in studies comparing Afro-Caribbean and African-American men with men of European descent (Slack *et al*, 1977; Morrison *et al*, 1981; Chaturvedi *et al*, 1993). In a subsequent study in Brent

Table 3.3 Diabetes prevalence by WHO criteria in Afro-Caribbeans and African-Americans

	Year	Sex	Age (years)	European	Black/Afro-Caribbean	Reference
Trinidad	1978	M&F	35–69	6%	12%	Beckles *et al*, 1986
USA	1980	M&F	40–64	10%	18%	Harris *et al*, 1987
Southall, UK	1989	M	40–64	5%	14%	McKeigue *et al*, 1991
Brent, UK	1991	M&F	40–64	5%	15%	Chaturvedi *et al*, 1993

(Chaturvedi *et al*, 1994), we found that the relatively favourable lipid pattern of Afro-Caribbean men compared with European men was maintained even in those with glucose intolerance. The favourable lipoprotein pattern in Afro-Caribbean men may be one reason for the low CHD mortality despite high prevalence of diabetes and hypertension in this group.

In contrast to South Asians, there is no evidence that Afro-Caribbean people tend to have a more central pattern of obesity than Europeans. Mean WHRs are no higher in Afro-Caribbean than in European men, although glucose intolerance is associated with higher WHRs in Afro-Caribbeans just as much as in Europeans or South Asians (Table 3.4) (McKeigue *et al*, 1991). The mean for waist–thigh ratio, an alternative measure of body fat distribution, is markedly lower in Afro-Caribbeans than in either of the two other ethnic groups. This emphasises the limitations of relying on one anthropometric index such as WHR to compare body fat pattern in groups with different physique. In any case it is clear that the high prevalence of NIDDM in Afro-Caribbeans is not part of a generalised syndrome of metabolic disturbances associated with central obesity, as it is in South Asians. The differences in triglyceride and HDL cholesterol levels between Afro-Caribbean and European men are in the opposite direction to the differences that we would predict from the hypothesis that dependent diabetes is but one manifestation of an insulin resistance syndrome.

Conclusion

The high rates of cardiovascular disease and NIDDM in migrants from South Asia and sub-Saharan Africa appear to reflect different patterns of susceptibility to the metabolic complications of obesity. Thus, South Asian populations develop high rates of CHD and diabetes in association with central obesity, whereas weight gain in African populations leads to high rates of hypertension, diabetes and stroke but not to coronary disease. In turn, these patterns of susceptibility probably result from past adaptations to survival under adverse conditions. The ability to deposit fat in visceral depots, for instance, may have

Table 3.4   Southall Study: mean obesity indices in men by ethnicity and glucose tolerance

	European		South Asian		Afro-Caribbean	
	GI	NG	GI	NG	GI	NG
N	48	1395	111	1056	352	158
BMI (kg/m^2)	28.2	25.7	28.2	25.4	26.5	25.8
Waist–hip ratio	0.98	0.93	0.99	0.97	1.00	0.93
Waist–thigh ratio	1.60	1.60	1.71	1.65	1.71	1.52

BMI: Body Mass Index; NG: normoglycaemic; GI: glucose-intolerant
Source; McKeigue *et al*, 1991

advantages under conditions of unreliable food supply and physically demanding work.

The experience of migrant populations is likely to be relevant to predicting the patterns of morbidity and mortality that will emerge in South Asia and West Africa as economic development continues in these regions of the world. Although no reliable information on cause-specific mortality in adults is available from West Africa, the high mortality from stroke and hypertension in recent migrants from West Africa suggests that rates of these diseases may already be high in urban populations in countries such as Nigeria and Ghana. The development of effective control strategies for cardiovascular disease and diabetes in these populations is limited by the lack of information on cause-specific mortality, and by uncertainties about the cost-effectiveness of possible interventions. Strategies for control of CHD which have been adopted in European countries are likely to be inappropriate for South Asian populations in whom the disease appears to be more closely related to the metabolic complications of obesity than in Europeans. For the low-income populations of black African descent who are most at risk of strokes and other hypertensive end-organ damage, programmes for the detection and management of hypertension may be a poor buy in comparison with other health interventions. Effective strategies for the control of obesity in the population would probably contribute more than any other measures to limiting the epidemic of cardiovascular disease and diabetes in native and migrant South Asian and African populations.

References

Adelstein AM. Some aspects of cardiovascular mortality in South Africa. *British Journal of Preventive and Social Medicine*, 1963; **17**: 29–40

Austin MA, King MC, Vranizan KM, Krauss RM. Atherogenic lipoprotein phenotype. A proposed genetic marker for coronary heart disease risk. *Circulation*, 1990; **82**: 495–506

Balarajan R, Bulusu L, Adelstein AM, Shukla V. Patterns of mortality among migrants to England and Wales from the Indian subcontinent. *British Medical Journal*, 1984; **289**: 1185–1187

Beckles GL, Miller GJ, Kirkwood BR, Alexis SD, Carson DC, Byam NT. High total and cardiovascular disease mortality in adults of Indian descent in Trinidad, unexplained by major coronary risk factors. *Lancet*, 1986; **i**: 1298–1301

Bhatnagar D, Anand IS, Durrington PN *et al.* Coronary risk factors in people from the Indian subcontinent living in west London and their siblings in India. Lancet, 1995; **345**: 405–409

Chadha SL, Radhakrishnan S, Ramachandran K, Kaul U, Gopinath N. Epidemiological study of coronary heart disease in urban population of Delhi. *Indian Journal of Medical Research*, 1990; **92**: 424–430

Chaturvedi N, McKeigue PM, Marmot MG. Resting and ambulatory blood pressure differences in Afro-Caribbeans and Europeans. *Hypertension*, 1993; **22**: 90–96

Chaturvedi N, McKeigue PM, Marmot MG. Relationship of glucose intolerance to coronary risk in Afro-Caribbeans compared with Europeans. *Diabetologia*, 1994; **37**: 765–772

Coon PJ, Rogus EM, Goldberg AP. Time course of plasma free fatty acid concentration in response to insulin: effect of obesity and physical fitness. *Metabolism*, 1992; **41**: 711–716

Danaraj TJ, Acker MS, Danaraj W, Ong WH, Yam TB. Ethnic group differences in coronary heart disease in Singapore: an analysis of necropsy records. *American Heart Journal*, 1959; **58**: 516–526

DeFronzo RA, Ferrannini E. Insulin resistance. A multifaceted syndrome responsible for NIDDM, obesity, hypertension, dyslipidemia, and atherosclerotic cardiovascular disease. *Diabetes Care*, 1991; **14**: 173–194

Dewan BD, Malhotra KC, Gupta SP. Epidemiological study of coronary heart disease in a rural community in Haryana. *Indian Heart Journal*, 1974; **26**: 68–78

Dowse GK, Gareeboo H, Zimmet PZ et al. High prevalence of NIDDM and impaired glucose tolerance in Indian, Creole and Chinese Mauritians. Mauritius Non-Communicable Disease Study Group. *Diabetes*, 1990; **39**: 390–396

Haenszel W, Kurihara M. Studies of Japanese migrants. I. Mortality from cancer and other diseases among Japanese in the United States. *Journal of the National Cancer Institute*, 1968; **40**: 43–68

Harris MI, Hadden WC, Knowler WC, Bennett PH. Prevalence of diabetes and impaired glucose tolerance and plasma glucose levels in U.S. population aged 20–74 yr. *Diabetes*, 1987; **36**: 523–534

Hughes K, Lun KC, Yeo PP. Cardiovascular diseases in Chinese, Malays and Indians in Singapore. I. Differences in mortality. *Journal of Epidemiology and Community Health*, 1990a; **44**: 24–28

Hughes K, Yeo PPB, Lun KC et al. Cardiovascular diseases in Chinese, Malays and Indians in Singapore. II. Differences in risk factor levels. *Journal of Epidemiology and Community Health*, 1990b; **44**: 29–35

Hughes LO, Cruickshank JK, Wright J, Raftery EB. Disturbances of insulin in British Asian and white men surviving myocardial infarction. *British Medical Journal*, 1989; **299**: 537–541

Jajoo UN, Kalantri SP, Gupta OP, Jain AP, Gupta K. The prevalence of coronary heart disease in rural population from central India. *Journal of the Association of Physicians of India*, 1988; **36**: 689–693

Keil JE, Sutherland SE, Knapp RG, Tyroler HA. Does equal socioeconomic status in black and white men mean equal risk of mortality? *American Journal of Public Health*, 1992; **82**: 1133–1136

Knowler WC, Pettitt DJ, Savage PJ, Bennett PH. Diabetes incidence in Pima Indians: contributions of obesity and parental diabetes. *American Journal of Epidemiology*, 1981; **113**: 144–156

McKeigue PM, Marmot MG. Mortality from coronary heart disease in Asian communities in London. *British Medical Journal*, 1988; **297**: 903

McKeigue PM, Marmot MG, Syndercombe Court YD, Cottier DE, Rahman S, Riemersma RA. Diabetes, hyperinsulinaemia and coronary risk factors in Bangladeshis in east London. *British Heart Journal*, 1988; **60**: 390–396

McKeigue PM, Shah B, Marmot MG. Relation of central obesity and insulin resistance with high diabetes prevalence and cardiovascular risk in South Asians. *Lancet*, 1991; **337**: 382–386

McKeigue PM, Pierpoint T, Ferrie JE, Marmot MG. Relationship of glucose intolerance and hyperinsulinaemia to body fat pattern in South Asians and Europeans. *Diabetologia*, 1992; **35**: 785–791

McKeigue PM, Ferrie JE, Pierpoint T, Marmot MG. Association of early-onset coronary heart disease in South Asian men with glucose intolerance and hyperinsulinemia. *Circulation*, 1993; **87**: 152–161

Miller GJ, Kotecha S, Wilkinson WH *et al.* Dietary and other characteristics relevant for coronary heart disease in men of Indian, West Indian and European descent in London. *Atherosclerosis*, 1988; **70**: 63–72

Miller GJ, Beckles GL, Maude GH *et al.* Ethnicity and other characteristics predictive of coronary heart disease in a developing country—principal results of the St James survey, Trinidad. *International Journal of Epidemiology*, 1989; **18**: 808–817

Morrison JA, Khoury P, Mellies M, Kelly K, Horvitz R, Glueck CJ. Lipid and lipoprotein distributions in black adults. The Cincinnati Lipid Research Clinic's Princeton School Study. *Journal of the American Medical Association*, 1981; **245**: 939–942

Office of Population Censuses and Surveys (OPCS). *Mortality and Geography: A Review in the Mid-1980s.* The Registrar-General's decennial supplement for England and Wales, series DS no 9. London: HMSO, 1990

Omar MA, Seedat MA, Dyer RB, Rajput MC, Motala AA, Joubert SM. The prevalence of diabetes mellitus in a large group of South African Indians. *South African Medical Journal*, 1985; **67**: 924–926

Ramachandran A, Jali MV, Mohan V, Snehalatha C, Viswanathan M. High prevalence of diabetes in an urban population in south India. *British Medical Journal*, 1988; **297**: 587–590

Ramachandran A, Snehalatha C, Dharmaraj D, Viswanathan M. Prevalence of glucose intolerance in Asian Indians—urban-rural difference and significance of upper-body adiposity. *Diabetes Care*, 1992; **15**: 1348–1355

Reaven GM. Banting Lecture. Role of insulin resistance in human disease. *Diabetes*, 1988; **37**: 1595–1607

Sarvotham SG, Berry JN. Prevalence of coronary heart disease in an urban population in northern India. *Circulation*, 1968; **37**: 939–953

Slack J, Noble N, Meade TW, North WR. Lipid and lipoprotein concentrations in 1604 men and women in working populations in north-west London. *British Medical Journal*, 1977; **2**: 353–357

Snehalatha C, Ramachandran A, Vijay V, Viswanathan M. Differences in plasma insulin responses in urban and rural Indians: a study in southern Indians. *Diabetic Medicine*, 1994; **11**: 445–448

Sorokin M. Hospital morbidity in the Fiji islands with special reference to the saccharine disease. *South African Medical Journal*, 1975; **49**: 1481–1485

Steinberg WJ, Balfe DL, Kustner HG. Decline in the ischaemic heart disease mortality rates of South Africans, 1968–1985. *South African Medical Journal*, 1988; **74**: 547–550

Tuomilehto J, Ram P, Eseroma R, Taylor R, Zimmet P. Cardiovascular diseases and diabetes mellitus in Fiji: analysis of mortality, morbidity and risk factors. *Bulletin of the World Health Organization*, 1984; **62**: 133–143

Worth RM, Kato H, Rhoads GG, Kagan A, Syme SL. Epidemiologic studies of coronary heart disease and stroke in Japanese men living in Japan, Hawaii and California: mortality. *American Journal of Epidemiology*, 1975; **102**: 481–490

Yki-Jarvinen H, Taskinen MR. Interrelationships among insulin's antipolytic and glucoregulatory effects and plasma triglycerides in nondiabetic and diabetic patients with endogenous hypertriglyceridemia. *Diabetes*, 1988; **37**: 1271–1278

Ziegler RG, Hoover RN, Pike MC *et al.* Migration patterns and breast cancer risk in Asian-American women. *Journal of the National Cancer Institute*, 1993; **85**: 1819–1827

Zimmet P, Taft P, Guinea A, Guthrie W, Thoma K. The high prevalence of diabetes on a Central Pacific island. *Diabetologia*, 1977; **13**: 111–115

Zimmet P, Taylor R, Ram P *et al.* Prevalence of diabetes and impaired glucose tolerance in the biracial (Melanesian and Indian) population of Fiji: a rural-urban comparison. *American Journal of Epidemiology*, 1983; **118**: 673–688

Discussion

K. Srinath Reddy

All India Institute of Medical Sciences, New Delhi, India

The second half of the twentieth century has witnessed the global spread of chronic disease epidemics, exemplified by coronary heart disease (CHD). While CHD mortality rates have shown a decline in recent years in developed countries, epidemics of CHD are occurring or accelerating in most developing countries. Hypertension, diabetes and cancer are also, similarly, becoming increasingly widespread in the global community. There is, however, wide-ranging variation in the nature of cardiovascular disease, cancers and the complications of diabetes, amongst the various ethnic groups in the world. While different stages of epidemiological transition may explain a part of this variance, the diversity of genetic–environment interactions is the factor which contributes most to this variability. The complex interplay of genetic and environmental influences raises interesting and intriguing issues of relative causal contribution to chronic diseases.

Migrant studies fortuitously offer us the opportunity of observing the role of environmental alteration in different ethnic groups. The occurrence of chronic disease in a relatively stable genetic pool confronted with the challenges of a new lifestyle is illustrative of the causal role played by the environment as well as the genetic contribution to the variability of responses to a common environmental change. Studies of migrants are also valuable in providing their countries of origin with a window into their own future, by revealing the effects of socio-economic and cultural changes that await them further along the path of development. McKeigue's excellent paper illustrates the many lessons that migrants offer in the area of chronic disease causation and control.

Migrants and cardiovascular disease

Studies of blood pressure patterns in unacculturated rural or nomadic communities and of urban migrants have revealed the rise of systolic and diastolic blood pressures and a rise in the prevalence of 'hypertension' which accompanies acculturation and lifestyle alteration (Poulter *et al*, 1990). It has also been observed that some unacculturated communities do not exhibit an age-related rise of blood pressure, while migration nullifies this protective phenomenon (Carvalho *et al*, 1989). That lifestyle is an important determinant of adult blood pressure and that an age-related rise of blood pressure is neither 'normal' nor 'inevitable' are lessons gleaned from these studies.

The effects of migration on CHD risk factors, morbidity and mortality are amongst the most interesting epidemiological insights provided by migrants. The Japan–Honolulu–San Francisco study provided strong evidence that lifestyle is a key determinant of CHD risk (Robertson *et al*, 1977). The recent studies in South Asian migrants, summarised by McKeigue, have further advanced our knowledge of the effects of genetic–environmental interaction on the risk of manifesting CHD (McKeigue *et al*, 1991; Enas and Mehta, 1995). The effects of migration on CHD have also been described recently by the Chinese (Li *et al*, 1994). The Chinese in Mauritius revealed higher CHD prevalence rates based on Q and ST abnormalities in the ECG (16.6% vs. 1.5% in males; 27.2% vs. 3.6% in females) and higher total blood cholesterol levels (5.3 mmol/l vs. 4.19 mmol/l in males; 5.27 mmol/l vs. 4.23 mmol/l in females) when compared to their Beijing counterparts.

CHD in South Asians

McKeigue describes the evidence denoting the enhanced risk of CHD which characterises the Indian diaspora, whatever the time or clime of migration. The pattern of excess and early mortality is not explained by the conventional risk factors of CHD, when mortality rates and risk profiles of South Asian migrants are compared with other ethnic groups in the countries of adoption. The hyperinsulinaemia–glucose intolerance–dyslipidaemia complex associated with central obesity (metabolic syndrome) reveals a stronger association with the risk of CHD in South Asians than in other population groups.

Does this reduce the relevance of the conventional risk factors in South Asians? Comparisons of risk profiles in rural and urban population groups in India as well as comparison of South Asians in the UK with ethnically similar communities in India do not suggest so. Community surveys in India have consistently revealed a two- to eight-fold excess of CHD prevalence in urban population groups in comparison to the rural communities. A recently completed community survey, initiated by the Indian Council of Medical Research (ICMR), revealed a two-fold excess of CHD prevalence in urban Delhi, in comparison with adjoining areas of rural Haryana (Reddy *et al*, unpublished data). Their risk profiles (anthropometric indices and blood lipids) are shown in Tables 3.5 and 3.6, in comparison with corresponding data from McKeigue's studies in London.

The rise in plasma cholesterol levels and ratios of total cholesterol to HDL cholesterol as the environment shifts from rural to urban India and further to London is striking. The rise in Body Mass Index (BMI) accompanying the rural–urban shift is again remarkable. South Asians in urban India as well as in London have higher waist–hip ratios (WHR) than Europeans. Rural–urban differences in WHR are less pronounced than observed for BMI. There is a five-fold excess of diabetes in the urban community in comparison with the rural

Table 3.5 Anthropometric measures: Delhi–London comparison

	Delhi (1994)		London (1991)	
	Rural	Urban	Asian	European
BMI				
Male	19.1	23.6	25.7	25.9
Female	20.3	25.2	27.0	25.2
WHR				
Male	0.947	0.993	0.98	0.94
Female	0.830	0.834	0.85	0.76

BMI = Body Mass Index (mean) (kg/m^2)
WHR = waist–hip ratio (mean)
Sources: Reddy KS (ICMR study) (unpublished results) – Delhi data; McKeigue et al, 1991—London data

Table 3.6 Blood lipids in South Asians and Caucasians: Delhi–London comparison

	Delhi (1994)		London (1991)	
	Rural	Urban	Asian	European
Cholesterol (mg/dl)				
Male	169.9	191.6	231.3	236.3
Female	165.6	193.5	230.5	243.2
Triglyceride (mg/dl)				
Male	146.1	161.5	173.0	148.0
Female	140.8	148.4	138.0	121.0
HDL cholesterol (mg/dl)				
Male	39.4	39.0	44.9	48.3
Female	41.9	43.4	53.4	61.1
Cholesterol/HDL ratio				
Male	4.55	5.06	5.15	4.89
Female	4.15	4.57	4.32	3.98

Sources: Reddy KS (ICMR study) (unpublished results)—Delhi data; McKeigue et al, 1991—London data

community (data not shown). The rise in BMI in urban Indians explains the high rate of diabetes better than WHR alone.

A recent comparison study of Punjabi migrants to the UK and their siblings in India also demonstrates that while both Indian groups have higher lipoprotein 'a' levels than the Caucasians in the UK, the migrant Indians have higher blood cholesterol and blood pressure levels than their siblings in India (Bhatnagar et al, 1995). Thus, while genetically determined variables like lipoprotein 'a' levels and factors such as the metabolic syndrome which may have 'genetic' or 'foetal programming' influences, possibly underlie the susceptibility of South Asians to

CHD, the acquisition or augmentation of conventional risk factors further enhances the risk of CHD. The confluence of the genetically determined or metabolically programmed factors and the environmentally acquired factors appears to make the Indian migrant especially vulnerable to CHD.

Variability of chronic disease in different migrant groups—genetic environmental interaction

The experience of Afro-Caribbean migrants to the UK, as described by McKeigue, illustrates the role of possible genetic factors in determining the nature of predominant vascular disease response to environmental challenges. Despite a high prevalence of non-insulin-dependent diabetes, this migrant group manifests stroke and not CHD as the main consequence of hypertension. The low levels of central obesity and the high levels of HDL cholesterol may be an important determinant of this response. These in turn may be genetically influenced, with a high level of physical activity also a probable protective contributor.

Thus, it would appear that (a) migrants moving from low-risk communities to high-risk communities acquire unfavourable risk profiles and vascular disease rates, principally due to environmental factors, and (b) the nature of dominant vascular disease which results from the environmental change is probably determined by genetic factors and/or foetal programming influences which enhance or decrease susceptibility to individual diseases.

Issues for investigation

The following questions need further elucidation in the context of chronic disease among migrants:

1. Is the gradient of relative risk, along the continuum of increasing risk factor levels, steeper for the migrant than for the non-migrant? Would a person migrating from a community with a mean cholesterol level of 170 mg% to a community with mean cholesterol level of 240 mg% share the same risk, at a cholesterol level of 230 mg%, as the non-migrant? Does a steeper slope exist for risk factors like cholesterol, blood pressure and BMI amongst the migrants?

2. Do the migrants who enter the higher socio-economic strata in the country of adoption differ in their risk profile and disease rates from the migrants who enter the lower socio-economic groups? To what extent do the socio-economic status-related differences in risk factors in the host country influence the effects of migration?

3. Do intrauterine growth patterns influence the nature and degree of response of migrants exposed to environmental change, i.e. is there a Barker effect?

4. How do migrants respond to preventive programmes in the host country? Does the tradition of moderate lifestyle prove conducive to their adoption of the preventive message, or does the temptation of consumer aspirations unleashed in the new environment prevail?

Public health implications for the home countries

McKeigue rightly emphasises the relevance of migrant experience for the countries of their origin. Given the same genetic susceptibility and the impending environmental changes which are attendant upon socio-economic transformation and the globalisation of economies and culture, these countries may soon replicate the chronic disease patterns now manifest in the migrants. This should alert policy-makers and public health activists to anticipate the emerging epidemics and plan for appropriate programmes of primordial and primary prevention, in which diet, nutrition and physical activity are major components. This may be the migrant's most valuable message to the families back home.

References

Bhatnagar D, Anand IS, Durrington PN *et al.* Coronary risk factors in people from the Indian subcontinent living in West London and their siblings in India. *Lancet*, 1995; **345**: 405–409

Carvalho JJ, Baruzzi RG, Howard PF *et al.* Blood pressure in four remote populations in the INTERSALT Study. *Hypertension*, 1989; **14**: 238–246

Enas EA, Mehta J. Malignant coronary artery disease in young Asian Indians. Thoughts on pathogenesis, prevention and therapy. Coronary Artery Disease in Asian Indians (CADI) Study. *Clinical Cardiology*, 1995; **18**: 131–135

Li N, Tuomilehto J, Dowse G, Virtala E, Zimmet P. Prevalence of coronary heart disease indicated by electrocardiogram abnormalities and risk factors in developing countries. *Journal of Clinical Epidemiology*, 1994; **47**: 599–611

McKeigue PM, Shah B, Marmot MG. Relation of central obesity and insulin resistance with high diabetes prevalence and cardiovascular risk in South Asians. *Lancet*, 1991; **337**: 382–386

Poulter NR, Khaw KT, Hopwood BE *et al.* The Kenyan Luo migration study: observations on the initiation of a rise in blood pressure. *British Medical Journal*, 1990; **300**: 967–972

Robertson TL, Kato H, Rhoads GG *et al.* Epidemiologic studies of coronary heart disease and stroke in Japanese men living in Japan, Hawaii and California. Incidence of myocardial infarction and death from coronary heart disease. *American Journal of Cardiology*, 1977; **39**: 239–243

4
Inequalities in diet and health

Eric Brunner

Department of Epidemiology and Public Health, University College London Medical School, London, UK

Since the nineteenth century, life expectancy at birth in England and Wales has risen from 44 to 74 years among boys, and from 48 to 79 years among girls. This dramatic increase in longevity is in small part the result of progress in medical science and improved access to health care, while the greater part is due to public health measures which have improved living and working conditions, and promoted the decline of infectious disease mortality (McKeown, 1995). Looking beyond these improvements in the mean level of health, to the distribution of health within populations, we lose the right to be self-congratulatory. Though there has in general been a decline in premature mortality in all social strata, the decline has been, and continues to be, distinctly uneven (Marmot, 1994). The role of diet and the food supply in generating these patterns, it is argued, is important but not well quantified. Diet not only influences health, but is itself influenced by numerous individual and social factors. Thus in epidemiological research diet cannot be classified only as an exposure, but also as an outcome variable when other factors such as socio-economic status are considered the exposure.

Health inequalities since World War II

National mortality data for England and Wales suggest that social class inequalities were at their narrowest at around the time of the 1951 census (Pamuk, 1985; Blane *et al*, 1996). This followed the introduction of Beveridge's welfare state, which included universal free health care after 1948, and a comprehensive system of welfare benefits. The nadir in social mortality differences also coincided with the period of wartime food rationing, which continued to have effects on the national diet for at least a decade after 1945. In Britain, trends in health inequality moved upwards during the 1970s. This has been documented

Diet, Nutrition and Chronic Disease: Lessons from Contrasting Worlds.
Edited by P. S. Shetty and K. McPherson © 1997 John Wiley & Sons, Ltd.

using occupational social class data, using two strata, manual and non-manual, to address the problem of change in the labour market over the decade (Marmot and McDowall, 1986). Between 1981 and 1991 health inequalities continued to widen and death rates actually rose among young adults in the most economically deprived areas of Britain (McLoone and Boddy, 1994; Phillimore et al, 1994). With increasing social polarisation, the re-emergence of tuberculosis was seen, almost exclusively among the poorest sections of society (Bhatti et al, 1995). In the USA, between 1960 and 1986, mortality rates widened among whites according to education level (Pappas et al, 1993); overall rates fell, but those with more education experienced the largest decline. It thus appears that despite the overall improvement in health of society, inequalities in health between socio-economic groups continue to persist.

The Whitehall studies

The first Whitehall study was set up by Reid and Rose at the London School of Hygiene & Tropical Medicine in 1967 to investigate risk factors for CHD. A total of 18 000 men working in London offices of the Civil Service completed a questionnaire on socio-demographic and behavioural factors and were given a cardiovascular examination at baseline. The cohort continues to be followed for mortality and its principal finding (Marmot et al, 1978) was a large stepwise inverse occupational gradient in coronary risk, which was contrary to the commonly held view that heart attacks occurred particularly among stressed senior executives (Figure 4.1). The coronary risk gradient was poorly explained by the three conventional risk factors: smoking, blood pressure and serum cholesterol. Rates of smoking varied in the expected way, but differences in smoking and in blood pressure, measured on a single occasion, accounted statistically for less than a third of the higher rates of disease observed in lower occupational groups. The few prospective studies which have evaluated reasons for socio-economic differences in CHD or total mortality have been able to explain less than half of class differences (Haan et al, 1987; Pocock et al, 1987). The likely reasons for this lack of explanatory power are both methodological and theoretical. Lifetime exposure to tobacco smoke is poorly estimated by obtaining a single self-report of smoking habits. Detailed measurement of current food intake in a large number of individuals requires considerable resources and, like smoking history, provides incomplete information about changes in dietary patterns over time. At the theoretical level, biomedical and psycho-social influences on health are seldom studied at the same time, and these factors, separately and interacting together, appear to be important.

In the first Whitehall study, serum cholesterol was a strong predictor of CHD in the entire study population (Davey Smith et al, 1992). However, mean cholesterol level showed a positive association with occupational grade in these men (Marmot et al, 1978); the higher the occupational grade, the higher the level

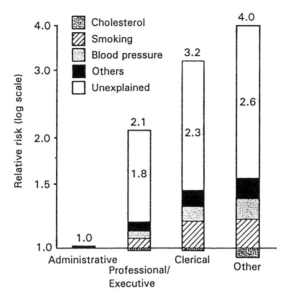

Figure 4.1   Socio-economic gradient in CHD. Age-standardised relative risk of coronary death at 7.5 year follow-up according to employment grade among 17 530 civil servants (The Whitehall study). Proportions that can be explained statistically by various risk factors are shown by the shaded areas. Source: Marmot *et al*, 1978.

of serum cholesterol. Differences in total cholesterol could not therefore account for the higher rates of CHD among the lower occupational grades. The pattern of serum cholesterol levels hence suggests that dietary fat intake might not be an important determinant of the distribution of coronary risk among occupational groups.

The Whitehall II cohort was established in 1985 to investigate additional—particularly dietary, metabolic and psycho-social—factors which might account for the unexplained magnitude of social gradients in CHD risk (Marmot *et al*, 1991). This study of 10 308 male and female civil servants found inverse gradients in the prevalence of ECG abnormalities in both sexes at the baseline that paralleled the findings in the original cohort. In the Whitehall II study population, mean cholesterol levels again did not appear to contribute to the expected occupational gradient in CHD risk. In both sexes, the mean cholesterol level at baseline was similar in each grade. Concentrations of serum apolipoprotein A1, the main structural protein of HDL cholesterol, did show an association with occupational grade (Brunner *et al*, 1993a), suggesting that characteristic disturbances of lipid metabolism were potentially identifiable and associated with lower occupational status. Some of the results of the second examination in 1991–1993 are presented here.

Obesity

Overweight is increasing in European and North American adults, and continues to be a public health issue for which no effective preventive or therapeutic solution has yet been identified (Kuczmarski et al, 1994; GB Department of Health Nutrition and Physical Activity Task Forces, 1995). Data from the Whitehall studies (I and II) illustrate the development of this problem, and its increasingly strong links with lower socio-economic status. The prevalence of obesity has increased markedly over the period of the two studies and is more common in women than men, and in both sexes more common among those in the lower occupational grades (Table 4.1).

Several data-sets have suggested that dietary fat intake is an important determinant of obesity (Prentice and Jebb, 1995). Total fat intake (both in grams or as a proportion of the total food energy) does not appear to be related to social status in men or women (Gregory et al, 1990). Other factors may be responsible for the observed social gradients in degree and distribution of obesity. Possible candidates are physical activity levels and food consumption patterns unrelated to overall fat content, but associated with a high energy density of the diet. The social gradient suggests also that inequalities in the psycho-social environment contribute to the excess of obesity in lower social strata.

Abdominal obesity and the metabolic syndrome

An abdominal or central fat distribution is well known to be a risk factor for non-insulin-dependent diabetes (NIDDM) and CHD in Europeans (Lapidus et al, 1984; Larsson et al, 1984) and South Asians (McKeigue et al, 1991). Evidence

Table 4.1   Body Mass Index and obesity in the Whitehall studies (age adjusted (40–59 years))

	Administrative	Professional/ executive	Clerical/support	Trend P
Whitehall				
Men: n	889	11 081	3232	
BMI	24.5(0.09)	24.7(0.03)	24.7(0.06)	0.15
Obesity	1.7(0.33)	1.9(0.09)	3.1(0.23)	<0.001
Whitehall II (phase 3)				
Men: n	2404	2300	334	
BMI	25.0(0.06)	25.2(0.07)	25.5(0.22)	<0.005
Obesity	6.6(0.51)	7.6(0.56)	10.1(1.65)	<0.05
Women: n	352	1006	821	
BMI	24.5(0.24)	25.4(0.14)	26.5(0.19)	0.0001
Obesity	11.3(1.78)	14.6(1.11)	18.8(1.48)	<0.05

BMI is given as mean (standard error) (kg/m^2). Prevalence of obesity (BMI > $30 \, kg/m^2$) is given as percentage (standard error)

from Whitehall II suggests that abdominal fatness, confirmed by the tendency to a higher waist–hip ratio, as well as overweight/obesity, is a feature of lower socio-economic status in men and women aged between 16 and 64 (Brunner *et al*, 1993b) (Figure 4.2).

A key metabolic correlate of central obesity is impaired glucose tolerance (WHO Study Group, 1985) which is associated with an increased likelihood of the development of NIDDM. An individual of given ethnicity with both a high waist–hip ratio and a high BMI is more likely to be glucose intolerant than an individual with one of these risk factors. Central obesity in Whitehall II subjects is linked with, in addition to impaired glucose tolerance, clustering of high plasma fibrinogen, high serum triglycerides and low levels of high-density lipoprotein (HDL) cholesterol. This metabolic syndrome or syndrome X (Reaven, 1993), is more common as one approaches lower employment grades in Whitehall II subjects (Figure 4.3).

In this and other populations (Heiss *et al*, 1980) HDL cholesterol, unlike total cholesterol, is related to socio-economic status. The causes of central obesity and the metabolic syndrome are not well understood. Diet, high alcohol consumption, low exercise levels and smoking appear to be involved to some degree. Sapolsky and Mott's work (1987) with non-human (non-smoking) primates suggests that psycho-social factors may also be involved. Their studies of Serengeti baboons are consistent with cardiovascular effects of position in the primate social hierarchy. The proposed mechanism involves chronic exposure to situations in which psycho-social stresses or demands exceed the individual's capacity to cope. The result is activation of the hypothalamic–pituitary–adrenal axis and increased

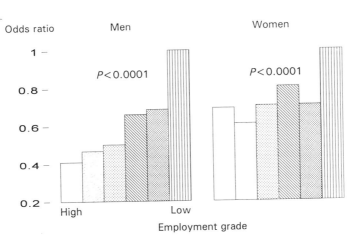

Figure 4.2   Central obesity by occupational status. Likelihood of being in top quintile of waist–hip ratio according to Civil Service employment grade. Whitehall II study, phase 3, 1991–1993, Europeans only. Adjusted for age, and menopausal status in women

E. Brunner

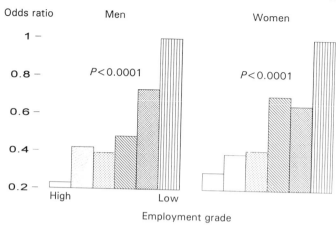

Figure 4.3 Clustering of metabolic syndrome variables by occupational status. Likelihood of being in top quintile of three or more of five metabolic syndrome variables (two-hour post-load glucose, HDL cholesterol (lower quintile), triglycerides, fibrinogen, waist–hip ratio) according to Civil Service employment grade. Whitehall II study, phase 3, 1991–1993, Europeans only. Adjusted for age, and menopausal status in women. P test for trend

corticotrophin-releasing hormone, adrenocorticotrophic hormone and cortisol secretion. This change in endocrine balance is associated with insulin resistance, diabetes, abdominal obesity, hypertriglyceridaemia and low HDL cholesterol level.

Role of diet in health inequalities

The reasons for the social class gradient in ill-health are not fully understood. Major British reviews (Townsend et al, 1992) concluded that it cannot be attributed to differences in medical care, but appears to relate to a combination of lifestyle and material conditions. There can be little doubt that diet is a factor in the poorer health expectations of individuals living in poverty. Dietary factors also appear to be important among those who are relatively, rather than absolutely, deprived. The main dietary factors likely to be relevant are caloric intake, fat quantity and quality, dietary antioxidants, micronutrient and fibre intakes.

Rates of diseases considered to have a dietary determinant in their causation, such as cardiovascular disease, several cancers (with the exception of breast cancer), musculo-skeletal disorders and cataract, are higher in lower socio-economic groups (Davey Smith, 1996). An inverse social gradient in disease incidence is an almost universal observation: 62 of the 66 main causes of death in men show the same inverse social trend (GB Department of Health Variations Sub-group, 1995). Also, several health-related behaviours have a social distribution consistent with their roles in attempting to explain the existence of social inequalities in health. Smoking is one of the most important behavioural factors, although an inverse social gradient in CHD is seen among those who never smoked in the Whitehall and other studies (Marmot *et al*, 1984; Hein *et al*, 1992). Psycho-social conditions of work environment have also been linked prospectively with increased risk of CHD morbidity in these studies (Bosma *et al*, 1996). Such 'stress-related' factors may exert their effects partly by dietary and other behavioural changes, or may operate by neuro-endocrine mechanisms which are independent of behavioural factors.

Social differences in diet

The 1986/1987 Dietary and Nutritional Survey of British Adults (Gregory *et al*, 1990) provides a high-quality data source for investigating social differences in diet. This comprises a representative sample of the adult population of England, Wales and Scotland, who completed a seven-day weighed intake record. Associations in energy, macronutrient and micronutrient intakes classified by social class of the head of household are summarised in Table 4.2.

As in the Caerphilly Heart Study (Fehily *et al*, 1984), which used a similar dietary method, men in manual occupations reported higher intakes of dietary energy, presumably reflecting higher levels of physical activity. In contrast, women in non-manual occupations in the British survey reported higher energy intakes. This finding may be due mainly to higher exercise levels, but in part is probably an artifact of differential rates of dietary under-reporting according to social class, which appears to be particularly high among women overall (Pryer *et al*, 1995).

Total and saturated fat intakes, as a proportion of dietary energy, were not

Table 4.2   Social differences in diet: dietary and nutritional survey of British adults 1986/1987

	Associations by social class of head of household	
	Men	Women
Energy	Inverse	Direct
Alcohol	Heterogeneous	Direct
Sugars	Direct	NS
Fibre	NS	Direct
Total/SFA	NS	NS
P:S ratio	Direct	Direct
Ca/Fe/Mg/K	Direct	Direct
Vitamin A/B/C	Direct	Direct

Key: Total/SFA: Total fat/saturated fatty acids; Ca: Calcium; Fe: Iron; Mg: Magnesium; K: Potassium; NS, not significant
Source: Gregory *et al*, 1990

associated with social class in the British survey. The mean polyunsaturated:saturated (P:S) ratio did vary according to social class, with men and women in higher social strata tending to report a higher P:S ratio. These data suggest that the amount of total and saturated dietary fat consumed may not play a major role in the excess coronary risk among adults of lower social status, while the lower polyunsaturated fatty acid intake may be important. This interpretation is supported by the findings of the National Survey of Health and Development, i.e. the 1946 birth cohort, which showed that saturated fat intake did not vary by education level among men (Braddon *et al*, 1988). Among women it was highest in those with university education. Although fat intakes appeared to be weakly associated with social position among adults in the 1980s, the micronutrient density of the diet differed markedly by social class. Vitamins A, B and C, and iron, magnesium, potassium, calcium and phosphorus were all present at higher levels in diets of those in higher social classes. The data on social differences in nutrition—similar fat intakes, but large differentials in micronutrient density—point to an effect of social differences in food consumption patterns. These are the product of a diverse combination of social, economic, cultural and personal factors.

Factors influencing dietary patterns

Recent decades have seen a myriad of changes in the food system of the rich nations. The retailing sector is a prominent example of this continuing transformation (see Lang, this volume), which has not brought uniform benefits to all levels of society. The increased availability of a great variety of raw and processed foods in large supermarkets has been at the cost of the loss of many small grocers shops which had offered local but restricted food choice to both urban and rural populations. Those without cars are particularly disadvantaged. The potential for persisting social differences in dietary patterns as a result of changes in food retailing is illustrated by a small study (Lobstein, 1995) carried out in North London (Table 4.3). A comparison of the costs of food shopping in two areas in 1995 showed that a basket of healthy food cost 41% more than a basket of less healthy food in the deprived area, as compared to 31% more in the affluent area. Cost differentials were shown to have increased substantially since the survey was initially conducted in 1988.

Poverty as a determinant of dietary intake is usually examined in the context of developing nations. With income levels in Britain becoming increasingly polarised, poverty may again be a major public health problem. Childhood poverty, defined as residence in a household with an income at or below Income Support level (Social Security Committee, 1995), was experienced by 29% of children in the UK in 1992. The implications for dietary intake, and current and future health are unclear.

While structural and other material influences are of great importance in relation to socio-economic variations, cultural factors also shape dietary patterns,

Table 4.3 Shopping basket survey, London—cost of two food baskets in two areas. Food Commission Surveys, 1988 and 1995

Basket	Deprived area	Affluent area
More healthy	£15.25	£14.87
Less healthy	£10.84	£11.30
1995 premium (%)	41	31
1988 premium (%)	20	16

Source: Lobstein, 1995

and these in turn are determinants of nutrient intakes. Perception of the nutritional quality of particular foods is one example of the way in which food selections may be made, independently of its nutrient composition. The epidemiological evidence from both food purchase and dietary intake surveys supports the observation that the countries of Europe and North America share a high-fat food culture. Three years after the 1984 COMA report (GB Department of Health Committee on Medical Aspects of Food Policy, 1984), which emphasised recommendations to reduce total and saturated fat intake, there were very low rates of compliance with those recommendations (Pryer et al, 1995). A high-fat food culture, once adopted, is apparently difficult to reverse. Although reluctant to reduce total fat intake, British adults appear willing to change the type of fat in their diet. Food purchase surveys show (GB Ministry of Agriculture, Fisheries and Food, 1990) that during the 1980s the population substituted polyunsaturated and partially hydrogenated seed oils for sources of saturated fatty acids, resulting in an approximately 60% increase in the P:S ratio. This modification in the national diet, and the decline in smoking rates, are the most distinct improvements in health-related behaviours that have accompanied the declining coronary heart disease mortality trends over this period (GB Department of Health, 1993). The recent change in fat quality of the British diet is significant because of the means by which it has been obtained. Health promotion directed at healthy adults with the aim of improving risk factor status can be moderately effective (Cutler et al, 1991; Imperial Cancer Research Fund OXCHECK Study Group, 1995). For example, a systematic review of single-factor trials of dietary advice demonstrates a modest net reduction in serum cholesterol of 0.22 mmol/l (95% confidence interval 0.05–0.39) after 9–18 months (Brunner et al, 1996).

Estimates of the cost-effectiveness of cholesterol-lowering using screening and dietary advice vary between £3000 (GB Department of Health, 1995) and £12 000 (Kristiansen et al, 1991) per life year gained, suggesting that such approaches may be costly. In comparison, the increase in P:S ratio appears to have occurred as a result of the combined effects of improved nutrition awareness together with changes in product availability and food-processing technology. The latter include the increased availability of polyunsaturated cooking oils and the development of palatable low-cost vegetable oil spreads.

Diet and health over the lifecourse

Dietary patterns are initially acquired in childhood. Tastes and preferences remain with the individual to some degree, though diet during life will be shaped by factors such as financial circumstances, food availability, novel products and nutritional beliefs, as outlined above. The sustained influence of childhood dietary pattern on eating habits in adults has been shown among men in Kuopio, Finland (Lynch *et al*, 1996). In this group, poor childhood socio-economic circumstances were associated with lower consumption of fruit and vegetables, and with lower vitamin C intakes, as adults (Figure 4.4).

A lifelong poor diet with a low dietary antioxidant intake among adults disadvantaged as children may be expected to increase the risks of cardiovascular disease and cancer in adult life (Rimm *et al*, 1996). Indirect evidence suggests, however, that the relation between childhood diet and adult health may not be straightforward. Data collected in the Carnegie Study, a pre-war survey of nutrition and health in English and Scottish children, show that the social class of the head of household and family expenditure on food were each directly associated with attained height and leg length (Gunnell *et al*, 1996; Davey Smith, 1996). Leg length in particular appears to be a good measure of early nutrition and growth (Leitch, 1951). Childhood circumstances showed the expected relation with growth, and longer leg length was associated with a smaller risk of cardiovascular mortality at the 57-year follow-up, but leg length showed no relationship with overall mortality, and had a direct association with cancer

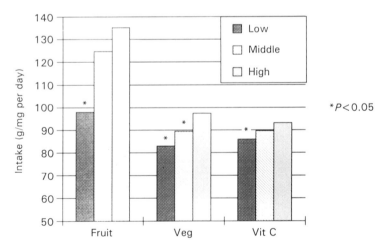

Figure 4.4 Childhood socio-economic circumstances and adult diet. Fruit, non-root vegetable and vitamin C intakes among Finnish men (Kuopio) according to childhood socio-economic circumstances (parental education and occupation and perceived level of wealth)

mortality in men. It appears that further studies over the whole lifecourse are required for a definition of an optimal diet in childhood.

Diet among civil servants in the Whitehall II study

The stepwise inverse occupational gradient in coronary risk observed in the first Whitehall study has been inadequately explained by the conventional risk factors (Marmot et al, 1978). Because the observed relation between occupational status and CHD risk was continuous, and not a threshold effect within this salaried group, the causes of the social gradient in risk appear to be relevant to the larger part of the population. The contribution of dietary explanations to this gradient are being investigated in Whitehall II, utilising data collected at the second examination of the cohort in 1991–1993. When incident disease has accumulated in the cohort, dietary factors will be examined as mediating variables in multivariate analysis of the association between employment grade and coronary events.

Preliminary results of the Whitehall II study presented here, where subjects completed a machine-readable semi-quantitative food frequency questionnaire (FFQ) (Willett et al, 1985) and a seven-day diet diary with estimated portion sizes (Braddon et al, 1988), are based on the results of 5494 men and 2445 women who completed the FFQ, and 275 men and 218 women whose diaries have been coded to date.

Low energy reporting

Reporting bias is an important consideration in dietary studies (Goldberg et al, 1991; Brunner et al, 1992), and this is particularly true when examining social variations. 'Low energy reporting' (LER) is defined as a reported energy intake of less than 1.2 times estimated basal metabolic rate (BMR) (Pryer et al, 1995), since the energy requirement for sedentary men and women in Western populations is estimated to be at least 1.55 times BMR (WHO, 1985). Energy intakes below 1.2 times BMR are rare, and habitual intakes of this order are unlikely to meet energy requirements. Some 36% of respondents of the Whitehall II cohort were classified as LERs (seven-day diary men: 32.4%, women: 37.6%; FFQ men: 38.9%, women: 32.6%). In comparison, 30% of men and 47% of women were LERs in the national survey which utilised a seven-day weighed intake method (Pryer et al, 1995). Low energy reporting or under-reporting may arise by the omission of food items from a diet record, or be the result of observation bias: the conscious or unconscious modification of diet during the recording period. Low energy reporting associated with the FFQ likewise may result from omission or underestimation of consumption frequency, which may again be conscious or unconscious. The Whitehall II data suggest that low energy reporting in one instrument is not always accompanied by low energy reporting on the other.

Increase in bodyweight is strongly associated with the prevalence of low energy reporting (Table 4.4); the seven-day diary performs better among men, whilst the food frequency questionnaire appears to provide less biased results among women. Low energy reporting is more common among subjects in lower employment grades. Among men, about 30% are LERs in top administrative grades while 50% are LERs in the clerical grade. Some 20% of women in the administrative grades are LERs on both dietary measures. The seven-day diary appears to be relatively demanding of lower-grade women, with about 55% appearing as LERs, compared to 35% on the FFQ. These findings are only to a small extent the result of the relative weight distribution across grades. Adjustment for BMI does not greatly reduce the differential in rates of low energy reporting (Table 4.4), which appear to be the result of cognitive factors.

Fat intake by employment grade

Three approaches were adopted in the analyses of mean total fat intakes by employment grade. First, all data were analysed without exclusions; second, LERs were excluded; and third, fat intakes were adjusted for energy intake after exclusion of subjects with energy intakes below 800 or above 4000 kcal/day. Though not a reference method, the seven-day diary may be taken as a more quantitative dietary method with which to compare the FFQ (Bingham *et al*, 1994). Among men, results for the seven-day diary excluding LERs and adjusting for energy suggest small inverse trends in mean total fat intake, with higher intakes in lower grades. In contrast, if all the data are used and dietary energy is not taken into account, no trend is evident. Among women, results excluding LERs and adjusting for energy do not show significant trends, while the data without exclusions indicate a direct relationship between occupational status and fat intake, an effect largely explained by the grade-related differential in low energy reporting.

Results obtained with the FFQ differ somewhat from those obtained with the seven-day diary. It should be noted that the latter is a sub-sample of the study

Table 4.4 Low energy reporting by relative weight. Whitehall II study, phase 3, 1991–1993 (available data)

	FFQ		Seven-day diary	
	Men ($n = 5485$)	Women ($n = 2493$)	Men ($n = 275$)	Women ($n = 218$)
Underweight (%)	22.1	18.8	12.5	15.4
'Normal' weight (%)	32.0	28.4	20.3	33.0
Overweight (%)	44.3	33.1	44.4	40.3
Obese (%)	64.4	49.5	50.0	56.3
Probability*	<0.0001	<0.0001	<0.0001	0.004

*Mantel–Haenszel χ^2 test for trend

population, and therefore differences in the results may be due to dietary method or to sampling. Among men, exclusion of LERs and adjustment for dietary energy suggest that there is, in contrast with the seven-day diary results, no difference in fat intake according to grade. The raw data, in contrast, show a direct association between grade and fat intake. For women, the energy-adjusted results for both dietary methods suggest no trend in fat intake, while excluding LERs yields an inverse gradient (Table 4.5).

Considering the evidence of reporting bias with respect to employment grade and relative weight, it may be that the analytical method involving the least bias is that utilising the largest sample size, the smallest number of exclusions, and regression adjustment for dietary energy intake as an attempt to control for bias due to low or high energy reporting. Results for mean saturated fatty acid intake and mean P:S ratio by grade are therefore presented from the FFQ data, excluding only those at the extremes of reported energy intake. For energy-adjusted saturated fatty acid intake by FFQ, statistically significant trends are not evident by grade, although there is a suggestion that lower-grade women, who tend to be more obese than their higher-grade counterparts, may tend towards a higher intake. Similar findings are seen for total fats. The mean P:S ratio is inversely related to grade, in contrast to the national data in 1986/87 which showed a direct association between social class and the P:S ratio (Gregory *et al*, 1990).

Dietary patterns and psycho-social determinants of disease

The psycho-social determinants of food intake deserve attention in order to support evidence-based approaches to health promotion. The relationship between perceived control over heart attack risk and a composite variable indicating a health-related dietary pattern was analysed. This variable was constructed using food type and frequency data from the FFQ. The measure of

Table 4.5 Low energy reporting by employment grade after adjustment for Body Mass Index. Whitehall II study, phase 3, 1991–1993 (available data)

Employment categorised by grade	FFQ		Seven-day diary	
	Men	Women	Men	Women
Unified grades 1–6 (%)	36.5	20.7	27.8	17.6
Unified grade 7 (%)	36.2	29.0	28.7	31.2
Senior executive officer (%)	39.4	27.3	27.0	14.1
Higher executive officer (%)	42.1	30.7	41.4	35.0
Executive officer (%)	44.7	32.5	28.6	53.9
Clerical (%)	46.1	35.1	47.9	55.2
Total N	5485	2443	275	218
Probability*	<0.0001	<0.0001	0.09	<0.0001

*Mantel–Haenszel χ^2 test for trend

E. Brunner

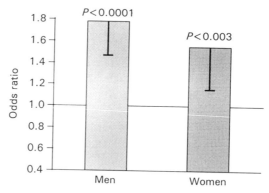

Figure 4.5 Coronary heart disease control beliefs and diet. Likelihood of meeting healthy eating criterion (usually use wholemeal/brown bread and reduced fat milk, and fresh fruit/vegetables daily or more) according to perceived level of control over heart attack risk. Food frequency questionnaire data adjusted for age and employment grade. Whitehall II study, phase 3, 1991–1993

control, which can be seen as a measure of fatalism or locus of control in relation to health (Pill and Stott, 1985), distinguishes between those who tend to believe their risk is largely a matter of fate, and those who believe their risk will be reduced by personal actions. The composite diet variable was constructed to summarise reported dietary pattern with reference to positive healthy eating messages (GB Department of Health Committee on Medical Aspects of Food Policy, 1994). Reported consumption in the FFQ of a reduced fat milk (skimmed or semi-skimmed), fresh fruit/vegetables (once or more per day), and lower extraction (wholemeal, granary or brown) breads yields a score of 1 on the diet indicator. If any of these three criteria was not met, the score was set to 0. Logistic regression analysis showed that the likelihood of being a healthy eater, as defined, is related to perception of control over heart attack risk independently of employment grade (Figure 4.5). Future analyses will compare food-based and nutrient-based approaches to the investigation of social differences in diet and health.

Conclusion

Persisting social inequalities in health accompany the substantial overall health gains of the twentieth century. There is a stepwise increase, rather than a threshold effect, in excess coronary mortality as social strata are descended. Chronic diseases with a dietary component in their aetiology, in particular cardiovascular disease, cancers of the gastro-intestinal tract, prostate, bladder and pancreas, non-insulin-dependent diabetes and cataract, have higher incidence rates in lower social strata. Breast cancer is unusual in that incidence is directly related to social status. It is unclear to what extent diet accounts for the inverse social gradients in chronic disease. Central obesity and accompanying metabolic disorders are strongly and inversely related to occupational status in the Whitehall II study. Major social differences in nutrient intake among British adults are seen in minerals (iron, magnesium, potassium and calcium), vitamins (retinol, B vitamins, ascorbic acid) and other antioxidants, while total fat intake shows little systematic social variation. Patterns of food consumption are the product of a diverse combination of economic, cultural and personal factors. European and North American countries have adopted a high-fat food culture which is resistant to change. Preliminary analyses of dietary data collected in the Whitehall II study add to the evidence that in recent years differences in total and saturated fatty acid intake are likely to have contributed little to the inverse social gradient in cardiovascular disease.

Acknowledgements

Dr Daryth Stallone carried out the analyses of the seven-day diary and the food frequency questionnaire. The Whitehall II study is supported by the Medical Research Council, British Heart Foundation, Health and Safety Executive and National Heart Lung and Blood Institute (2ROI HL36310), Agency for Health Care Policy Research (5ROI HS06516), Institute for Work and Health, Ontario, and the John D. and Catherine T. MacArthur Foundation Research Network on Successful Midlife Development. The diet component of the study was funded by the Ministry of Agriculture, Fisheries and Food and Department of Health.

References

Bhatti N, Law MR, Morris JK, Halliday R, Moore-Gillon J. Increasing incidence of tuberculosis in England and Wales: a study of the likely causes. *British Journal of Medicine*, 1995; **310**: 967–969

Bingham SA, Gill C, Welch A *et al*. Comparison of dietary assessment methods in nutritional epidemiology: weighed records versus 24 h recalls, food frequency questionnaires and estimated-diet records. *British Journal of Nutrition*, 1994; **72**: 619–643

Blane D, Brunner E, Wilkinson R. The evolution of public health policy: an anglocentric view of the last fifty years. In: Blane D, Brunner E, Wilkinson RG, eds. *Health and Social Organization: Towards a Health Policy for the the 21st Century*. London: Routledge, 1996, p 1

Bosma HJ, Marmot MG, Hemingway H, Nicholson A, Brunner EJ, Stansfeld SA. Low job control and the risk of coronary heart disease in the Whitehall II study. *British Medical Journal* (in press)

Braddon FE, Wadsworth ME, Davies JMC, Cripps HA. Social and regional differences in food and alcohol consumption and their measurement in a national birth cohort. *Journal of Epidemiology and Community Health*, 1988; **42**: 341–349

Brunner EJ, Sharma A, Pryer JA, Elliott P, Marmot MG. Effects of reporting bias in the dietary and nutritional survey of British adults on the estimation of nutrient–blood lipid relationships. 4th European Conference on Nutritional Epidemiology, Berlin, 1992 (Abstract)

Brunner EJ, Marmot MG, White IR *et al*. Gender and employment grade differences in blood cholesterol, apolipoproteins and haemostatic factors in the Whitehall II study. *Atherosclerosis*, 1993a; **102**: 195–207

Brunner EJ, Nicholson A, Marmot MG. Trends in central obesity and insulin resistance across employment grades: the Whitehall II Study. *Journal of Epidemiology and Community Health*, 1993b; **47**: 404–405 (Abstract)

Brunner EJ, White IR, Thorogood M, Bristow A, Curle D, Marmot MG. Can dietary interventions in the population change diet and cardiovascular risk factors? An assessment of effectiveness utilizing a meta-analysis of randomized controlled trials. *American Journal of Public Health* (in press)

Cutler JA, Grandits GA, Grimm RH, Thomas HE, Billings JH, Wright NH. Risk factor changes after cessation of intervention in the Multiple Risk Factor Intervention Trial. The MRFIT Research Group. *Preventive Medicine*, 1991; **20**: 183–196

Davey Smith G, Shipley MJ, Marmot MG, Rose G. Plasma cholesterol concentration and mortality: the Whitehall Study. *Journal of the American Medical Association*, 1992; **267**: 70–76

Davey Smith G. The 4th Lord Rayner Lecture. Down at heart: the meaning and implications of inequalities in cardiovascular disease. London: Royal College of Physicians, 1996 (in press)

Fehily AM, Phillips KM, Yarnell JWG. Diet, smoking, social class, and body mass index in the Caerphilly heart disease study. *American Journal of Clinical Nutrition*, 1984; **40**: 827–833

Goldberg GR, Black AE, Jebb SA *et al.* Critical evaluation of energy intake data using fundamental principles of energy physiology: 1. Derivation of cut-off limits to identify under-recording. *European Journal of Clinical Nutrition*, 1991; **45**: 569–581

Great Britain Committee on Medical Aspects of Food. Panel on Diet in Relation to Cardiovascular Disease. *Diet and Cardiovascular Disease.* London: HMSO, 1984

Great Britain Committee on Medical Aspects of Food Policy. Cardiovascular Review Group. *Nutritional Aspects of Cardiovascular Disease.* London: HMSO, 1994

Great Britain Department of Health. *The Health of the Nation: One Year on—A Report on the Progress of the Health of the Nation.* London: HMSO, 1993

Great Britain Department of Health. *Assessing the Options in the CHD and Stroke Key Area.* London: Department of Health, 1995

Great Britain Department of Health Nutrition and Physical Activity Task Forces. *Obesity: Reversing the Increasing Problem of Obesity in England.* London: Department of Health, 1995

Great Britain Department of Health Variations Sub-group of the Chief Medical Officer's Health of the Nation Working Group. *Variations in Health: What Can the Department of Health and the NHS Do?* London: HMSO, 1995

Great Britain Ministry of Agriculture, Fisheries and Food. *Household Food Consumption and Expenditure 1989.* Annual report of the National Food Survey Committee. London: HMSO, 1990

Gregory J, Foster K, Tyler H, Wiseman M. The *Dietary and Nutritional Survey of British Adults: A Survey of the Dietary Behaviour, Nutritional Status and Blood Pressure of Adults Aged 16 to 64 Living in Great Britain.* London: HMSO, 1990

Gunnell DJ, Frankel S, Nanchahal K, Braddon FEM, Davey Smith G. Lifecourse exposure and later disease: a follow-up study based on a survey of family diet and health in pre-war Britain (1937–39). *Public Health*, 1996; **110**: 85–94

Haan M, Kaplan GA, Camacho T. Poverty and health. Prospective evidence from the Alameda County study. *American Journal of Epidemiology*, 1987; **125**: 989–998

Hein HO, Suadicani P, Gyntelberg F. Ischaemic heart disease incidence by social class and form of smoking: the Copenhagen male study—17 years' follow-up. *Journal of Internal*

Medicine, 1992; **231**: 477–483

Heiss G, Haskell W, Mowery R, Criqui MH, Brockway M, Tyroler HA. Plasma high-density lipoprotein cholesterol and socioeconomic status. The Lipid Research Clinics Program Prevalence Study. *Circulation*, 1980; **62** (Suppl IV): 108–115

Imperial Cancer Research Fund OXCHECK Study Group. Effectiveness of health checks conducted by nurses in primary care: final results of the Oxcheck Study. *British Medical Journal*, 1995; **310**: 1099–1104

Kristiansen IS, Eggen AE, Thelle DS. Cost effectiveness of incremental programmes for lowering serum cholesterol concentration: is individual intervention worth while? *British Medical Journal*, 1991; **302**: 1119–1122

Kuczmarski RJ, Flegal KM, Campbell SM, Johnson CL. Increasing prevalence of overweight among US adults. *Journal of the American Medical Association*, 1994; **272**: 205–211

Lapidus L, Bengtsson C, Larsson B, Pennert K, Rybo E, Sjostrom L. Distribution of adipose tissue and risk of cardiovascular disease and death: a 12 year follow up of participants in the population study of women in Gothenburg, Sweden. *British Medical Journal*, 1984; **289**: 1261–1263

Larsson B, Svardsudd K, Welin L, Wilhelmsen L, Bjorntorp P, Tibblin G. Abdominal adipose tissue distribution, obesity, and risk of cardiovascular disease and death: 13 year follow up of participants in the study of men born in 1913. *British Medical Journal*, 1984; **288**: 1401–1404

Leitch I. Growth and health. *British Journal of Nutrition*, 1951; **5**: 142–151

Lobstein T. The increasing cost of a healthy diet. *Food Magazine*, 1995; **31**: 17

Lynch JW, Kaplan GA, Salonen JT. Why do poor people behave badly: variation in adult health behaviours and psychosocial characteristics by stages of the socioeconomic lifecourse. *Social Science Medicine*, 1996 (in press)

Marmot MG. Social differentials in health within and between populations. *Daedalus*, 1994; **123**: 197–216

Marmot MG, McDowall ME. Mortality decline and widening social inequalities. *Lancet*, 1986; **2**: 274–276

Marmot MG, Rose G, Shipley M, Hamilton PJS. Employment grade and coronary heart disease in British civil servants. *Journal of Epidemiology and Community Health*, 1978; **32**: 244–249

Marmot MG, Shipley MJ, Rose G. Inequalities in death—specific explanations of a general pattern. *Lancet*, 1984; **i**: 1003–1006

Marmot MG, Davey Smith G, Stansfeld S *et al*. Health inequalities among British Civil Servants: the Whitehall II study. *Lancet*, 1991; **337**: 1387–1393

McKeigue PM, Shah B, Marmot MG. Relation of central obesity and insulin resistance with high diabetes prevalence and cardiovascular risk in South Asians. *Lancet*, 1991; **337**: 382–386

McKeown T. The medical contribution. In: Davey B, Gray A, Seale C, eds. *Health and Disease*, 2nd edn. Buckingham: Open University Press, 1995, pp 182–190

McLoone P, Boddy FA. Deprivation and mortality in Scotland, 1981 and 1991. *British Medical Journal*, 1994; **309**: 1465–1470

Pamuk ER. Social class inequality in mortality from 1921 to 1972 in England and Wales. *Population Studies*, 1985; **39**: 17–31

Pappas G, Queen S, Hadden W, Fisher G. The increasing disparity in mortality between socioeconomic groups in the United States, 1960 and 1986. *New England Journal of Medicine*, 1993; **329**: 103–109

Phillimore P, Beattie A, Townsend P. Widening inequality of health in northern England, 1981–91. *British Medical Journal*, 1994; **308**: 1125–1128

Pill R, Stott NHC. Choice or chance: further evidence on ideas of illness and responsibility for health. *Social Science Medicine*, 1985; **20**: 981–991

Pocock SJ, Shaper AG, Cook DG, Phillips AN, Walker M. Social class differences in ischaemic heart disease in British men. *Lancet*, 1987; **ii**: 197–201

Prentice AM, Jebb SA. Obesity in Britain: gluttony or sloth? *British Medical Journal*, 1995; **311**: 437–439

Pryer JA, Brunner EJ, Elliott P, Nichols R, Dimond H, Marmot MG. Who complied with COMA 1984 dietary fat recommendations among a nationally representative sample of British adults in 1986–7 and what do they eat? *European Journal of Clinical Nutrition*, 1995; **49**: 718–728

Reaven GM. Role of insulin resistance in human disease (syndrome X): an expanded definition. *Annual Review of Medicine*, 1993; **44**: 121–131

Rimm EB, Ascherio A, Giovannucci E, Spiegelman D, Stampfer MJ, Willett WC. Vegetable, fruit, and cereal fiber intake and risk of coronary heart disease among men. *Journal of the American Medical Association*, 1996; **275**: 447–451

Sapolsky RM, Mott GE. Social subordinance in wild baboons is associated with suppressed high density lipoprotein-cholesterol concentrations: the possible role of chronic social stress. *Endocrinology*, 1987; **121**: 1605–1610

Social Security Committee. *First Report on Low Income Statistics: Low Income Families 1989–92*. London: HMSO, 1995

Townsend P, Davidson N, Whitehead M. *Inequalities in Health: The Black Report; The Health Divide*. London: Penguin, 1992

Willett WC, Sampson L, Stampfer MJ et al. Reproducibility and validity of a semiquantitative food frequency questionnaire. *American Journal of Epidemiology*, 1985; **122**: 51–65

World Health Organization. *Energy and protein requirements. Report of a Joint FAO/WHO/UNU Expert Consultation*. WHO Technical Report No 724. Geneva: World Health Organization, 1985

World Health Organization Study Group. *Diabetes Mellitus: Report of a WHO Study Group*. WHO Technical Report No 727. Geneva: World Health Organization, 1985

Discussion

Elizabeth Dowler

Human Nutrition Unit, London School of Hygiene & Tropical Medicine, UK

In addressing inequalities in diet and health, as Eric Brunner has suggested, the fundamental issues are clear enough. Do poor people eat badly? If they do, why do they eat badly? And, we might add, does it matter? These are simple questions but they yield no simple answers. In fact, responses are often burdened by unconsidered prejudice. One part of the problem has been getting appropriate data; but another lies in defining what is meant by 'poor people' and by 'eating badly'. In non-industrialised countries, poverty in the urban and rural sectors is widely recognised as being associated with inadequate dietary intakes and general food insecurity (FAO/WHO, 1994). In industrialised societies, by contrast, the association between low socio-economic status and poor health or dietary intakes has only intermittently found its way onto the public health agenda.

Most nutritional studies in industrialised societies use occupational social class to differentiate populations—sometimes reducing these categories simply to 'manual' or 'non-manual'. National surveys on individuals have only recently been published with nutrient data by other socio-economic indicators, such as employment status, education level, tenure or receipt of state benefits. In the UK, for instance, as we have heard, men and women who are unemployed, or claiming benefits, or who come from manual social classes, have lower intakes of many vitamins and minerals (particularly calcium, iron, carotene and vitamin C) than those who are employed or from non-manual occupations. This finding has been shown in cross-sectional studies in a number of industrialised countries (Riches, 1997), and in the UK similar findings have emerged from surveys of pre-school and school-aged children as well (Department of Health, 1989; Gregory et al, 1995). In addition, the UK annual National Household Food Survey has shown for a number of years that nutrients per head are less likely to be adequate in households with three or more children, or headed by a lone parent, or from the lowest income group (those claiming state benefits) (MAFF, 1995). However, few surveys, large- or small-scale, have differentiated nutrient intakes or food patterns using the deprivation indices employed by those who analyse mortality differentials.

In terms of foods eaten, the same surveys mentioned above show that members of poorer households are less likely to eat the kinds of foodstuffs recommended for health: fruit, fresh salads, lean meat and oily fish, or drink fruit juice (although they are more likely to eat bread and potatoes) than people from richer households, and are more likely to consume whole milk, hard fats, sugar and meat products.

Whether this evidence constitutes 'eating badly' is a moot point. I have referred to the likelihood that nutrient intakes are less adequate, in terms of the achieved percentage reference values, and I do not need to point out that reference values are probability statements, about the risk that groups in the population are, or are not, obtaining sufficient quantities of a nutrient to avoid future health risks. A 'poor diet' is in some ways as difficult to define unequivocally as 'the poor'. Richer people also have intakes below the reference levels for many nutrients, and they, too, eat more fat and sugar than may be good for them. The case therefore needs to be made that it is those on the lowest incomes, or living in the most difficult circumstances, who are the least likely to eat enough to avoid ill-health: their food and nutrition security are in the greatest jeopardy. We need evidence that characterises both the social inequality and the nutritional risk. We need to be able to distinguish the effects of sociological aspects of class from cumulative life risks. Which groups of people are at risk, what is the nature of their poverty or social position, and what forces constrain them to remain poor? How large are these different groups, and how are their numbers likely to change in the future, and why? Secondly, what is the nature of the nutritional risk involved, the likely consequence of reduced or, conversely, of excessive intakes of nutrients or dietary components? We know that health risks accumulate over time, with accumulation of negative, or low, social factors—what is the role of diet in these processes? Thirdly, what are the consequences of limited dietary variety—which is a regular feature of food poverty the world over? What factors contribute to diets being monotonous and of poor quality? How do these factors differ between, say, single older people living on inadequate pensions, and young families headed by an unemployed parent? I think in the UK we have gone some way to answering a number of these questions (though not, perhaps, far enough in characterising or enumerating groups, or mapping their location and geographical distribution). To some extent, therefore, we have also been able to elaborate potential responses at local and national levels.

Eric Brunner's paper has covered much of the general evidence on this topic, as well as giving details from the Whitehall studies. These studies make an important contribution not only because they have linked low nutrients and less healthy dietary patterns with health outcomes (which few other studies do), but also because they avoid the debate about what poverty is, and demonstrate variations in nutrient intake and dietary patterns across employment grades. What gives rise to these differences? Income is clearly part of the answer—having enough to meet basic needs, and also to provide a sense of security. Will Hutton (1996) has described what he calls the '30:30:40 society' in Britain today (not so different from other places): 40% of the population who are in secure jobs or financial circumstances; 30% who have no hope of either; and 30% who are in part-time, or insecure, or casual employment and could readily slide into the second group. The combination of an income sufficient to live a reasonable life and security in obtaining it is crucial, but it is hard to quantify for epidemiological/nutritional surveys. The Whitehall study has, however, made some progress towards this.

Yet all the participants in Whitehall I and II were, by definition, gainfully employed. What of those who are not, whether long-term or shifting unemployed, or those who are 'economically inactive' and living on low pensions? State or private provision varies from country to country, but most have a basic, minimal amount which entitled citizens may claim. Many in the UK live in these circumstances for some time; and the numbers who do so have increased over the past two decades; in 1994 about 10 million people lived on income support (in 5.6 million households). The levels of all state benefits in the UK have fallen relative to the prevailing cost of living, and entitlement has been reduced. This growth in insecurity and income inequality has been paralleled by widely documented mortality and health differentials. Indeed, Wilkinson (e.g. 1994; 1995) has regularly and explicitly argued the connection between inequality and mortality in the *British Medical Journal* over the past five years, although he has never mentioned the role of food in mediating these differentials.

Furthermore, the Whitehall studies have shown a gradation of health and nutrition differentials with no evidence of a threshold effect, and other studies such as McLoone and Boddy (1994) have shown health differentials graded across postcode sectors. Again, the participants are employed, even if on very different wage levels and with different degrees of job status and personal control. Our own recent small-scale study (Dowler and Calvert, 1995) showed that nutrient intakes were much less likely to be adequate (in terms of reference intakes) in the long-term unemployed living on means-tested benefits, particularly where automatic deductions were made from those benefits for rent or fuel debt recovery. This finding was largely independent of smoking. In some ways such findings should not surprise us: state benefits are intended to provide for short-term basic subsistence needs only. If money is taken off these benefits (and this happens to about one in five claimants in Britain today), something in the domestic budget has to be cut, and it is usually food.

References

Department of Health. *The Diets of British Schoolchildren.* London: HMSO, 1989

Dowler E, Calvert C. *Nutrition and Diet in Lone-parent Families in London.* London: Family Policy Studies Centre, 1995

FAO/WHO. *International Conference on Nutrition: Final Report of the Conference, Rome, December 1992.* Rome: FAO, and Geneva: WHO, 1994

Gregory JR, Collins DL, Davies PSW, Hughes JM, Clarke PC. *National Diet and Nutrition Survey: Children Aged 1.5 to 4.5 Years.* London: HMSO, 1995

Hutton W. *The State We're In.* London: Vantage Press, 1996

McLoone P, Boddy FA. Deprivation and mortality in Scotland, 1981–1991. *British Medical Journal,* 1994; **309**: 1465–1470

Riches G (ed). *First World Hunger: Food Security and Welfare Politics.* London: MacMillan, 1997

Wilkinson RG (editorial). Divided we fall: the poor pay the price of increased social inequality with their health. *British Medical Journal,* 1994; **308**: 1113–1114

Wilkinson RG. Commentary: a reply to Ken Judge: mistaken criticisms ignore overwhelming evidence. *British Medical Journal,* 1995; **311**: 1285–1287

5
Dietary fats and non-communicable diseases

W. C. Willett

Harvard School of Public Health, Boston, MA, USA

During the past two decades, major reviews and official recommendations on diet and health in affluent countries have consistently emphasised a reduction in dietary fat, usually as the highest nutritional priority. Typically, the goal has been to reduce fat intake to 30% of energy or less. The anticipated benefits of fat reduction have been lower rates of coronary heart disease (CHD) and several important cancers, as well as a reduced prevalence of obesity. In this overview the evidence supporting these anticipated benefits from a reduction in total fat intake is briefly reviewed, acknowledging that the literature on each of the specific topics is vast. Some consideration is given to specific types of fat, again without being able to do full justice to the extensive literature.

Dietary fat and coronary heart disease (CHD)

A central pillar of support for the classical diet–heart hypothesis has been the study by Keys and colleagues (1970) demonstrating a correlation between national *per capita* saturated fat intake and rates of coronary heart disease. Although this correlation continues to be used to demonstrate both the existence and the magnitude of this relationship, Keys himself noted that the correlation was likely to be overstated. If the effect of saturated fat is mediated by serum cholesterol, the influence of saturated fat on serum cholesterol in metabolic studies can explain less than half of the regression slope relating saturated fat to CHD mortality rates. Thus, either saturated fat acts by additional mechanisms or other factors, confounding variables, explain most of the effects attributed to saturated fat. In the same study, Keys (1970) also found little association between total fat intake and CHD risk; notably he observed that the areas with both the

Diet, Nutrition and Chronic Disease: Lessons from Contrasting Worlds.
Edited by P. S. Shetty and K. McPherson © 1997 John Wiley & Sons, Ltd.

lowest CHD rate (Crete) and the highest rate (Finland) consumed approximately 40% of energy from fat. Thus, international comparisons do not implicate fat *per se* in the aetiology of CHD and may be misleading in terms of the relationship of saturated fat intake to CHD risk.

Migrant studies have also been used to support a causal relation between saturated fat intake and CHD risk. The classic investigation has been the Ni-Ho-San study (Table 5.1), in which dietary factors were assessed among Japanese men living in Japan, Hawaii and San Francisco (Kato *et al*, 1973); rates of CHD varied almost three-fold among these groups. The first point to note is that the consumption of saturated fat attributed to Japanese men in San Francisco (26% of energy, with total fat intake being 37% of energy) is almost certainly a gross error; 16–17% is probably a better estimate given US diets at that time. Also, other striking differences existed in risk factors for CHD, particularly the three-fold greater prevalence of obesity among Japanese men living in San Francisco, and the low intake of alcohol (the best established nutritional risk factor for CHD). Underlying the contrasts in obesity, but not measured, are almost certainly large differences in physical activity. Although this study demonstrates the general importance of lifestyle factors in the aetiology of CHD, these types of extremely confounded data cannot be used to support specifically an effect of fat or saturated fat.

In addition to the epidemiological observations noted above, the classic diet–heart hypothesis has rested heavily on the repeated observation that serum total cholesterol levels predict CHD risk, and that reductions in serum cholesterol decrease risk (Shepherd *et al*, 1995). Serum cholesterol has thus functioned as a surrogate marker of risk in hundreds of metabolic studies. These studies, summarised as equations by Keys (1984) and Hegsted (1986), indicated that, compared with carbohydrates, saturated fats and dietary cholesterol increase and polyunsaturated fat decreases serum cholesterol, whereas monounsaturated fat has no influence. These widely used equations, while valid for total cholesterol, are of questionable relevance in the prediction of CHD risk, with the recognition that the high-density lipoprotein cholesterol fraction (HDL) is strongly and inversely related to CHD risk, and that the ratio of total cholesterol to HDL is a much better predictor of CHD than serum cholesterol alone (Castelli *et al*, 1983;

Table 5.1 Ni-Ho-San study

	Japan	Hawaii	California
Saturated fat (%E)	8	23	26
Cholesterol (mg/day)	464	545	533
Alcohol (%E)	8.9	3.7	2.5
Serum cholesterol	181	218	228
> 120% relative weight (%)	22	56	63

E = energy. Source: Kato *et al*, 1973

Mensink and Katan, 1987; Ginsberg et al, 1990; Mensink and Katan, 1992). After accounting for the total cholesterol/HDL ratio, serum cholesterol is not related to CHD risk (Stampfer et al, 1991).

Substitution of carbohydrate for saturated fat tends to reduce HDL as well as total and low-density lipoprotein (LDL) cholesterol; thus, the ratio does not change appreciably (Mensink and Katan, 1987; Ginsberg et al, 1990; Mensink and Katan, 1992). Substituting monounsaturated fat for saturated fat reduces LDL without affecting HDL, providing an improved ratio (Mensink and Katan, 1992). Thus, the evidence from metabolic studies examining cholesterol fractions rather than just total serum cholesterol would predict that replacing saturated fat by carbohydrate would have no effect on CHD, and replacing overall fat (which also includes unsaturated fats) by carbohydrate without altering the composition of the fat would actually increase risk.

The use of surrogate endpoints, such as blood lipid fractions, to evaluate the effect of dietary fats on CHD risk is always treacherous because dietary factors may influence risk, either favourably or unfavourably, by other mechanisms. Questions have been raised as to whether the reductions in HDL resulting from a high carbohydrate diet have the same adverse effect as reductions caused by other factors (Brinton et al, 1991). Although this is difficult to resolve directly, other factors that influence HDL levels, including alcohol, oestrogens, obesity, smoking, exercise, and medications, affect CHD risk in the predicted direction (Manntari et al, 1990; Sacks and Willett, 1991). Studies relating diet to clinical endpoints are clearly desirable.

Surprisingly, few prospective cohort studies have examined the relationships of dietary total or saturated fat to CHD incidence. Those that are available are summarised in Table 5.2 (Willett and Lenart, 1996). In the most detailed study published to date, the Western Electric Study (Shekelle et al, 1981), a weak positive association was seen with intake of dietary cholesterol and an inverse association was observed with polyunsaturated fat; no relation was seen with saturated fat. Little or no relation was seen between saturated fat intake and CHD risk in other published studies, but these studies have not been sufficiently large or rigorous to exclude a modest association. The relation between fat intake and risk of CHD has recently been examined in a population of nearly 50 000 male health professionals, which provides by far the statistically most powerful examination of this issue (unpublished data). In age-adjusted analyses a strong and highly significant association between both total and saturated fat intake was observed, indicating that substantial variation in saturated fat existed in this population and that the dietary questionnaire was sufficiently precise to predict disease. However, after adjusting for standard risk factors and dietary fibre, no relation remained with total or saturated fat. Although a small effect could not be excluded, the findings were not compatible with the magnitude of association predicted by the international correlation between saturated fat intake and CHD risk.

Table 5.2 Prospective cohort studies of dietary factors in relation to risk of coronary heart disease

Study	Population	Dietary method	CHD cases	Energy	Saturated fat	Poly	Diet chol.	Lipid score*	Fibre	Fish	Alcohol	Comments
Morris et al (1977)	337 UK bank clerks	7-day record, weighted	45	↓	0	–	0	–	↓	–	–	Trend of ↓ risk with high P/S ratio
Shetkelle et al (1981 and 1985)	1900 US men	Diet history interview	~200 CHD deaths	–	0	↓	↑	↑	–	↓	–	
Garcia-Palmieri et al (1980)	8218 Puerto Rican men	24-hour recall	163	↓	0	0	0	–	–	–	↓	Inverse relation with starch intake
Gordon et al (1981) Dawber et al (1982)	895 Framingham men	24-hour recall	51	↓	0	0	0	–	–	–	↓	No association with egg intake
McGee et al (1984)	7088 Honolulu men	24-hour recall	309	↓	↑†	0	↑	–	–	–	↓	Dietary fat values were divided by calories
Kromhout et al (1982, 1984, 1985)	857 Zutphen men (Dutch)	Diet history interview	30 CHD deaths	↓	0	0	0	–	↓	↓	0	Inverse relation with fibre not significant when divided by calories
Kushi et al (1985)	1001 Irish and Boston men	Diet history interview	110 CHD deaths	0	↑†	0	0	↑	↓	–	–	Dietary fat values were divided by calories
Snowdon et al (1984)	25 153 US Seventh Day Adventists	28-item frequency questionnaire	1599	–	–	0	–	–	–	–	–	Positive association with meat intake (RR = 1.5)

Reference	Population	Dietary method	Events								Conclusions
Khaw et al (1987)	California men and women	24-hour recall	65 CHD deaths	0	—	—	0	—	→	0	Vegetarians have lower CHD mortality
Burr et al (1982)	10 943 Welsh vegetarians	Short food frequency questionnaire	585	—	—	—	—	—	—	0	
Lapidus et al (1986)	1462 Swedish women	24-hour recall	28 infarctions →	—	—	—	—	—	—	—	
Norell et al (1986)	10 966 Swedish men and women	?	800 CHD deaths —	—	—	—	—	—	→	—	
Fraser et al (1992)	31 208 Seventh Day Adventists	65-item food frequency questionnaire	463 incident CHD deaths —	—	—	—	—	→	—	—	Those consuming nuts several times per week had significantly lower risk of fatal and non-fatal CHD. Inverse relationship for fibre is whole wheat bread vs. white bread consumption. Attempted to control for food habits associated with increased nut intake

(continued overleaf)

Table 5.2 (*continued*)

Study	Population	Dietary method	CHD cases	Energy	Saturated fat	Poly	Diet chol.	Lipid score*	Fibre	Fish	Alcohol	Comments
Fehily et al (1993)	2512 men from South Wales	50-item food frequency questionnaire	148	↓	0	–	–	–	0	–	↓	Total fibre intake lower in those having an incident IHD event, but not independent of total calories
Goldbourt et al (1993)	10059 Israeli civil service men	Short dietary questionnaire	1089 CHD deaths	–	↑†	↓†	–	–	–	–	–	Independent dietary influence on CHD rates not strong. No difference in CHD for those surviving concentration camps and others from Europe
Dolecek (1992)	6250 men from usual care group from MRFIT	24-hour dietary recall	175 CHD deaths	–	↓†	↓†	–	–	–	↓†	–	Inverse association between polyunsaturated fat intake and CHD marginally significant

*Lipid score refers to Keys or Hegsted scores for predicting serum cholesterol
↓ = inverse association; ↑ = positive association; 0 = no statistically significant association; – = no information
† Expressed as % of total calories

Ideally, the relation between fat intake and CHD incidence could be resolved by randomised trials. Unfortunately, trials of sufficient size and duration are difficult to conduct. Also, in some trials, multiple interventions have been used, making any conclusion about a particular component unclear. In the two studies usually cited to support the diet–heart hypothesis, the Los Angeles VA study (Dayton et al, 1969), and the non-randomised Finnish hospital study (Turpeinen et al, 1979), fat intakes in the intervention group were high because extremely high levels of polyunsaturated fat were used to replace saturated fat. Other trials, including secondary intervention studies, have generally seen little benefit from fat reduction, but reductions in both serum cholesterol levels and CHD risk have been found when unsaturated fats were used to replace saturated fat. The most dramatic benefits were seen in the recent report by de Lorgeril et al (1994) in which monounsaturated fat and linolenic acid replaced saturated fat, along with other changes in diet. Thus, these studies, allowing for the limitations in design, do not allow a distinction between beneficial effects of unsaturated fats and adverse effects of saturated fat. They do not provide support for a reduction in fat *per se*.

Understanding of the interrelationships between dietary fats, blood lipids and CHD risk has been further complicated by evidence that the oxidative modification of LDL cholesterol plays a critical role in the development of atherosclerosis (Steinberg and Witztum, 1990). LDL particles formed on a diet high in monounsaturated fat in the form of olive oil appear to be relatively resistant to oxidation, even when compared to diets high in saturated fat or carbohydrates (Reaven et al, 1993; Berry et al, 1995). Also, experimental evidence suggests that lipid-soluble antioxidants such as vitamin E can block the oxidative modification of LDL. Within Europe, countries with higher blood antioxidant levels have lower rates of CHD (Gey et al, 1987), and vitamin E supplements have been inversely associated with CHD risk (Rimm et al, 1993; Stampfer et al, 1993). As liquid vegetable oils, particularly those that are minimally processed, are the primary source of vitamin E in our diets, reduction of these fats could have adverse effects on CHD risk. Soybean oil may be an exception because it is highly polyunsaturated, yet its primary form of vitamin E, gamma-tocopherol, is rapidly excreted and poorly incorporated into tissues and lipoproteins. Thus, diets high in soybean oil, the major fat in the US diet, might result in LDL particularly susceptible to oxidation.

The optimal amount of polyunsaturated fat intake in the diet remains uncertain. The earlier metabolic studies predicting total serum cholesterol (Keys, 1984; Hegsted, 1986) suggested that intakes should be maximised, and the American Heart Association recommended intakes to 10% of energy (compared with US averages of about 3% in the 1950s and 6% at present). However, in more recent metabolic studies, the benefits of polyunsaturated fat have been less clear (Mensink and Katan, 1992) and concerns have arisen from animal studies in which omega-6 polyunsaturated fat (typically corn oil) has promoted tumour growth (Welsch, 1992), and the possibility that high intakes of omega-6 relative to omega-3 fatty acids might promote coronary thrombosis (Renaud *et al*, 1970; Leaf and Weber, 1988). Evidence that higher intake of *N*-3 fatty acids from fish prevents myocardial infarction remains mixed (Kromhout *et al*, 1985; Vollset *et al*, 1985; Burr *et al*, 1989; Ascherio *et al*, 1995; Morris *et al*, 1995). In reducing thrombosis, polyunsaturated fats involving both *N*-6 and *N*-3 series have been hypothesised to decrease the threshold for ventricular fibrillation (Siscovick *et al*, 1995), which might account for some of the discordant findings between incidence and mortality from CHD.

Most epidemiological studies of diet and heart disease conducted until recently have failed to distinguish between the natural *cis* and the *trans* isomers of unsaturated fatty acids, possibly contributing to the inconsistent findings. *Trans* fatty acids are formed by the partial hydrogenation of liquid vegetable oils in the production of margarine and vegetable shortening and can account for as much as 40% of these products. Intake of partially hydrogenated vegetable fats (which increased from nothing in 1900 to a peak of about 5.5% of total fat in about the 1960s) has closely paralleled the epidemic of CHD during this century, in contrast to intake of animal fat, which has steadily declined over this period (Booyens and Louwrens, 1986). *Trans* fatty acids increase LDL and decrease HDL (Booyens and Louwrens, 1986; Mensink and Katan, 1990; Nestel *et al*, 1992; Zock and Katan, 1992; Judd *et al*, 1994; Sundram *et al*, 1995), as well as raise Lp(a), another lipid fraction implicated in CHD aetiology (Mensink *et al*, 1992; Nestel *et al*, 1992). On a gram-for-gram basis and compared with *cis*-unsaturated fat, *trans* fatty acids have approximately twice the adverse effect on the ratio of total to HDL cholesterol as do saturated fats. Positive associations between intake of *trans* fatty acids and CHD have been seen among regions in the Seven Countries Study (Kromhout *et al*, 1995), in a prospective study of US women (Willett *et al*, 1993), a case-control study of men and women (Ascherio *et al*, 1994), and a cross-sectional angiographic study (Siguel and Lerman, 1993). In a multi-centre European case-control study, adipose tissue levels of *trans* fatty acids were by far the lowest in Spain, which was also the country with the lowest CHD rates (Aro *et al*, 1995). In the same study, the risk of CHD within countries was 40–50% higher among individuals with the highest *trans* fatty acid levels, but this did not attain statistical significance. No association was seen in a study of sudden death, but the number of cases was so small that the confidence interval for the relative risk included the association seen in all other studies (Roberts *et al*, 1995).

Dietary fat and cancer

Another major justification for decreasing dietary fat has been anticipated reductions in the risk of cancers of the breast, colon and rectum, and prostate (US National Research Council, 1989; Prentice and Sheppard, 1990). The primary evidence has been that countries with low fat intake, also the less affluent areas, have had low rates of these cancers (Armstrong and Doll, 1975; Prentice and Sheppard, 1990). These correlations have been primarily with animal fat and meat intake, rather than with vegetable fat consumption. The hypothesis that fat intake increases breast cancer risk has been supported by animal models (Freedman *et al*, 1990; Ip, 1990), although no association was seen in a very large study that did not use an inducing agent (Appleton and Landers, 1985). Moreover, energy restriction profoundly decreases incidence of breast cancer in animal studies (Appleton and Landers, 1985; Ip, 1990; Welsch, 1992), which has accounted for the effect of fat in some, although not all, experiments.

In most case-control studies, no association between fat intake and breast cancer was observed, although a weak positive association (RR = approx 1.07 for 40% vs. 30% of energy from fat) was seen in the pooled data from 12 such studies (Howe *et al*, 1990). However, the case-control studies are now of diminishing relevance as data from six large prospective studies, including 3400 cases among 280 000 women, have been reported (Mills *et al*, 1989; Howe *et al*, 1991; Graham *et al*, 1992; Kushi *et al*, 1992; Willett *et al*, 1992; Van den Brandt *et al*, 1993); in none of these studies was the risk of breast cancer significantly elevated among those with the highest fat intake. The investigators of the large prospective studies have recently published a pooled analysis of the collective findings (Hunter *et al*, 1996); this enabled a detailed examination of dietary fat over a wide range of intakes. From 15% to more than 45% of energy from fat, no variation in risk of breast cancer was observed. However, at less than 15% of energy from fat, a statistically significant and more than two-fold excess risk was seen. Thus, over the wide range of fat intake consumed by middle-aged women in these studies, dietary fat does not appear to influence breast cancer risk. Effects of fat intake at an early period in life could not, however, be excluded.

Ecological studies have suggested a possible protective effect of monounsaturated fat, or olive oil specifically, relative to other types of dietary fat. Greek women with approximately 40% of energy from fat, mainly as olive oil (Gerber, 1991; Trichopoulou *et al*, 1993), have had breast cancer rates only about one-third those of US women, who have consumed about 35–40% of energy from fat until recently (Willett, 1994). Breast cancer rates are also low in Spain and southern Italy, where olive oil consumption is high (WHO, 1993). Although these ecological relationships could be confounded by other factors, the combined evidence from animal (Cohen *et al*, 1986; US National Research Council, 1989; Weisburger and Wynder, 1991; Weisburger, 1992) and epidemiologic observations led Cohen and Wynder (1990) to hypothesise that monounsaturated fatty acids play a protective role in breast carcinogenesis.

Recent case-control and cohort studies have provided additional support for the hypothesis that monounsaturated fat or olive oil may reduce breast cancer risk. In a case-control study conducted in Spain, Martin-Moreno *et al* (1994) found no overall association between fat intake and breast cancer risk; however, consumption of olive oil was associated with a reduction in risk (RR = 0.66, 95%

confidence interval (CI) 0.46–0.97). In a large case-control study from Greece (Trichopoulou *et al*, 1995), a similar lack of overall association with fat intake was seen but the risk of breast cancer was 25% lower in women consuming olive oil more than once per day (RR = 0.75, CI 0.57–0.98). In another Spanish case-control study (Landa *et al*, 1994), women in the highest third of mono-unsaturated fat intake had reduced risk of breast cancer (RR = 0.30, 95% CI 0.1–0.8). In the only published study to control one type of fat for another, we observed in the 1984–1988 analysis of the Nurses' Health Study a significant inverse association between monounsaturated fat and breast cancer risk (RR = 0.70, CI 0.54–0.91), but no relation with saturated fat intake (Willett *et al*, 1992).

Associations between animal fat consumption and colon cancer incidence have been seen more consistently (Whittemore *et al*, 1990; Willett *et al*, 1990; Giovannucci *et al*, 1995), although not in all studies (Phillips and Snowdon, 1983), whereas little relation has been seen with vegetable fat. Positive associations with animal fat have also been observed for adenomatous polyps, a precursor lesion (Giovannucci *et al*, 1992). However, in case-control studies a positive association between total energy intake and risk of colon cancer was generally observed, which now appears to be the result of reporting bias because inverse associations have been found in all prospective studies. In a pooled analysis of case-control studies that controlled for total energy intake, no relation between total or saturated fat intake and colon cancer risk was seen (G. Howe, personal communication). Associations between red meat consumption and colon cancer have been even stronger than the effect of fat in some analyses (Willett *et al*, 1990; Giovannucci *et al*, 1995), suggesting that relationships with red meat may be due to other components of cooked flesh, such as heat-induced carcinogens (Gerhardsson de Verdier *et al*, 1991) or the high content of readily available iron (Babbs, 1990).

Like breast and colon cancer, prostate cancer rates are much higher in affluent than in developing countries (Armstrong and Doll, 1975). More detailed epidemiological studies are few; in subsets of several case-control studies, men with prostate cancer reported higher fat intake than did controls (Graham *et al*, 1983; Kolonel *et al*, 1988). In a large case-control study (Whittemore *et al*, 1995) and two recent prospective studies, positive associations were seen between intake of animal fat and red meat (Giovannucci *et al*, 1994; Le Marchand *et al*, 1994).

Dietary fat and body fatness

Overweight is an important cause of morbidity and mortality, and fat reduction has often been proposed as a method for controlling weight. There are several reasons to believe that the fat composition of the diet may increase obesity. Fat is the most energy-dense nutrient; thus, to the extent that food intake is regulated by volume, total energy intake may be greater on a high-fat diet. Also, texture and flavour may be enhanced by higher amounts of fat in the diet, leading to overeating. The metabolic cost of storing fat is less than that of storing energy from carbohydrate, which may also increase obesity on diets higher in fat. In addition, Flatt (1985) has suggested that the body regulates carbohydrate stores, but not fat stores, so that body fat may be proportional to the percentage of energy from dietary fat.

Population differences in weight do not appear to be due primarily to fat intake. Southern European countries with relatively low fat intake have higher rates of obesity than Northern European countries (Seidell, 1994). Among 65 counties in China, no correlation was seen between bodyweight and fat intake, which varied from about 6 to 25% of energy (Chen *et al*, 1990). Within the USA, a decline in fat intake has been accompanied by a major increase in obesity. Inconsistent associations have been observed in cross-sectional and prospective studies within countries, but such observations are particularly prone to distortion because subjects may alter their diets because of their weight. In randomised trials of fat reduction, the optimal way to study the relationship between dietary and body fat, modest weight reductions are typically seen in the short term (Lissner *et al*, 1987; Schaefer *et al*, 1995). However, in randomised studies lasting a year or longer, reductions in fat to 20–25% of energy have typically had only up to a 1.8 kg effect on overall long-term bodyweight (National Diet–Heart Study Group, 1968; Boyd *et al*, 1990; Sheppard *et al*, 1991) (Table 5.3). In a trial among obese women, a reduction in fat intake to 17% of energy reduced weight by only 2.6 kg, and no appreciable effect on waist/hip ratio or percentage body fat was observed (Kasim *et al*, 1993).

Although most of the longer-term studies have shown little if any effect on fat reduction, they have generally been biased toward finding an effect because the intervention group received intensive counselling to heighten consciousness about food intake, whereas the control group received no such support. Very few studies have compared groups with comparable intensities of intervention. In a pilot trial to the National Diet–Heart Study (1968), two levels of fat composition of the diet were given in a double-blind manner by providing the foods themselves. After approximately one year, only a 0.8 kg difference in weight was seen. In a recent 18-month study, a low-fat diet was compared with a low-calorie

Table 5.3   Long-term trials of fat reduction and bodyweight

Study	Length of trial (months)	N	% Fat Control	Intervention	Difference in weight (kg)
National Diet–Heart Study (1968)	12–20	900	35	30	−0.8
Sheppard *et al* (1991)	24	276	38	20	−1.8
Boyd *et al* (1990)	12	206	37	21	−1.0
Kasim *et al* (1993)	12	72	36	17	−2.6

diet (Jeffery *et al*, 1995); both groups received similar levels of intervention. Weight losses were seen in both groups at six months, but after 18 months of intervention both groups had regained their weight and no significant differences between groups were seen at any time. In a study of weight loss with carefully controlled total caloric intakes, a non-significantly greater weight loss was seen among subjects fed 20% compared with those fed 10, 30, or 40% of energy from fat (Powell *et al*, 1994). This finding indicates that the theoretically more efficient metabolism of fat does not seem to be important in realistic situations. One possible explanation for only a transient effect of dietary fat composition on body fat could be that the compliance with fat reduction in the longer-term studies is also only transient. However, this does not seem likely in the double-blind National Diet–Heart Study (1968) in which the food was provided. Also, in the longer-term studies, there was biochemical evidence of substantial compliance with low fat intake, specifically depressed HDL-cholesterol levels, which was sustained even when weight loss was not (Lee-Han *et al*, 1988; Kasim *et al*, 1993). Very low fat intakes, for example less than 10% of energy, in conjunction with a high volume of bulky food as consumed by some traditional societies, may induce weight loss (Shintani *et al*, 1991), but long-term studies are needed. However, available evidence suggests that reductions in dietary fat composition over the ranges currently recommended are not likely to have sustained and substantial effects on body fatness.

Summary and conclusions

What can we now say about dietary fat and health? As noted in the executive summary of the US National Research Council's Report (1989), but generally ignored, there is little evidence that dietary fat *per se* is associated with risk of CHD. Metabolic and epidemiological data suggest that decreasing intake of *trans* fats will reduce the incidence of CHD. Metabolic data, intervention studies, and indirect epidemiological data support a reduction in saturated fats, particularly from dairy sources, to as low as feasible, if these are replaced by unsaturated fats. However, these effects will probably be modest and considerably less than that predicted by international correlations. The effect of substituting carbohydrates for saturated fat is unclear; metabolic studies would predict no benefit. Definitive data are not available on the optimal intake of polyunsaturated and monounsaturated fats, but the metabolic data as well as the experience of Southern European populations suggest that consuming a substantial proportion of energy as monounsaturated fat would be desirable. Available evidence also suggests that overall fat reduction would have little effect on breast cancer risk, although reducing red meat intake may well decrease the incidence of colon and prostate cancer. Thus, there is presently no clear evidence that reducing total fat intake to 30% of energy or even 20% has any health benefit. This does not mean that some benefit might not eventually be shown, but the effect is likely to be small at most. Thus, it appears that the nutrition community has vastly oversold the importance of reducing total fat in the diet.

Finally, the possibility exists that our torch-and-spear crusade to pursue every nubbin and ripple of fat in the diet might actually create harm. Potential adverse consequences include adverse effects on blood lipids if unsaturated as well as saturated and *trans* fats are reduced, and decreased antioxidant intake and increased oxidisability of LDL-cholesterol. There is a question of loss of credibility, too. Perhaps most importantly, the intense focus on dietary fat *per se* diverts attention from more important aspects of lifestyle, such as increasing physical activity and the consumption of vegetables and fruits.

References

Appleton BS, Landers RE. Oil gavage effects on tumor incidence in the national toxicology program's 2-year carcinogenesis bioassay. In: Poirier LA, Newberne PM, Pariza MW, eds. *Advances in Experimental Medicine and Biology*, 1985; **206**: 99–104

Armstrong B, Doll R. Environmental factors and cancer incidence and mortality in different countries, with special reference to dietary practices. *International Journal of Cancer*, 1975; **15**: 617–631

Aro A, Kardinaal AFM, Salminen I *et al*. Adipose tissue isomeric trans fatty acids and risk of myocardial infarction in nine countries: the EURAMIC study. *Lancet*, 1995; **345**: 273–278

Ascherio A, Hennekens CH, Buring JE, Master C, Stampfer MJ, Willett WC. Trans fatty acids intake and risk of myocardial infarction. *Circulation*, 1994; **89**: 94–101

Ascherio A, Rimm EB, Stampfer MJ, Giovannucci E, Willett WC. Dietary intake of marine n-3 fatty acids, fish intake and the risk of coronary disease among men. *New England Journal of Medicine*, 1995; **332**: 977–982

Babbs CF. Free radicals and the etiology of colon cancer. *Free Radical Biology and Medicine*, 1990; **8**: 191–200

Berry EM, Eisenberg S, Friedlander Y *et al*. Effects of diets rich in monounsaturated fatty acids on plasma lipoproteins—the Jerusalem Nutrition Study. *Nutrition and Metabolism in Cardiovascular Diseases*, 1995; **5**: 55-62

Booyens J, Louwrens CC. The Eskimo diet. Prophylactic effects ascribed to the balanced presence of natural *cis* unsaturated fatty acids and to the absence of unnatural *trans* and *cis* isomers of unsaturated fatty acids. *Medical Hypotheses*, 1986; **21**: 387–408

Boyd NF, Cousins M, Beaton M, Kriukov V, Lockwood G, Tritchler D. Quantitative changes in dietary fat intake and serum cholesterol in women: results from a randomized controlled trial. *American Journal of Clinical Nutrition*, 1990; **52**: 470–476

Brinton EA, Eisenberg S, Breslow JL. Increased apo A-I and apo A-II fractional catabolic rate in patients with low high density lipoprotein-cholesterol levels with or without hypertriglyceridemia. *Journal of Clinical Investigation*, 1991; **87**: 536–544

Burr ML, Sweetnam PM, Vegetarianism, dietary fiber, and mortality. *American Journal of Clinical Nutrition*, 1982; **36**: 873–877

Burr ML, Fehily AM, Gilbert JF *et al*. Effects of changes in fat, fish, and fibre intakes on death and myocardial reinfarction: diet and reinfarction trial (DART). *Lancet*, 1989; **ii**: 757–761

Castelli WP, Abbott RD, McNamara PM. Summary estimation of cholesterol used to predict coronary heart disease. *Circulation*, 1983; **67**: 730–734

Chen J, Campbell C, Junyao L, Peto R. *Diet, Lifestyle and Mortality of 65 Chinese Counties*. Oxford: Oxford University Press, 1990

Cohen LA, Wynder EI. Do dietary monounsaturated fatty acids play a protective role in carcinogenesis and cardiovascular disease? *Medical Hypotheses*, 1990; **31**: 83–89

Cohen LA, Thompson DO, Maeura Y, Choi K, Blank ME, Rose DP. Dietary fat and mammary cancer. I. Promoting effects of different dietary fats on N-nitrosomethylurea-induced rat mammary tumorigenesis. *Journal of the National Cancer Institute*, 1986; **77**: 33–42

Dawber TR, Nickerson RJ, Brand FN, Pool J. Eggs, serum cholesterol, and coronary heart disease. *American Journal of Clinical Nutrition*, 1982; **36**: 617–625

Dayton S, Pearce ML, Hashimoto S, Dixon WJ, Tomiyasu U. A controlled clinical trial of a diet high in unsaturated fat in preventing complications of atherosclerosis. *Circulation*, 1969; **40** (suppl II): 1

de Lorgeril M, Renaud S, Mamelle N *et al*. Mediterranean alpha-linolenic acid-rich diet in secondary prevention of coronary heart disease. *Lancet*, 1994; **343**:1454–1459

Dolecek TA. Epidemiological evidence of relationships between dietary polyunsaturated fatty acids and mortality in the multiple risk factor intervention trial. *Proceedings of the Society for Experimental Biology and Medicine*, 1992; **200**: 177–182

Fehily AM, Yarnell JW, Sweetnam PM, Elwood PC. Diet and incident ischaemic heart disease: the Caerphilly study. *British Journal of Nutrition*, 1993; **69**: 303–314

Flatt JP. Energetics of intermediary metabolism. In: Garrow JS, Halliday D, eds. *Substrate and Energy Metabolism in Man*. London: John Libbey, 1985: 58–69

Fraser GE, Sabate J, Beeson WL, Strahan TM. A possible protective effect of nut consumption on risk of coronary heart disease. The Adventist Heath Study. *Archives of Internal Medicine*, 1992; **152**: 14, 16–24

Freedman LS, Clifford C, Messina M. Analysis of dietary fat, calories, body weight, and the development of mammary tumors in rats and mice: a review. *Cancer Research*, 1990; **50**: 5710–5719

Garcia-Palmieri MR, Sorlie P, Tillotson J, Costas R, Cordero E, Rodriguez M. Relationship of dietary intake to subsequent coronary heart disease incidence: the Puerto Rico Heart Health Program. *American Journal of Clinical Nutrition*, 1980; **33**: 1818–1827

Gerber M. Olive oil and cancer. In: Giacosa A, Hill MJ, eds. *The Mediterranean Diet and Cancer Prevention. Proceedings of a Workshop Organised by European Cancer Prevention Organization and the Italian League against Cancer in Consenza, Italy, 28–30 June 1991*. Andover: European Cancer Prevention Organization, 1991

Gerhardsson de Verdier M, Hagman U, Peters RK, Steineck G. Meat, cooking methods and colorectal cancer: a case-referent study in Stockholm. *International Journal of Cancer*, 1991; **49**: 520–525

Gey KF, Brubacher GB, Stahelin HB. Plasma levels of antioxidant vitamins in relation to ischemic heart disease and cancer. *American Journal of Clinical Nutrition*, 1987; **45(s)**: 1368–1377

Ginsberg HN, Barr SL, Gilbert A *et al*. Reduction of plasma cholesterol levels in normal men on an American Heart Association Step 1 diet or a Step 1 diet with added monounsaturated fat. *New England Journal of Medicine*, 1990; **322**: 574–579

Giovannucci E, Stampfer MJ, Colditz GA, Rimm EB, Willett WC. Relationship of diet to risk of colorectal adenoma in men. *Journal of the National Cancer Institute*, 1992; **84**: 91–98

Giovannucci E, Rimm EB, Stampfer MJ, Colditz GA, Ascherio A, Willett WC. Intake of fat, meat, and fiber in relation to risk of colon cancer in men. *Cancer Research*, 1994; **54**: 2390–2397

Giovannucci E, Rimm EB, Ascherio A, Stampfer MJ, Colditz GA, Willett WC. Alcohol, low-methionine-low-folate diets, and risk of colon cancer in men. *Journal of the National Cancer Institute*, 1995; **87**: 265–273

Goldbourt U, Yaari S, Medalie JH. Factors predictive of long-term coronary heart disease mortality among 10,059 male Israeli civil servants and municipal employees: a 23-year mortality follow-up in the Israeli Ischemic Heart Disease Study. *Cardiology*, 1993; **82**: 100–121

Gordon T, Kagan A, Garcia-Palmieri M *et al*. Diet and its relation to coronary heart disease and death in three populations. *Circulation*, 1981; **63**: 500–515

Graham S, Haughey B, Marshall J *et al*. Diet in the epidemiology of carcinoma of the prostate gland. *Journal of the National Cancer Institute*, 1983; **70**: 687–692

Graham S, Zielezny M, Marshall J *et al*. Diet in the epidemiology of postmenopausal breast cancer in a New York State cohort. *American Journal of Epidemiology*, 1992; **136**: 1327–1337

Hegsted DM. Serum-cholesterol response to dietary cholesterol: a re-evaluation. *American Journal of Clinical Nutrition*, 1986; **44**: 299–305

Howe GR, Hirohata T, Hislop TG *et al*. Dietary factors and risk of breast cancer: combined analysis of 12 case-control studies. *Journal of the National Cancer Institute*, 1990; **82**: 561–569

Howe GR, Friedenreich CM, Jain M, Miller AB. A cohort study of fat intake and risk of breast cancer. *Journal of the National Cancer Institute*, 1991; **83**: 336–340

Hunter DJ, Spiegelman D, Adami HO *et al*. Cohort studies of fat intake and the risk of breast cancer–a pooled analysis. *New England Journal of Medicine*, 1996; **334**: 356–361

Ip C. Quantitative assessment of fat and calorie as risk factors in mammary carcinogenesis in an experimental model. In: *Recent Progress on Nutrition and Cancer*. New York: Wiley-Liss Inc, 1990, pp 107–117

Jeffery RW, Hellerstedt WL, French SA, Baxter JE. A randomized trial of counseling for fat restriction versus calorie restriction in the treatment of obesity. *International Journal of Obesity and Related Metabolic Disorders*, 1995; **19**: 132–137

Judd JT, Clevidence BA, Muesing RA, Wittes J, Sunkin ME, Podczasy JJ. Dietary trans fatty acids: effects of plasma lipids and lipoproteins of healthy men and women. *American Journal of Clinical Nutrition*, 1994; **59**: 861–868

Kasim SE, Martino S, Kim PN *et al*. Dietary and anthropometric determinants of plasma lipoproteins during a long-term low-fat diet in healthy women. *American Journal of Clinical Nutrition*, 1993; **57**: 146–153

Kato H, Tillotson J, Nichaman MZ, Rhoads GG, Hamilton HB. Epidemiologic studies of coronary heart disease and stroke in Japanese men living in Japan, Hawaii and California: serum lipids and diet. *American Journal of Epidemiology*, 1973; **97**: 372–385

Keys A, ed. *Coronary Heart Disease in Seven Countries*. American Heart Association Monograph Number 29. *Circulation* 1970; **41, 42** (suppl I): 1–211

Keys A. Serum-cholesterol response to dietary cholesterol. *American Journal of Clinical Nutrition*, 1984; **40**: 351–359

Khaw KT, Barret-Connor E. Dietary fiber and reduced ischemic heart disease mortality rates in men and women: a 12-year prospective study. *American Journal of Epidemiology*, 1987; **126**: 1093–1102

Kolonel LN, Yoshizawa CN, Hankin JH. Diet and prostatic cancer: a case-control study in Hawaii. *American Journal of Epidemiology*, 1988; **127**: 999–1012

Kromhout D, de Lezenne Coulander C. Diet, prevalence and 10-year mortality from coronary heart disease in 871 middle-aged men. The Zutphen Study. *American Journal of Epidemiology*, 1984; **119**: 733–741

Kromhout D, Bosschieter EB, de Lezenne Coulander C. Dietary fibre and 10-year mortality for coronary heart disease, cancer and all causes. The Zutphen Study. *Lancet*, 1982; **ii**: 518–522

Kromhout D, Bosschieter EB, de Lezenne Coulander C. The inverse relation between fish consumption and 20-year mortality from coronary heart disease. *New England Journal of Medicine*, 1985; **312**: 1205–1209

Kromhout D, Menotti A, Bloemberg B *et al.* Dietary saturated and *trans* fatty acids and cholesterol and 25-year mortality from coronary heart disease: the Seven Countries Study. *Preventive Medicine*, 1995; **24**: 308-315

Kushi LH, Lew RA, Stare FJ *et al.* Diet and 20-year mortality from coronary heart disease: the Ireland–Boston Diet–Heart study. *New England Journal of Medicine*, 1985; **312**: 811–818

Kushi LH, Sellers TA, Potter JD *et al.* Dietary fat and postmenopausal breast cancer. *Journal of the National Cancer Institute*, 1992; **84**: 1092–1099

Landa MC, Frago N, Tres A. Diet and the risk of breast cancer in Spain. *European Journal of Cancer Prevention*, 1994; **3**: 313–320

Lapidus L, Andersson H, Bengtsson C, Bosaeus I. Dietary habits in relation to incidence of cardiovascular disease and death in women: a 12-year follow-up of participants in the population study in Gothenburg, Sweden. *American Journal of Clinical Nutrition*, 1986; **44**: 444–448

Leaf A, Weber PC. Cardiovascular effects of n-3 fatty acids. *New England Journal of Medicine*, 1988; **318**: 549–557

Lee-Han H, Cousins M, Beaton M *et al.* Compliance in a randomized clinical trial of dietary fat reduction in patients with breast dysplasia. *American Journal of Clinical Nutrition*, 1988; **48**: 575–586

Le Marchand L, Kolonel LN, Wilkens LR, Myers BC, Hirohata T. Animal fat consumption and prostate cancer: a prospective study in Hawaii. *Epidemiology*, 1994; **5**: 276–282

Lissner L, Levitsky DA, Strupp BJ, Kalkwarf HJ, Roe DA. Dietary fat and the regulation of energy intake in human subjects. *American Journal of Clinical Nutrition*, 1987; **46**: 886–892

Manntari M, Huttunen JK, Koskinen P *et al.* Lipoproteins and coronary heart disease in the Helsinki Heart Study. *European Heart Journal*, 1990; **11** (suppl H): 26h–31h

Martin-Moreno JM, Willett WC, Gorgojo L *et al.* Dietary fat, olive oil intake and breast cancer risk. *International Journal of Cancer*, 1994; **58**: 774–780

McGee DL, Reed DM, Yano K, Kagan A, Tillotson J. Ten-year incidence of coronary heart disease in the Honolulu Heart Program: relationship to nutrient intake. *American Journal of Epidemiology*, 1984; **119**: 667–676

Mensink RP, Katan MB. Effect of monounsaturated fatty acids versus complex carbohy-drates on high-density lipoprotein in healthy men and women. *Lancet*, 1987; **i**: 122–125

Mensink RP, Katan MB. Effect of dietary *trans* fatty acids on high-density and low-density lipoprotein cholesterol levels in healthy subjects. *New England Journal of Medicine*, 1990; **323**: 439–445

Mensink RP, Katan MB. Effect of dietary fatty acids on serum lipids and lipoproteins: a meta-analysis of 27 trials. *Arteriosclerosis and Thrombosis*, 1992; **12**: 911–919

Mensink RP, Zock PL, Katan MG, Hornstra G. Effect of dietary *cis* and *trans* fatty acids on serum lipoprotein [a] levels in humans. *Journal of Lipid Research*, 1992; **33**: 1493–1501

Mills PK, Beeson WL, Phillips RL, Fraser GE. Dietary habits and breast cancer incidence among Seventh-day Adventists. *Cancer*, 1989; **64**: 582–590

Morris JN, Marr JW, Clayton DG. Diet and heart: a postscript. *British Medical Journal*, 1977; **2**: 1307–1314

Morris MC, Manson JE, Rosner B, Buring JE, Willett WC, Hennekens CH. Fish consumption and cardiovascular disease in the Physicians' Health Study: A prospective study. *American Journal of Epidemiology*, 1995; **142**: 166–175

[National Diet–Heart Study Research Group]. The National Diet–Heart Study Final Report. *Circulation*, 1968; **37(s)**: 1–154

Nestel P, Noakes M, Belling B *et al*. Plasma lipoprotein and Lp[a] changes with substitution of elaidic acid for oleic acid in the diet. *Journal of Lipid Research*, 1992; **33**: 1029–1036

Norell SE, Ahlbom A, Feyching M, Pedersen NL. Fish consumption and mortality from coronary heart disease. *British Medical Journal of Clinical Research and Education*, 1986; **293**: 426

Phillips RL, Snowdon DA. Association of meat and coffee use with cancers of the large bowel, breast, and prostate among Seventh-Day Adventists: preliminary results. *Cancer Research*, 1983; **43(s)**: 2403s–2408s

Powell JJ, Tucker L, Fisher AG, Wilcox K. The effects of different percentages of dietary fat intake, exercise, and calorie restriction on body composition and body weight in obese females. *American Journal of Health Promotion*, 1994; **8**: 442–448

Prentice RL, Sheppard L. Dietary fat and cancer: consistency of the epidemiologic data, and disease prevention that may follow from a practical reduction in fat consumption. *Cancer Causes and Control*, 1990; **1**: 81–97

Reaven P, Parthasarathy S, Grasse BJ, Miller E, Steinberg D, Witztum JL. Effects of oleate-rich and linoleate-rich diets on the susceptibility of low density lipoprotein to oxidative modification in mildly hypercholesterolemic subjects. *Journal of Clinical Investigation*, 1993; **91**: 668–676

Renaud S, Kuba K, Goulet C, Lemire Y, Allard C. Relationship between fatty-acid composition of platelets and platelet aggregation in rat and man. Relation to thrombosis. *Circulation Research*, 1970; **26**: 553–564

Rimm EB, Stampfer MJ, Ascherio A, Giovannucci E, Colditz GA, Willett WC. Vitamin E consumption and the risk of coronary heart disease among men. *New England Journal of Medicine*, 1993; **328**: 1450–1456

Roberts TL, Wood DA, Riemersma RA, Gallagher PJ, Lampe FC. *Trans* isomers of oleic and linoleic acids in adipose tissue and sudden cardiac death. *Lancet*, 1995; **345**: 278–282

Sacks FM, Willett WC. More on chewing the fat—The good fat and the good cholesterol. *New England Journal of Medicine*, 1991; **325**: 1740–1742

Schaefer EJ, Lichtenstein AH, Lamon-Fava S *et al*. Body weight and low-density lipoprotein cholesterol changes after consumption of a low-fat ad libitum diet. *Journal of the American Medical Association*, 1995; **274**: 1450–1455

Seidell JC. Obesity in Europe—prevalences and consequences for use of medical care. *Pharmacoeconomics* 1994; **5** (suppl 1): 38–44

Shekelle RB, Shryock AM, Paul O *et al*. Diet, serum cholesterol, and death from coronary heart disease: The Western Electric Study. *New England Journal of Medicine*, 1981; **304**: 65–70

Shekelle RB, Missell L, Paul O, Shryock AM, Stamler J. Fish consumption and mortality from coronary heart disease (letter). *New England Journal of Medicine*, 1985; **313**: 820

Shepherd J, Cobbe SM, Ford I *et al*. Prevention of coronary heart disease with pravastatin in men with hypercholesterolemia. West of Scotland Coronary Prevention Study Group. *New England Journal of Medicine*, 1995; **333**: 1301–1307

Sheppard L, Kristal AR, Kushi LH. Weight loss in women participating in a randomized trial of low-fat diets. *American Journal of Clinical Nutrition*, 1991; **54**: 821–828

Shintani TT, Hughes CK, Beckham S, O'Connor HK. Obesity and cardiovascular risk intervention through the ad libitum feeding of traditional Hawaiian diet. *American*

Journal of Clinical Nutrition, 1991; **6**: 1647s–1651s.

Siguel EN, Lerman RH. Trans fatty acid patterns in patients with angiographically documented coronary artery disease. *American Journal of Cardiology*, 1993; **71**: 916–920

Siscovick DS, Raghunathan TE, King I *et al*. Dietary intake and cell membrane levels of long-chain n-3 polyunsaturated fatty acids and the risk of primary cardiac arrest. *Journal of the American Medical Association*, 1995; **274**: 1363–1367

Snowdon DA, Phillips RL, Fraser GE. Meat consumption and fatal ischemic heart disease. *Preventive Medicine*, 1984; **13**: 490–500

Stampfer MJ, Sacks FM, Salvini S, Willett WC, Hennekens CH. A prospective study of cholesterol, apolipoproteins, and the risk of myocardial infarction. *New England Journal of Medicine*, 1991; **325**: 373–381

Stampfer MJ, Hennekens CH, Manson JE, Colditz GA, Rosner B, Willett WC. Vitamin E consumption and risk of coronary disease in women. *New England Journal of Medicine*, 1993; **328**: 1444–1449

Steinberg D, Witztum JL. Lipoproteins and atherogenesis: current concepts. *Journal of the American Medical Association*, 1990; **264**: 3047–3052

Sundram K, Anisah I, Hayes KC, Jeyamalar R, Pathmanathan R. *Trans*-18:1 raises cholesterol more than *cis*-mono or saturated fats in humans (abstract). *Federation of American Societies for Experimental Biology (FASEB) Journal*, 1995; **9**: 2549

Trichopoulou A, Toupadaki N, Tzonou A. The macronutrient composition of the Greek diet: estimates derived from six case-control studies. *European Journal of Clinical Nutrition*, 1993; **47**: 549–558

Trichopoulou A, Katsouyanni K, Stuver S *et al*. Consumption of olive oil and specific food groups in relation to breast cancer risk in Greece. *Journal of the National Cancer Institute*, 1995; **87**: 110–116

Turpeinen O, Karvonen MJ, Pekkarinen M, Miettinen M, Elosuo R, Paavilainen E. Dietary prevention of coronary heart disease: the Finnish Mental Hospital Study. *International Journal of Epidemiology*, 1979; **8**: 99–118

US National Research Council—Committee on Diet and Health. *Diet and Health: Implications for Reducing Chronic Disease Risk*. Washington DC: National Academy Press, 1989

Van den Brandt PA, Van't Veer P, Goldbohm RA *et al*. A prospective cohort study on dietary fat and the risk of postmenopausal breast cancer. *Cancer Research*, 1993; **53**: 75–82

Vollset SE, Heuch I, Bjelke E. Fish consumption and mortality from coronary heart disease (letter). *New England Journal of Medicine*, 1985; **313**: 820–821

Weisburger JH. Mechanisms of macronutrient carcinogenesis. In: Miccozi MS, Moon TE, eds. *Macronutrients: Investigating Their Role in Cancer*. New York: Marcel Dekker, 1992, pp 3–31

Weisburger JH, Wynder EL. Dietary fat intake and cancer. *Hematology/Oncology Clinics of North America*, 1991; **5**: 7–23

Welsch CW. Relationship between dietary fat and experimental mammary tumorigenesis: A review and critique. *Cancer Research*, 1992; **52** (suppl 7): 2040S–2048S

Whittemore AS, Wu-Williams AH, Lee M *et al*. Diet, physical activity and colorectal cancer among Chinese in North America and China. *Journal of the National Cancer Institute*, 1990; **82**: 915–926

Whittemore AS, Kolonel LN, Wu AH *et al*. Prostate cancer in relation to diet, physical activity, and body size in blacks, whites, Asians in the United States and Canada. *Journal of the National Cancer Institute*, 1995; **87**: 652–661

Willett WC. Diet and health: What should we eat? *Science*, 1994; **264**: 532–537

Willett WC, Lenart EB. Diet in the prevention of coronary heart disease. In: Manson JE,

Ridker PM, Gaziani M, Hennekens CH, eds. *Prevention of Myocardial Infarction.* Oxford University Press, 1996

Willett WC, Stampfer MJ, Colditz GA, Rosner BA, Speizer FE. Relation of meat, fat, and fiber intake to the risk of colon cancer in a prospective study among women. *New England Journal of Medicine*, 1990; **323**: 1664–1672

Willett WC, Hunter DJ, Stampfer MJ *et al.* Dietary fat and fiber in relation to risk of breast cancer: An eight year follow-up. *Journal of the American Medical Association*, 1992; **268**: 2037–2044

Willett WC, Stampfer MJ, Manson JE *et al.* Intake of *trans* fatty acids and risk of coronary heart disease among women. *Lancet*, 1993; **341**: 581–585

World Health Organization. *Food and Health Indicators in Europe.* (Preliminary software issued by the WHO Regional Office for Europe, Copenhagen, September, 1993) 1993

Zock PL, Katan MB. Hydrogenation alternatives: effects of *trans* fatty acids and stearic acid versus linoleic acid on serum lipids and lipoproteins in humans. *Journal of Lipid Research*, 1992; **33**: 399–410

Discussion

W. Philip T. James

Rowett Research Institute, Aberdeen, UK

Professor Walter Willett presents an intriguing story which seems to exonerate dietary fat from much of the blame for coronary heart disease (CHD), cancers and obesity. Only *trans* fatty acids seem to be important. These views are powerfully put both in the scientific press and in the public media. The *trans* fatty acid story does have biological validity (Wahle and James, 1993), but not as the crucial factor in Western CHD rates (GB Department of Health, 1995a). When there are huge public health issues as well as financial interests vested in the fats and oils business we must get the message right.

I would argue that, in policy terms, Professor Willett's analyses are limited for two reasons. First, the analyses place far too great an emphasis on the validity of his and other cohort studies, valuable though they are. These studies are far less powerful than supposed because of error problems and inter-individual variation. Secondly, his analyses neglect the need to rely on a variety of clinical, physiological and animal evidence when deciding on public health policy.

First let us deal with total dietary fat and CHD. I am unaware of any expert committee specifying a powerful causal link between total fat intake and CHD whatever the other lifestyle factors; this has been true since Keys' days, but a policy suggesting a low-fat diet may then emerge as a strategy to reduce saturated fat intake. A high total fat intake may also contribute rather than being crucial to

CHD in three possible ways: (a) by inducing obesity (see below); (b) by promoting thrombosis, through its effects on factor VII activation (Miller *et al*, 1989); and (c) by modifying the hepatic responses to alterations in the intake of different fatty acids.

Professor Willett's neglect of the role of saturated fatty acids in promoting CHD has made me understand the common misinterpretation of epidemiological data! Thus, almost all cohort studies fail to show a relationship between CHD and saturated fatty acid intakes despite their crucial importance. This stems from two problems—unrecognised errors in dietary methodology and the fundamental importance of gene–nutrient interactions. This interaction is reflected in cholesterol levels: an intermediate marker of inter-individual responsiveness without which the link between saturated fats and CHD would only be seen in cross-country analyses (Keys, 1980) and then only if there are not major confounding factors, e.g. antioxidant intake (Gey, 1995). The data have to be interpreted in relation to a biologically plausible mechanism, because the accepted link between dietary saturated fat and serum cholesterol is lost in cohort studies and obscured in cross-cultural studies (Keys and Kimura, 1970). Cohort studies should therefore be treated with caution if they produce negative findings because it is impossible for cohort studies to demonstrate a causal and important relationship when the inter-individual variation in responsiveness to the dietary factor is large and when there are other confounding factors.

The issue of measurement error is also crucial. Plummer and Clayton (1993) and Plummer *et al* (1994) have now dealt with this in great detail and have highlighted the way that random measurement error can markedly attenuate a dose–response relationship within cohorts. A food frequency questionnaire, for example, has many in-built errors which I suspect will produce false positive as well as false negative results. There is the usual neglect of portion size, systematic and random under- and over-reporting, scaling bias, and very substantial errors in converting these data into nutrient intakes with food compositional tables. Few studies test the reproducibility of the measurement and rarely is the measurement repeated in cohort studies and this repetition used in adjusting the regression relationship. The validation process is also often in error even when the 'gold standard' is, for example, the weighed food intake. Yet recently we have had to cast considerable doubt on the usefulness of this weighed intake technique, particularly in weight-conscious women who tend to under-report their true intake. This is a very serious problem because when we recalculated the UK Adult Dietary Survey and imposed a generous allowance for daily variations in intake, we still found about two-thirds of women were under-reporting compared with the expected intakes estimated from these women's predicted basal metabolic rates and assuming light physical activity (James and Ralph, 1995). Thus, I would be astonished if US nurses (and perhaps professional men) do not overwhelmingly under-report, perhaps selectively, their intake.

Statistical problems abound: where correlations between the reference dietary assessment technique and the true habitual intake lie between 0.25 and 0.5 as for fat, then Plummer and Clayton (1993) calculate that three to six times as many subjects need to be included in the calibration study as the number of cases of disease, e.g. CHD or breast cancer, found in the main cohort study which uses the crude questionnaire system! This is rarely if ever done, and few epidemiologists dare integrate the sequential errors involved in these large prospective studies: too much money and prestige, I suppose, may be involved! Plummer and Clayton (1993) highlight the value of a biomarker which can give a reference point for estimating the errors in different approaches to estimating the diet. They conclude that without a biomarker it is all too easy to become overconfident about the dietary methodology: they describe the implications for cohort and case-control studies as involving 'a substantial amount of faith' and where the use of dietary methodology 'is often statistically naive'.

With CHD the dietary factors can now be seen in context (Scottish Office, 1993), but with cancer the problems escalate because of the usual absence of intermediate biological markers of risk. Since inter-individual differences in responsiveness to diet apply to every nutrient studied, it is fundamentally wrong to neglect the biology of carcinogenesis, the data on the fat promotion of induced cancers in animals, the role of fat in obesity (see below) and the value of cross-cultural rather than cohort or case-control studies.

Obesity emerges in every country with, on average, fat intakes over 15% energy, but energy density may be the real key to passive overconsumption of energy (Stubbs et al, 1995) which readily leads to slow weight gain in an inactive society (GB Department of Health, 1995b). Most middle-aged women in affluent societies are restrained eaters who strive to remain thin, so the failure to demonstrate a relationship between fat intake (measured very inaccurately) and weight gain in an inactive weight-obsessed society is to be expected. Animal data clearly show not only the crucial roles of inactivity and high-fat diets, but the individual propensity to weight gain in the genetically prone—a feature also shown in adults (Heitmann et al, 1995). Therapeutic trials with different slimming diets are irrelevant to the issue, and trials of low-fat diets will have only modest effects if energy density is neglected, if inactivity persists and if there is, as seems increasingly clear, a re-setting of appetite control as weight gain occurs.

I conclude that Professor Willett is dominated in his thinking by cohort studies and by the data on the value of extra virgin olive oil, rich in phytoprotectants, in explaining the preservation of low CHD and cancer rates in Greeks who were, in practice, very active (Christakis et al, 1965), but are now increasingly obese. On these bases I believe it unwise to alter our recommendations for a low-fat diet.

References

Christakis G, Severinghaus EL, Maldonado Z, Kafatos FC, Hashim SA. Crete: A study in the metabolic epidemiology of coronary heart disease. *The American Journal of*

Cardiology, 1965; **15**: 320–332

Gey F. Ten-year retrospective on the antioxidant hypothesis of arteriosclerosis: threshold plasma levels of antioxidant micronutrients related to minimum cardiovascular risk. *Journal of Nutritional Biochemistry*, 1995; **6**: 206–236

Great Britain Department of Health. Committee on Medical Aspects of Food Policy. Cardiovascular Review Group. *Nutritional Aspects of Cardiovascular Disease*. Report on Health and Social Subjects No. 46. London: HMSO, 1995a

Great Britain Department of Health. *Obesity: Reversing the increasing problem of obesity in England*. A Report from the Nutrition and Physical Activity Task Forces. London: Department of Health, 1995b

Heitmann BL, Lissner L, Sørensen TIA, Bengtsson C. Dietary fat intake and weight gain in women genetically predisposed for obesity. *American Journal of Clinical Nutrition*, 1995; **61**: 1213–1217

James WPT, Ralph A. Matching nutrition knowledge to nutritional needs. In: Wahlqvist M et al, eds. *Nutrition in a Sustainable Environment*. London: Smith-Gordon, 1995: 73–86

Keys A. Seven Countries: *A Multivariate Analysis of Death and Coronary Heart Disease*. Cambridge, MA: Harvard University Press, 1980

Keys A, Kimura IN. Diets of middle-aged farmers in Japan. *American Journal of Clinical Nutrition*, 1970; **23**: 212–223

Miller GJ, Cruickshank JK, Ellis LJ et al. Fat consumption and factor VII coagulant activity in middle-aged men. An association between dietary and thrombogenic coronary risk factor. *Atherosclerosis*, 1989; **78**: 19–24

Plummer M, Clayton D. Measurement error in dietary assessment: an investigation using covariance structure models. *Statistics in Medicine*, 1993; **12**: 925–935; 937–948

Plummer M, Clayton D, Kaaks R. Calibration in multi-centre cohort studies. *International Journal of Epidemiology*, 1994; **23**: 419–426

Scottish Office. *Scotland's Health: A Challenge to Us All. The Scottish Diet*. Report of a Working Party to the Chief Medical Officer for Scotland. Edinburgh: Scottish Office Home and Health Department, 1993

Stubbs RJ, Ritz P, Coward WA, Prentice AM. Covert manipulation of the ratio of dietary fat to carbohydrate and energy density: effect on food intake and energy balance in free-living men eating ad libitum. *American Journal of Clinical Nutrition*, 1995; **62**: 330–337

Wahle KWJ, James WPT. Isomeric fatty acids and human health. *European Journal of Clinical Nutrition*, 1993; **47**: 828–839

6
Diet and large bowel cancer

Sheila A. Bingham and John H. Cummings

Dunn Clinical Nutrition Centre, Cambridge, UK

Large bowel cancer arises in epithelial cells lining the colon and rectum. Healthy cells start to proliferate, progress through abnormal crypts with dysplastic cells to polyps which grow and eventually undergo malignant transformation with tissue invasion and metastasis (Morson, 1974). Associated with these phenotypic changes are a series of genetic abnormalities (Table 6.1). The first of these was shown by Herrera *et al* (1986) in a case report of a patient in whom deletion of the long arm of chromosome 5 was associated with multiple colonic polyps, synchronous colon carcinomas, mental subnormality and other developmental abnormalities. A number of exciting discoveries have been made since, particularly by Vogelstein's group (Solomon *et al*, 1987; Kinzler *et al*, 1991; Nishisho *et al*, 1991) and by Bodmer (Bodmer *et al*, 1987) and there are now several well established chromosomal abnormalities found in colorectal cancer (CRC) (Aaltonen *et al*, 1993; Peltomaki *et al*, 1993). Genes are involved in the control of cell growth, cell differentiation and DNA repair, and these genetic studies have shown that a single gene defect does not lead to CRC, although the 5q21 abnormality found in familial adenomatous polyposis (FAP) is particularly associated with a hereditary form of colonic polyps. A number of gene defects are collectively needed to produce the varying stages in the cycle from normal epithelium, through polyp formation, tumour growth and metastasis (Vogelstein *et al*, 1988; Fearon, 1992) and it is possible that these originate from a single clone of stem cells (Griffiths *et al*, 1989; Fuller *et al*, 1990).

Epidemiology

Colorectal cancer is prevalent in industrialised countries with Western-style diets, although it is now appearing with increasing frequency in South America, Japan, Singapore and other countries of the Far East (Parkin *et al*, 1992). It is

Diet, Nutrition and Chronic Disease: Lessons from Contrasting Worlds.
Edited by P. S. Shetty and K. McPherson © 1997 John Wiley & Sons, Ltd.

Table 6.1   Genetic abnormalities in colo-rectal cancer

Chromosome	Gene	Tumours with mutations (%)	Action of gene
2	hMSH2	12–28	DNA mismatch repair
3	hMLH2	35–45	Tumour suppressor
	APC		
5q	MCC		
12	Ki-ras	50	Oncogene
17p	p53	75+	Tumour suppressor
18q	DCC	70+	Tumour suppressor

Sources: Bodmer et al, 1987; Solomon et al, 1987; Kinzler et al, 1991; Nishisho et al, 1991; Aaltonen et al, 1993; Peltomaki et al, 1993

essentially a disease of the elderly, with incidence rising rapidly after the age 50 and a cumulative risk of up to 7% in some populations by age 74. Evidence for an environmental agent in the aetiology of CRC comes from several sources, principally the world-wide variation in rates, time trends within populations, migrant studies and associations with diet (Tomatis, 1990).

The dietary epidemiology of CRC has been summarised in a number of recent reviews (Bingham, 1990). In epidemiological studies, cancers of the colon and rectum are sometimes separated because there is uncertainty as to whether they have different aetiologies. They probably share a common aetiology, although there are differences in patterns of distribution of tumours of the colon and rectum amongst populations and also between sexes. For example, recto-sigmoid tumours are commoner in Western industrialised nations, whereas in countries with low rates of CRC, right-sided colonic lesions tend to predominate. There is also the observation that rectal cancer is more strongly associated with alcohol consumption, particularly beer drinking (IARC, 1988; Riboli et al, 1991).

In cross-sectional studies the principal dietary associations with CRC are fat and meat which increase risk, and with cereal foods, fruit and vegetables, which reduce risk. The results of case-control studies, of which more than 50 have been published, are less consistent, possibly due to methodological problems with these studies. The majority, however, show an increased risk for meat consumption, particularly with red meat, but not with fish and other seafood. Dairy products and eggs show no risk, but vegetables and fruit are consistently protective. Non-starch polysaccharide (NSP) intakes tend to be lower in populations with increased risk of CRC but 'fibre' intake data are notoriously unreliable and poorly obtained (Bingham, 1990). If starch intakes are taken into account (Cassidy et al, 1994) then the protective effect is clearer. A review of over 30 case-control studies looking at 'dietary fibre' intakes and CRC showed a significant protective effect which was mostly associated with fruit and vegetable consumption (Bingham, 1990). More recently, energy intake and bodyweight have been shown to be associated with increased CRC risk in males, while increased levels of physical activity may be protective (Gerhardsson *et al*, 1986; 1988; 1990).

Mechanisms of diet-induced carcinogenesis

Given the role of genetic factors in CRC, how can the dietary epidemiology be reconciled with events occurring at a cellular and metabolic level? Carcinogenesis is a multi-stage process, the initiation of which is almost certainly due to DNA damage. Potential DNA damaging agents in the large intestine include heterocyclic amines (HAA), *N*-nitrosocompounds (NOC), and free radicals. Adducts include O^6-methyl-guanine, 8-hydroxy guanine, and HAA adducts. DNA damage alone, however, is clearly not enough to lead to a chromosomal abnormality because there are active DNA repair mechanisms going on in the cell all the time. As yet, not much attention has been paid to these DNA repair mechanisms and it is possible that diet may play an important part here.

Dietary fat intake

In the 1970s, fat intake was considered to be the principal risk factor for CRC and the proposed mechanism was through an effect on bile acid metabolism (Hill *et al*, 1971; 1975). Secondary bile acids were known promoters in mouse models, and deoxycholic acid was shown in epidemiological studies to be related to risk of CRC (Hill *et al*, 1975). High faecal bile acid concentrations and greater amounts of deoxycholate were associated with increased risk. Subsequent studies, however, indicated that the epidemiological findings were not so clear (Setchell *et al*, 1987). Recently the bile acid/fat theory has received new impetus with the observation that bile acids may stimulate cell proliferation in the colon through the action of diacylglycerol (DAG), which activates protein kinase C (PKC) (Guillem *et al*, 1987; Reddy *et al*, 1994). Bile acids stimulate phospholipid turnover in cell membranes resulting in release of DAG. DAG is one of two intracellular messengers which increase the affinity of PKC for calcium and render it active at physiological levels, phosphorylating serine and threonine residues in many target organs. Phorbol esters are well known promoters which resemble DAG, but are not degraded. The fatty acid composition of DAG is modified by intake of dietary lipid, and it is possible that a change in the type of DAG may affect activation of PKC. Increased levels of PKC have been shown in colonic tumour tissue (Guillem *et al*, 1987) and DAG production from phosphatidylcholine is enhanced in human fermentation systems by the presence of deoxycholic acid (Morotomi *et al*, 1990). In physiological studies, increase in dietary fat was shown to increase colonic fat and bile acid levels, an effect which is thought to be ameliorated by dietary calcium supplements (Newmark *et al*, 1984; Welberg *et al*, 1991). Diets which reduce deoxycholate levels in faecal water, such as high-resistant starch diets, lead to reduced cell proliferation in the human colon (van Munster *et al*, 1994). Reduction of dietary fat, therefore, must remain a strong component of the strategy for bowel cancer prevention in Western countries.

In animal studies, fat acts very clearly as a promoter of large bowel cancer. Fat is also a major contributor to energy intake in many diets. Energy restriction has a powerful effect in reducing tumorigenesis at most sites by mechanisms such as reduced growth in tissues, alteration of carcinogen metabolism, and reduction in oxidative damage to DNA. The dietary restrictions required for this effect must be in excess of 10% of the total intake. Increased tumorigenesis is not clearly demonstrated with increased intake, because rodents will not voluntarily ingest excess energy (Rogers *et al*, 1993). There is some debate as to whether high-fat diets or high-energy diets are more important. No significant effects of total fat intake were seen on either initiation or promotion of azoxymethane-induced tumours of the large intestine of rats, while energy intake was significantly associated (Clinton *et al*, 1992). In contrast, independent effects of fat and energy were seen with a significant increase in the number of azoxymethane-induced tumours in animals fed high-fat (as corn oil) ad libitum diets, compared with animals fed low-fat ad libitum, low-fat restricted, and high-fat restricted diets (Steinbach *et al*, 1993).

Protein and meat intakes

Meat and protein are probably the most consistently observed dietary factors that increase risk of CRC. There are a number of possible ways in which meat and protein may increase risk:

- Heterocyclic amines produced during cooking.
- *N*-Nitroso compounds; amines and amides from protein fermentation serve as a nitrosatable substrate.
- Ammonia accumulates in the colon on high-meat diets, promotes and enhances cell proliferation.
- Induction of bile acid degrading enzymes.
- Source of iron.
- Source of sulphur.

For protein to have an effect on large bowel function, it is not unreasonable to suppose that it must first reach this organ before being metabolised by the resident flora. The human large intestine receives 6–24 g of protein each day from the upper gut. Some of this is from endogenous sources, such as gut enzymes and mucus, but the major part is dietary in origin (Gibson *et al*, 1976; Chacko and Cummings, 1988; Silvester and Cummings, in press). The amount of dietary protein that reaches the colon is primarily dependent upon the amount in the diet, although the physical form of the protein is also important. Figure 6.1 shows

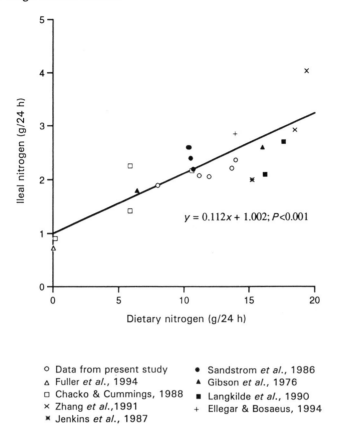

$$y = 0.112x + 1.002; P<0.001$$

o Data from present study • Sandstrom *et al.*, 1986
Δ Fuller *et al.*, 1994 ▲ Gibson *et al.*, 1976
□ Chacko & Cummings, 1988 ■ Langkilde *et al.*, 1990
× Zhang *et al.*,1991 + Ellegar & Bosaeus, 1994
✳ Jenkins *et al.*, 1987

Figure 6.1 Relationship between dietary and ileal nitrogen excretion. Meta-analysis of nine studies (Silvester and Cummings, in press)

the combined results of several studies which have looked at protein digestibility in the upper gut in relation to its sources, cooking and physical form. Meat protein does not have a digestibility different from cheese, even when grilled at high temperature, and the association of meat-eating with bowel cancer is mainly with red and processed meat (Willett *et al*, 1990), suggesting that this may not entirely be due to meat-eaters having higher protein intakes.

Cooking meat leads to the formation of a number of carcinogenic substances of which heterocyclic amines (HAA) such as imidazoquinoline (IQ), methyl IQ and phenyl imidazopyridine (PhIP) are strongly mutagenic in *in vitro* assays (Felton *et al*, 1986; Gross, 1990; Sugimura *et al*, 1994). PhIP has attracted particular attention because it tends to be the most abundant, and colon tumours that are produced from it in rats have a high frequency of microsatellite instability which is similar to that seen in human inherited and sporadic CRC (Canzian *et al*, 1994).

The production of these compounds is enhanced during cooking at high temperatures for long periods. However, grilling and frying meat do not lead to particularly large amounts of HCA being formed (Silvester, 1996). Frying chicken, beef, pork or fish for 6 minutes on either side at 200°C gave levels of MeIQ and PhIP of < 3.1 ng/g and daily intakes of around 1 μg. Average intakes in US diets are of the same order, and comparisons between the amount required for carcinogenicity in animals and amounts found in diets suggest that the relative contribution of HAA to colon cancer incidence may be small, i.e. 0.25% of all colon cancers (Layton et al, 1995). There are species differences between humans and rodents and direct extrapolation from rodent experiments to human risks may be misleading.

Some base substitutions which are seen in CRC are characteristic of alkylating agents such as NOCs. Although NOCs have not usually been associated with CRC, they are found in human faeces (Rowland et al, 1991). Preformed NOCs occur in food, but technological changes in the production of what were once major sources of NOC in the diet, i.e. beer and nitrite-cured meat products, have halved dietary consumption of volatile nitrosamines to about 0.5 μg per day. The major non-dietary exogenous source is tobacco, the mainstream smoke from one cigarette containing up to 65 μg of volatile nitrosamines and the sidestream smoke 1000 μg (Preussman, 1984). Endogenous formation of NOCs does, however, occur, since the colonic lumen is rich in amines and amides produced primarily by bacterial decarboxylation of amino acids, and in the presence of a nitrosating agent these can be N-nitrosated to a large variety of NOCs. Nitrosated amides are direct-acting carcinogens, tending to produce tumours nearer to the site where they are produced, whereas nitrosated amines require hydroxylation via cytochrome P450 enzymes and can initiate tumours at distal sites (Shuker, 1989). Endogenous nitrate production must occur since nitrate excretion exceeds that consumed in food and water (Witter et al, 1982). Wagner et al (1983) showed that nitrate synthesis is enhanced during immunostimulation, while Stuehr and Marletta (1985) showed that nitrite and nitrate are produced by macrophages. Studies with ^{15}N established that the source is dietary arginine, and increased arginine from protein might be expected to increase urine nitrate excretion, an effect demonstrated in animals (Mallett et al, 1988; Ward et al, 1989). Nitric oxide from stimulated macrophages in the large bowel mucosa, together with nitrite produced from reduced nitrate diffusing into the gut, are available for the formation of NOCs.

Human faecal samples contain negligible amounts of volatile NOCs (Archer et al, 1981), but Rowland et al (1991), using chemiluminescence, detected an average of 13 μg per sample on a low (11 mg) nitrate diet which increased to 60 μg per sample when given a 300 mg supplement of nitrate per day. High-protein diets have also been shown to increase urine N-nitrosoproline excretion in animals. In a recent study Bingham et al (1996) determined the effect of red meat consumption on faecal NOC excretion in healthy subjects. The study was done under

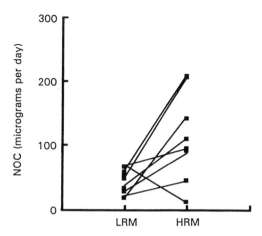

Figure 6.2   Total faecal NOC (μg/day) on low red meat (LRM) and high red meat (HRM) diets in eight volunteers (Bingham *et al*, 1996)

metabolically controlled conditions, and subjects ate either 60 g per day or 600 g per day of fried beef, chicken and pork. Figure 6.2 shows that faecal NOC excretion increased from 40 ± 7 to 113 ± 25 μg/day—a range of exposure similar to that seen with cigarette smoke. There was no reduction in NOC excretion when bran was added to the diet. In other studies, NOC excretion was increased by high-meat diets but feeding resistant starch had no effect (Silvester, 1996). Thus NOC can be formed in the colon and provides a possible link between protein intakes and the risk of CRC.

Protective factors

The major dietary protective factors are fruit, vegetables and 'fibre'. There are a number of components in fruit and vegetables which may protect against CRC, including:

- non-starch polysaccharides (NSP);
- antioxidant micronutrients (vitamins C, E, folate, calcium and selenium);
- ʊ3 and ʊ6 fatty acids;
- glucosinolates and other sulphur compounds;
- phenols and flavonoids;
- lignans and isoflavonoids (e.g. genstein); and
- salicylates.

Wattenburg (1971) was the first to show that minor constituents of vegetables have a profound effect on intestinal P450 activity. Indoles present in brassicae as glucosinolates, such as indole 3 carbinol, were identified in brussels sprouts, cabbage and cauliflower and found to induce both small intestinal and hepatic P450 hydroxylase (Loub et al, 1975). Despite this activity, which is associated with carcinogen activation, Wattenburg (1985) proposed a classification of the numerous constituents of fruits and vegetables, based on their ability to prevent carcinogenesis. Examples were vitamin C, which inhibits NOC formation, and blockers, for example phenols and isothiocyanates, which have effects on p450 enzyme activity.

Glucosinolates and other sulphur compounds

Vegetables contain a wide range of sulphur compounds, usually conjugated in foods as glucosinolates. Broccoli contains indoles, which have been shown to increase large bowel tumour production (Pence et al, 1986). Sulphoraphane was also recently identified from broccoli and shown to be an inducer of quinone reductase and glutathione transferase (GST) (Zhang et al, 1992). In rats, diallyl sulphide in garlic induces GST, and suppresses colon tumours induced by dimethyl hydrazine, but in another model it enhances hepatocarcinogenesis. The related diallyl disulphide was, however, an inhibitor of colon carcinogenesis (Wargovich, 1987; Sparnins et al, 1988; Takahashi et al, 1992). There is much current interest in constituents of vegetables and fruit that can act as chemopreventers.

Flavonoids and phenols

A very large class of natural compounds, widespread in plants mainly as the glycosides, are the flavonoids. At least 1 g per day of flavonoids is present in human food, with tea and wine containing large quantities. Flavonoids have strong antioxidant properties because they are metal ion chelators, scavengers of superoxide, and are able to terminate lipid peroxidation chain reactions (Yang and Wang, 1993). Rutin and quercitin have been known for some time to be mutagenic, but more recent studies suggest they are protective in animal models. Green tea, and to a lesser extent black tea, has consistently been shown to inhibit carcinogenesis in the lung, oesophagus, forestomach, liver, duodenum and small intestine, in addition to the large bowel (Yang and Wang, 1993). The effect of black tea, which is more commonly consumed by humans in Western societies, has not been investigated for chemoprevention in bowel cancer, and there is inconclusive epidemiological support for a role for black tea drinking in large bowel cancer prevention. Tea polyphenols also alter p450 enzyme activity (Khan et al, 1992; Mukhtar et al, 1992) and have been found to inhibit hyperproliferation, colonic abnormalities and tumour incidence in mice, regardless of the level of fat in the diet (Deschner et al, 1991; 1993). Simpler polyphenols, such as caffeic and ferulic acids, are able to block N-nitrosamine formation (Kuenzig et al, 1984). Other flavonoids, the isoflavones, are inhibitory in animal models of breast cancer and have also been suggested to be important in the genesis of bowel cancer (Setchell and Adlercreutz, 1988; Barnes *et al*, 1990).

Dietary fibre

The hypothesis that 'dietary fibre prevents large bowel cancer' must be credited largely to Burkitt, who in 1971 described the epidemiology of CRC and suggested an association between dietary fibre intake and large bowel function. The strength of Burkitt's hypothesis was the suggestion that fibre could prevent bowel cancer, through its capacity to 'regulate the speed of transit, bulk and consistency of stool . . .', to dilute carcinogens and to alter microbial metabolism (Burkitt, 1971). The notion that fibre might protect against bowel cancer was not entirely new. In 1960, Higginson and Oettlé had reported their studies of cancer incidence in Bantu and Cape Coloured races of South Africa. In order to explain the lack of bowel cancer in Bantu compared to other races they said that it was 'difficult to avoid suspecting the diet . . .' and that '. . . in the Bantu a large amount of roughage is normally consumed, and constipation in the Western sense is rare' (Higginson and Oettlé, 1960). Oettlé expanded on this in 1964 saying that in the Bantu 'stools are bulkier and more frequent, and the complaint of constipation may indicate no more than that the frequency of bowel movements has fallen to two or less per day. The use of regular enemas and purges is widespread. These practices would dilute any carcinogens and might shorten the duration of exposure ...' (Oettlé, 1964). Bremner (1964) stated that the roughage content of the Bantu diet, together with their greater use of aperients and greater physical exercise, might explain their low incidence of rectal cancer. Trowell, who also worked in Africa, noted in his book *Non-Infective Disease in Africa* (1960) that the African was rarely constipated, consumed a bulky diet and that this might explain the rarity of Western-type bowel diseases. In India, Malhotra (1967) was intrigued by the geographical distribution of gut cancer across the continent. He felt that diet must have something to do with it, and wrote, in relation to the fact that bowel cancer was much more common in South India than in North India, 'one explanation that might be likely is the difference in the cellullose and fibre content in the diets of the South Indians as compared to those of the North Indians'.

These observations from contrasting worlds have led to a rapid expansion of research into diet and CRC. Today Burkitt's theory must be seen as an oversimplification but nevertheless much credit is due to him; few scientists have had such an impact on nutrition research in the latter part of this century. Burkitt was probably correct in associating bowel habit with CRC risk, although he did not really collect the relevant data. This has now been done (Cummings *et al*, 1992) and Figure 6.3 shows the relationship. A mean daily stool weight of around 100 g is associated with high risk of CRC which falls to about one-third of the risk at 200 g/day. However, the idea that dietary fibre is the protective factor in the diet has proved to be more elusive. Burkitt neither defined nor measured fibre,

S. A. Bingham and J. H. Cummings

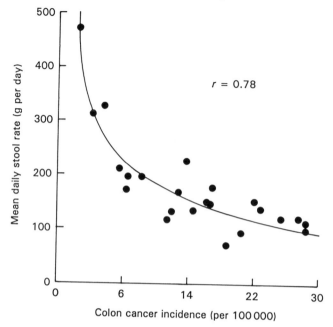

Figure 6.3   Relation between average daily stool weight and colon cancer incidence in 23 population groups from 12 countries (Cummings *et al*, 1992)

and thus left a legacy which has led to much confusion and debate. If Burkitt's idea was that a type of diet characterised by high dietary fibre was protective then he was probably on the right lines. We know today that CRC risk is lowest in populations eating diets high in fruits, vegetables and cereals, and low in meat and fat. More problematic is determining of the role of 'fibre' itself. Leaving aside problems of definition and analysis (Englyst and Hudson, 1993) the balance of epidemiological studies suggests a protective effect for 'fibre' against CRC (Bingham, 1990; Trock *et al*, 1990).

Cross-sectional studies show low risk of CRC in populations with high dietary fibre intakes but a number of anomalies in this relationship occur; for example, the Japanese have similar intakes of dietary fibre measured as NSP to people in the UK (Kuratsune *et al*, 1986; Bingham, 1990) but a much lower risk of CRC. Case-control studies provide more consistent evidence for a protective effect of fibre (Howe *et al*, 1992) whilst cohort studies are bedevilled by oversimplified dietary intake methods and poor dietary fibre analytical techniques. As yet, no study has been reported using NSP.

What makes the fibre story so much more credible is that a number of potential mechanisms exist whereby it can protect against CRC. Central to our understanding of this is fermentation, in which carbohydrate is metabolised by the indigenous anaerobic flora with the production of various gases, short-chain fatty acids—acetate, propionate and butyrate—and stimulation of bacterial biomass (Cummings, 1983). The following are mechanisms whereby fermentation may lead to protection against colorectal cancer:

- Fermentation—butyrate production—differentiating agent.
- Laxative effects—dilution and adsorption of potential carcinogen.
- Suppression of bacterial enzymes such as nitro-reductase, β-glucuronidase.
- Reduced secondary bile acids.
- Increased N uptake into bacteria.

Butyrate is an important molecule in large intestinal epithelial cell function. In addition to providing an energy source and being trophic to the mucosa, butyrate acts to control cell growth and differentiation. This it does through the arrest of early cell growth, induction of differentiation, stimulation of cytoskeletal organisation and alteration in gene expression. The slowing or arrest of cell growth is seen in many cell lines, including ovarian cells (D'Anna et al, 1980), hepatoma (van Wijk et al, 1981), colon (Kim et al, 1980; Tsao et al, 1982; Dexter et al, 1984; Chung et al, 1985; Whitehead et al, 1986; Gamet et al, 1992; Gibson et al, 1992), pancreas (Bloom et al, 1989), cervix (Dyson et al, 1992), prostate (Reese et al, 1985; Halgunset et al, 1988) and breast (Guilbaud et al, 1990). Changes in cell growth are associated with differentiation, as indicated, for example, by the expression of alkaline phosphatase (Morita et al, 1982; Gum et al, 1987; Kim et al, 1994).

The effect of butyrate on differentiation is related to the control of gene expression. Toscani et al (1988; 1990) have shown with Swiss 3T3 cells that the arrest of cell growth and differentiation is associated with a specific reduction of c-myc, p53, thymidine kinase and induction of c-fos and aP2. These events ultimately lead to adipocyte differentiation in Swiss 3T3 cells, when combined with either insulin or dexamethasone. Butyrate alters the expression of many genes, including EGF receptors in hepatocytes (Gladhaug et al, 1988; Gladhaug and Christoffersen, 1989; Gladhaug et al, 1989), metallothionein in hepatoma cells (Birren and Herschman, 1986), oestrogen, prolactin and EGF receptors in breast tissue cells (De Fazio et al, 1992; Ormandy et al, 1992) and many others. In CRC cells a number of changes in gene expression have been observed (Wice et al, 1985; Saini et al, 1990; Bates et al, 1992; Gibson et al, 1992; Souleimani and Asselin, 1993; Gibson et al, 1994; 1995b). The induction of differentiation in tumour cell lines is associated with changes in cytoskeletal architecture and adhesion properties of cells (Malik et al, 1987; Higgins and Ryan, 1989; Wilson and Weiser, 1992).

A number of cellular mechanisms have been suggested for the action of butyrate (Kruh et al, 1992; 1995). The best known is the effect on histone acetylation which has been shown in many cell types. Smith (1986) has demonstrated that by inhibiting histone deacetylase, butyrate allows hyper-acetylation of histones to occur. In turn, this 'opens up' the DNA structure, facilitating access of DNA repair enzymes. In an animal study in which wheat bran was fed, Boffa *et al* (1992) demonstrated that butyrate levels in the colonic lumen are positively related to colonic epithelial cell histone acetylation and inversely related to cell proliferation. Butyrate thus appears to be able to modulate DNA synthesis *in vivo*. Increase in histone acetylation may not be the entire explanation for the specificity of butyrate in modulating gene expression. Evidence is now accumulating that butyrate acts by a mechanism that involves specific regulatory DNA sequences. Butyrate moderates the expression of two related genes BRF1 and BRF2 (butyrate response factor genes) which are members of the TIS 11 family of primary response genes, and are associated with neoplastic growth (Bustin *et al*, 1994).

Other possible mechanisms of action include inhibition of chromatin protein phosphorylation and hypermethylation of DNA. Recently, Paraskeva and colleagues (Hague *et al*, 1993; 1995) have suggested that butyrate causes apoptosis. In cell lines from colorectal cancers and polyps, sodium butyrate in 1–4 mmol/l concentrations induced apoptosis, while tumour growth factor alpha did not. Apoptosis in the colon may therefore be triggered as cells migrate up the crypt and are exposed to luminal growth factors.

Other mechanisms whereby fermentation may protect against CRC include the laxative properties of fermentation which is associated with increased bulk of material in the large intestine and thus dilution of any potentially DNA-damaging substances. Some forms of dietary fibre provide a surface for bacteria and for the adsorption of various organic substances. Fermentation has also been shown to affect bile acid metabolism and in particular reduce the amounts of deoxycholic acid in faecal water (van Munster *et al*, 1993).

Other carbohydrates

Whilst the study of dietary fibre in the large intestine has led to the identification of a number of possible mechanisms whereby fermentation may protect against this cancer, the inconsistencies in the epidemiological associations have led to the search for other dietary components which may stimulate fermentation. It is now clear that dietary fibre is not the only fermented carbohydrate in the human large intestine, and that significant amounts of resistant starch and oligosaccharides also reach the large bowel. Few studies have related these substances to CRC risk, although Cassidy *et al* (1994) have shown, in a cross-sectional epidemiological study, that CRC risk is reduced in populations with high total starch intake. Even less work has been done on the role of oligosaccharides, which are known to stimulate selectively the growth of bifidobacteria in the large intestine (Gibson *et al*, 1995a). Feeding probiotic organisms such as bifidobacteria reduces CRC in animal models (Reddy and Rivenson, 1993). The recognition of other fermentable carbohydrates means epidemiological studies of diet and CRC risk need to be redone looking at risk in relation to the entire fermentable carbohydrate content of the diet and not just dietary fibre.

Conclusion

Large bowel cancer is one of the commonest causes of cancer death in Western countries, and is now emerging in many other parts of the world. It is, above all other cancers, the one for which there is most evidence of diet being involved in its causation and its prevention. Furthermore, the genetic abnormalities associated with these tumours are better defined than for many of the other common cancers, and thus it offers one of the greatest hopes for a public health prevention strategy through dietary modification.

Acknowledgements

Unilever (Vlaardingen) is thanked for its support for this work.

References

Aaltonen LA, Peltomaki P, Leach FS *et al*. Clues to the pathogenesis of familial colorectal cancer. *Science*, 1993; **260**(5109): 812–816
Archer, MC, Saul RL *et al*, eds. *Analysis of Nitrate, Nitrite and Nitrosamines in Human Feces*. Banbury Report No. 7. New York: Cold Spring Harbor Laboratory, 1981
Barnes S, Grubbs C *et al*. Soybeans inhibit mammary tumours in models of breast cancer. In: Pariza MW *et al*, eds. *Mutagens and carcinogens in the diet*. New York: Wiley Liss, 239–253
Bates SE, Currier SJ, Alvarez M, Fojo AT. Modulation of P-glycoprotein phosphorylation and drug transport by sodium butyrate. *Biochemistry*, 1992; **31**: 6366–6372
Bingham SA. Mechanisms and experimental and epidemiological evidence relating dietary fibre (non-starch polysaccharides) and starch to protection against large bowel cancer. *Proceedings of the Nutrition Society*, 1990; **49**: 153–171
Bingham SA, Pignatelli B, Pollock JR *et al*. Does increased endogenous formation of N-nitrosocompounds in the human colon explain the association between red meat and colon cancer? *Carcinogenesis*, 1996; **17**: 515–523
Birren BW, Herschman HR. Regulation of the rat metallothionen-I gene by sodium butyrate. *Nucleic Acids Research*, 1986; **14**: 853–867
Bloom EJ, Siddiqui B, Hicks JW, Kim YS. Effect of sodium butyrate, a differentiating agent, on cell surface glycoconjugates of a human pancreatic cell line. *Pancreas*, 1989; **4**: 59–64
Bodmer WF, Bailey CJ, Bodmer J *et al*. Localization of the gene for familial adenomatous polyposis on chromosome 5. *Nature*, 1987; **328**: 614–616
Boffa LC, Lupton JR, Mariani MR *et al*. Modulation of colonic epithelial cell proliferation, histone acetylation, and luminal short chain fatty acids by variation of dietary fiber (wheat bran) in rats. *Cancer Research*, 1992; **52**: 5906–5912
Bremner CG. Ano-rectal disease in the South African Bantu. 1. Bowel habit and physiology. *Suid-Afrikaanse Tydskrif vir Chirurgie* 1964; **2**: 119–123
Burkitt DP. Epidemiology of cancer of the colon and rectum. *Cancer*, 1971; **28**: 3–13
Bustin SA, Nie XF, Barnard RC *et al*. Cloning and characterisation of ERF-1, a member of the Tis11 family of early-response genes. *DNA and Cell Biology*, 1994; **13**: 449–459
Canzian F, Ushijama T, Serikawa T, Wakabayashi K, Sugimura T, Nagao M. Instability of microsatellites in rat colon tumours induced by heterocyclic amines. *Cancer*

Research, 1994; **54**: 6315–6317

Cassidy A, Bingham SA, Cummings JH. Starch intake and colorectal cancer risk: an international comparison. *British Journal of Cancer*, 1994; **69**: 937–942

Chacko A, Cummings JH. Nitrogen losses from the human small bowel: obligatory losses and the effect of physical form of food. *Gut*, 1988; **29**: 809–815

Chung YS, Song IS, Erickson RH, Sleisenger MH, Kim YS. Effect of growth and sodium butyrate on brush border membrane-associated hydrolases in human colorectal cancer cell lines. *Cancer Research*, 1985; **45**: 2976–2982

Clinton SK, Imrey PB, Mangian HJ, Nandkumar S, Visek WJ. The combined effects of dietary fat, protein and energy intake on azoxymethane-induced renal and intestinal carcinogenesis. *Cancer Research*, 1992; **52**: 857–865

Cummings JH. Fermentation in the human large intestine: evidence and implications for health. *Lancet*, 1983; **i**: 1206–1209

Cummings JH, Bingham SA, Heaton KW, Eastwood MA. Fecal weight, colon cancer risk and dietary intake of non-starch polysaccharides (dietary fiber). *Gastroenterology*, 1992; **103**: 1783–1789

D'Anna JA, Tobey RA, Gurley LR. Concentration-dependent effects of sodium butyrate in Chinese hamster cells: cell-cycle progression, inner histone acetylation, histone H1 dephosphorylation and induction of an H1-like protein. *Biochemistry*, 1980; **19**: 2656–2671

De Fazio A, Chiew Y-E, Donoghue C, Lee CS, Sutherland RL. Effect of sodium butyrate on estrogen receptor and epidermal growth factor receptor gene expression in human breast cancer cell lines. *Journal of Biological Chemistry*, 1992; **267**: 18008–18012

Deschner EE, Ruperto JF *et al.* Quercitin and rutin as inhibitors of AOM-induced colonic neoplasia. *Carcinogenesis*, 1991; **12**: 1193–1196

Deschner EE, Ruperto JF, Wong GY, Newmark HL. The effect of dietary quercitin and rutin on AOM-induced colonic epithelial abnormalities in mice fed a high fat diet. *Nutrition and Cancer*, 1993; **20**: 199–204

Dexter DL, Lev R, McKendall GR, Mitchell P, Calabres P. Sodium butyrate-induced alteration of growth properties and glycogen levels in cultured human colon carcinoma cells. *Histochemical Journal*, 1984; **16**: 137–149

Dyson JED, Daniel J, Surrey CR. The effect of sodium butyrate on the growth characteristics of human cervix tumour cells. *British Journal of Cancer*, 1992; **65**: 803–808

Englyst HN, Hudson GJ. Dietary fiber and starch: classification and measurement. In: Spiller GA, ed. *CRC Handbook of Dietary Fiber in Human Nutrition*, 2nd edition. Boca Raton: CRC Press, 1993: 53–71

Fearon EF. Genetic alterations underlying colorectal tumorigenesis. In: *Tumour Suppressor Genes, the Cell Cycle and Cancer*. London: Imperial Cancer Research Fund, 1992: 119–136

Felton JS, Knize MG, Shen NH *et al.* The isolation and identification of a new mutagen from fried ground beef: 2-amino-1-methyl-6-phenylimidazo[4,5-b]pyridine (PhIP). *Carcinogenesis*, 1986; **7**: 1081–1086

Fuller CE, Davies RP, Williams GT, Williams ED. Crypt restricted heterogeneity of goblet cell mucus glycoprotein in histologically normal human colonic mucosa: a potential marker of somatic mutation. *British Journal of Cancer*, 1990; **61**: 382–384

Gamet L, Daviaud D, Denis-Pouxviel C, Remesy C, Murat JC. Effects of short-chain fatty acids on growth and differentiation of the human colon-cancer cell line HT29. *International Journal of Cancer*, 1992; **52**: 286–289

Gerhardsson M, Norell SE, Kiviranta H, Pedersen NL, Ahlbom A. Sedentary jobs and colon cancer. *American Journal of Epidemiology*, 1986; **123**: 775–780

Gerhardsson M, Floderus B, Norell SE. Physical activity and colon cancer risk. *International Journal of Epidemiology*, 1988; **17**: 743–746

Gerhardsson deVerdier M, Steineck G, Hagman U, Rieger A, Norell SE. Physical activity and colon cancer: a case-referent study in Stockholm. *International Journal of Cancer*, 1990; **46**: 985–989

Gibson JA, Sladen GE, Dawson AM. Protein absorption and ammonia production: the effects of dietary protein and removal of the colon. *British Journal of Nutrition*, 1976; **35**: 61–65

Gibson PR, Moeller I, Kagelari O, Folino M, Young GP. Contrasting effects of butyrate on the expression of phenotypic markers of differentiation in neoplastic and non-neoplastic colonic epithelial cells *in vitro*. *Journal of Gastroenterology and Hepatology*, 1992; **7**: 165–172

Gibson PR, Rosella O, Rosella G, Young GP. Butyrate is a potent inhibitor of urokinase secretion by normal colonic epithelium *in vitro*. *Gastroenterology*, 1994; **107**: 410–419

Gibson GR, Beatty ER, Wang X, Cummings JH. Selective stimulation of bifidobacteria in the human colon by oligofructose and inulin. *Gastroenterology*, 1995a; **108**: 975–982

Gibson P, Folino M, McKintyre A, Rosella O, Finch C, Young G. Dietary modulation of colonic mucosal urokinase activity in rats. *Journal of Gastroenterology and Hepatology*, 1995b; **10**: 324–330

Gladhaug IP, Christoffersen T. n-butyrate and dexamethasone synergistically modulate the surface expression of epidermal growth factor receptors in cultured rat hepatocytes. *FEBS Letters*, 1989; **243**: 21–24

Gladhaug IP, Refsnes M, Sand TE, Christofferson T. Effects of butyrate on epidermal growth factor receptor binding, morphology, and DNA synthesis in cultured rat hepatocytes. *Cancer Research*, 1988; **48**: 6560–6564

Gladhaug IP, Refsnes M, Christoffersen T. Regulation of hepatocyte epidermal growth factor receptors by n-butyrate and dimethyl sulfoxide: sensitivity to modulation by the tumor promoter TPA. *Anticancer Research*, 1989; **9**: 1587–1592

Griffiths DF, Sacco P, Williams D, Williams GT, Williams ED. The clonal origin of experimental large bowel tumours. *British Journal of Cancer*, 1989; **59**: 385–387

Gross GA. Simple methods for quantifying mutagenic heterocyclic aromatic amines in food products. *Carcinogenesis*, 1990; **11**: 1597–1603

Guilbaud NF, Gas N, Dupont MA, Valette A. Effects of differentiation-inducing agents on maturation of human MCF-7 breast cancer cells. *Journal of Cellular Physiology*, 1990; **145**: 162–172

Guillem JG, O'Brian CA, Fitzer CJ et al. Studies on protein kinase C and colon carcinogenesis. *Archives of Surgery*, 1987; **122**: 1475–1478

Gum JR, Kam WK, Byrd JC, Hicks JW, Sleisinger MH, Kim YS. Effects of sodium butyrate on human colonic adenocarcinoma cells. Induction of placental-like alkaline phosphatase. *Journal of Biological Chemistry*, 1987; **262**: 1092–1097

Hague A, Manning AM, Hanlon KA, Huschtscha LI, Hart D, Paraskeva C. Sodium butyrate induces apoptosis in human colonic tumour cell lines in a p53-independent pathway: implications for the possible role of dietary fibre in the prevention of large bowel cancer. *International Journal of Cancer*, 1993; **55**: 498–505

Hague A, Elder DJ, Hicks DJ, Paraskeva C. Apoptosis in colorectal tumour cells: induction by the short chain fatty acids butyrate, propionate and acetate and by the bile salt deoxycholate. *International Journal of Cancer*, 1995; **60**: 400–406

Halgunset J, Lamvik T, Espevik T. Butyrate effects on growth, morphology and fibronectin production in PC-3 prostatic carcinoma cells. *The Prostate*, 1988; **12**: 65–77

Herrera L, Kakati S, Gibas L, Pietrzak E, Sandberg AA. Gardner syndrome in a man with an interstitial deletion of 5q. *American Journal of Medical Genetics*, 1986; **25**: 473–476

Higgins PJ, Ryan MP. Cytoarchitecture of ras oncogene-expressing tumor cells: butyrate modulation of substrate adhesion, cytoskeletal actin content and subcellular microfilament distribution. *International Journal of Biochemistry*, 1989; **21**: 1143–1151

Higginson J, Oettlé AG. Cancer incidence in the Bantu and 'Cape Colored' races of South Africa: report of a cancer survey in the Transvaal (1953–55). *Journal of the National Cancer Institute*, 1960; **24**: 589–671

Hill MJ, Drasar BS, Hawksworth G, Aries V, Crowther JS, Williams RE. Bacteria and aetiology of cancer of the large bowel. *Lancet*, 1971; **i**: 95–100

Hill MJ, Drasar BS, Williams RE. Faecal bile acids and clostridia in patients with cancer of the large bowel. *Lancet*, 1975; **i**: 535–539

Howe GR, Benito E, Castelleto R. Dietary intake of fibre and decreased risk of cancers of the colon and rectum: evidence from combined analysis of 13 case-controlled studies. *Journal of the National Cancer Institute*, 1992; **84**: 1887–1896

IARC Working Group on the Evaluation of Carcinogenic Risks to Humans. Alcohol drinking. *IARC Monographs on Carcinogenic Risks to Humans*, 1988; **44**: 1–416

Khan SG, Katiyar SK, Agarwal R, Mukhtar H. Enhancement of antioxidant and phase II enzymes by oral feeding of green tea polyphenols in drinking water to SKH-1 hairless mice: possible role in cancer chemoprevention. *Cancer Research*, 1992; **52**: 4040–4052

Kim YS, Tsao D, Siddiqui B *et al.* Effects of sodium butyrate and dimethylsulfoxide on biochemical properties of human colon cancer cells. *Cancer*, 1980; **45**: 1185–1192

Kim YS, Gum JR *et al.* Colonocyte differentiation and proliferation: overview and the butyrate-induced transcriptional regulation of oncodevelopmental placental-like alkaline phosphatase gene in colon cancer cells. In: Binder HJ, Cummings JH, Soergel KH, eds. *Short Chain Fatty Acids*. Lancaster: Kluwer Academic Publishers, 1994: 119–134

Kinzler KW, Nilbert MC, Su LK *et al.* Identification of FAP locus genes from chromosome 5q21. *Science*, 1991; **253**: 661–665

Kruh J, Defer N, Tichonicky L. Action moleculaire et cellulaire du butyrate. *Comptes Rendus des Séances de la Societé de Biologie*, 1992; **186**: 12–25

Kruh J, Defer N *et al.* Effects of butyrate on cell proliferation and gene expression. In: Cummings JH, Rombeau JL, Sakata T, eds. *Physiological and Clinical Aspects of Short Chain Fatty Acids*. Cambridge: Cambridge University Press, 1995: 275–288

Kuenzig W, Chau J, Norkus K *et al.* Caffeic and ferulic acid as blockers of nitrosamine formation. *Carcinogenesis*, 1984; **5**: 309–313

Kuratsune M, Honda T, Englyst HN, Cummings JH. Dietary fiber in the Japanese diet as investigated in connection with colon cancer risk. *Japanese Journal of Cancer Research*, 1986; **77**: 736–738

Layton DW, Bogen KT, Knize MG, Hatch FT, Johnson VM, Felton JS. Cancer risk of heterocyclic amines in cooked foods: an analysis and implications for research. *Carcinogenesis*, 1995; **16**: 39–52

Loub WD, Wattenberg LW, Davis DW. Aryl hydrocarbon hydroxylase induction in rat tissue by naturally occurring indoles of cruciferous plants. *Journal of the National Cancer Institute*, 1975, **54**: 985–988

Malhotra SL. Geographical distribution of gastrointestinal cancers in India with special reference to causation. *Gut*, 1967; **8**: 361–372

Malik H, Nordenberg J, Novogrodsky A, Fuchs A, Malik Z. Chemical inducers of differentiation, dimethylsulfoxide, butyric acid and dimethylthiourea, induce selective ultrastructural patterns in B16 melanoma cells. *Biology of the Cell*, 1987; **60**: 33–39

Mallett AK, Walters DG, Rowland IR. Protein-related differences in the excretion of nitrosoproline and nitrate by the rat—possible modification of de novo nitrate synthesis. *Food Chemistry and Toxicology*, 1988; **26**: 831–835

Morita A, Tsao D, Kim YS. Effect of sodium butyrate on alkaline phosphatase in HRT-18, a human rectal cancer cell line. *Cancer Research*, 1982; **42**: 4540–4545

Morotomi M, Guillem JG, LoGerfo P, Weinstein IB. Production of diacylglycerol, an activator of protein kinase C, by human intestinal microflora. *Cancer Research*, 1990; **50**: 3595–3599

Morson B. The polyp cancer sequence in the large bowel. *Proceedings of the Royal Society of Medicine*, 1974; **67**: 451–457

Mukhtar H, Wang ZY, Katiyar SK, Agarwal R. Tea components: antimutagenic and anticarcinogenic effects. *Preventive Medicine*, 1992; **21**: 351–360

Newmark HL, Wargovich MJ, Bruce WR. Colon cancer and dietary fat, phosphate and calcium: a hypothesis. *Journal of the National Cancer Institute*, 1984; **72**: 1323–1325

Nishisho I, Nakamura Y, Miyoshi Y *et al.* Mutations of chromosome 5q21 genes in FAP and colorectal cancer patients. *Science*, 1991; **253**: 665–669

Oettlé AG. Cancer in Africa, especially in regions south of the Sahara. *Journal of the National Cancer Institute*, 1964; **33**: 383–439

Ormandy CJ, de Fazio A, Kelly PA, Sutherland RL. Coordinate regulation of oestrogen and prolactin receptor expression by sodium butyrate in human breast cancer cells. *Biochemical & Biophysical Research Communications*, 1992; **182**: 740–745

Parkin DM, Muir CS, Whelan SL *et al. Cancer Incidence in Five Continents*, Vol VI. Lyon: IARC, 1992

Peltomaki P, Aaltonen LA, Sistonen P *et al.* Genetic mapping of a locus predisposing to human colorectal cancer. *Science*, 1993; **260**: 810–812

Pence BC, Buddingh F, Yang SP. Multiple dietary factors in the enhancement of dimethylhyrazine carcinogenesis: main effect of indole-3-carbinol. *Journal of the National Cancer Institute*, 1986; **77**: 269–276

Preussman R. Occurrence and exposure to N-nitroso compounds. In: O'Neil I, ed. *Evaluation of Carcinogenic Risk to Humans*. Lyon: IARC, 1984: 3–15

Reddy BS, Rivenson A. Inhibitory effect of *Bifidobacterium longum* on colon, mammary and liver carcinogenesis induced by 2-amino-3-methylimidazo[4,5-f] quinoline, a food mutagen. *Cancer Research*, 1993; **53**: 3914–3918

Reddy BS, Simi B, Engle A. Biochemical epidemiology of colon cancer: effect of types of dietary fiber on colonic diacylglycerols in women. *Gastroenterology*, 1994; **106**: 883–889

Reese DH, Gratzner HG, Block NL, Politano VA. Control of growth, morphology and alkaline phosphatase activity by butyrate and related short-chain fatty acids in the retinoid-responsive 9-1C rat prostatic adenocarcinoma cell. *Cancer Research*, 1985; **45**: 2308–2313

Riboli E, Cornee J, Macquart-Moulin G, Kaaks R, Casagrande C, Guyader M. Cancer and polyps of the colorectum and lifetime consumption of beer and other alcoholic beverages. *American Journal of Epidemiology*, 1991; **134**: 157–166

Rogers AE, Zeisel SH, Groopman J. Diet and carcinogenesis. *Carcinogenesis*, 1993; **14**: 2205–2217

Rowland IR, Granli T, Bockman OC, Key PE, Massey RC. Endogenous N-nitrosation in man assessed by measurement of apparent total N-nitroso compounds in faeces. *Carcinogenesis*, 1991; **12**: 1395–1401

Saini K, Steele G, Thomas P. Induction of carcinoembryonic-antigen-gene expression in human colorectal carcinoma by sodium butyrate. *Biochemical Journal*, 1990; **272**: 541–544

Setchell KDR, Street JM *et al.* Faecal bile acids. In: Setchell KDR, Kritchevsky D, Nair PP, eds. *The Bile Acids*. New York: Plenum, 1987: 441–571

Setchell KDR, Adlercreutz H, eds. *Mammalian Lignans and Phyto-oestrogens. Recent Studies on Their Formation, Metabolism and Biological Role in Health and Disease. Role of the Gut Flora in Toxicity and Cancer*. London: Academic Press, 1988

Shuker DE. Detection of adducts arising from human exposure to NOC. *Cancer Surveys*, 1989; **8**: 475–487

Silvester KR. Role of meat and starch in colorectal cancer. PhD Thesis, Cambridge University, 1996

Silvester KR, Cummings JH. Factors determining protein digestion: effect of source, amount and of resistant starch, studied in human ileostomates. *Nutrition & Cancer*, in press

Smith PJ. n-Butyrate alters chromatin accessibility to DNA repair enzymes. *Carcinogenesis*, 1986; **7**: 423–429

Solomon E, Voss R, Hall V *et al*. Chromosome 5 allele loss in human colorectal carcinomas. *Nature*, 1987; **328**: 616–618

Souleimani A, Asselin C. Regulation of C-fos expression by sodium butyrate in the human colon carcinoma cell line Caco-2. *Biochemical & Biophysical Research Communications*, 1993; **193**: 330–336

Sparnins VL, Barany G, Wattenberg LW. Effects of organosulphur compounds from garlic and onions on benzo(a)pyrene-induced neoplasia and glutathione-S-transferase activity in the mouse. *Carcinogenesis*, 1988; **9**: 131–134

Steinbach G, Kumar SP, Reddy BS, Lipkin M, Holt PR. Effects of caloric restriction and dietary fat on epithelial cell proliferation in the rat. *Cancer Research*, 1993; **53**: 2745–2749

Stuehr DJ, Marletta MA. Mammalian nitrate biosynthesis: mouse macrophages produce nitrite and nitrate in response to *Escherichia coli* lipopolysaccharide. *Proceedings of the National Academy of Sciences of the USA*, 1985; **82**: 7738–7742

Sugimura T, Nagao M, Wakabayashi K. Heterocyclic amines in cooked foods: candidates for causation of common cancers. *Journal of the National Cancer Institute*, 1994; **86**: 2–4

Takahashi S, Hakoi K, Yada H, Hirose M, Ito N, Fukushima S. Enhancing effect of diallyl sulfide on hepatocarcinogenesis and inhibitory actions of the related diallyl disulfide on colon and renal carcinogenesis in rats. *Carcinogenesis*, 1992; **13**: 1513–1518

Tomatis L, ed. *Cancer: Causes, Occurrence and Control*. IARC Scientific Publications No. 100. Lyon: IARC, 1990

Toscani A, Soprano DR, Soprano KJ. Molecular analysis of sodium butyrate-induced growth arrest. *Oncogene Research*, 1988; **3**: 223–238

Toscani A, Soprano DR, Soprano KJ. Sodium butyrate in combination with insulin or dexamethasone can terminally differentiate actively proliferating Swiss 3T3 cells into adipocytes. *Journal of Biological Chemistry*, 1990; **265**: 5722–5730

Trock B, Lanza E, Greenwald P. Dietary fiber, vegetables and colon cancer. Critical review and meta analysis of the epidemiologic evidence. *Journal of the National Cancer Institute*, 1990; **82**: 650–661

Trowell HC. *Non-Infective Diseases in Africa*. London: Edward Arnold, 1960

Tsao D, Morita A, Bella A Jr, Luu P, Kim YS. Differential effects of sodium butyrate, dimethyl sulfoxide and retinoic acid on membrane-associated antigen, enzymes and glycoproteins of human rectal adenocarcinoma cells. *Cancer Research*, 1982; **42**: 1052–1058

van Munster IP, Nagengast FM, Tangerman A. The effect of resistant starch on fecal bile acids, cytotoxicity and colonic mucosal proliferation. *Gastroenterology*, 1993; **104**: A460

van Munster IP, Tangerman A, Nagengast FM. The effect of resistant starch on colonic fermentation, bile acid metabolism and mucosal proliferation. *Digestive Diseases and Sciences*, 1994; **39**: 834–842

van Wijk R, Tichonicky L, Kruh J. Effect of sodium butyrate on the hepatoma cell cycle: possible use for cell synchronization. *In Vitro*, 1981; **17**: 859–862

Vogelstein B, Fearon ER, Hamilton SR. Genetic alterations during colorectal-tumor development. *New England Journal of Medicine*, 1988; **319**: 525–532

Wagner DA, Young VR, Tannenbaum SR. Mammalian nitrate biosynthesis: incorporation of 15NH3 into nitrate is enhanced by endotoxin treatment. *Proceedings of the National Academy of Sciences of the USA*, 1983; **80**: 4518–4521

Ward JM, Coates ME, Walker R. Influence of dietary protein and gut microflora on endogenous synthesis of nitrate and N-nitrosamines in the rat. *Food Chemistry and Toxicity*, 1989; **27**: 49–59

Wargovich MJ. Diallyl sulfides, a flavor component of garlic (*Allium sativum*), inhibits dimethylhyrazine-induced colon cancer. *Carcinogenesis*, 1987; **8**: 487–489

Wattenberg LW. Chemoprevention of cancer. *Cancer Research*, 1985; **45**: 1–8

Wattenberg LW. Studies of polycyclic hydrocarbon hydroxylases of the intestine possibly related to cancer. Effect of diet on benzpyrene hyroxylase activity. *Cancer*, 1971; **28**: 99–102

Welberg W, Kleibeuker JH, Van der Meer R, Mulder NH, De Vries E. Calcium and the prevention of colon cancer. *Scandinavian Journal of Gastroenterology*, 1991; **26**: 52–59

Whitehead RH, Young GP, Bhathal PS. Effects of short chain fatty acids on a new human colon carcinoma cell line (LIM1215). *Gut*, 1986; **27**: 1457–1463

Wice BM, Trugnan G, Pinto M *et al.* The intracellular accumulation of UDP-N-acetyl hexosamines is concomitant with the inability of human colon cancer cells to differentiate. *Journal of Biological Chemistry*, 1985; **260**: 139–146

Willett WC, Stampfer MJ, Colditz GA, Rosner BA, Speizer FE. Relation of meat, fat and fiber intake to the risk of colon cancer in a prospective study among women. *New England Journal of Medicine*, 1990; **323**: 1664–1672

Wilson JR, Weiser MM. Colonic cancer cell (HT29) adhesion to laminin is altered by differentiation: adhesion may involve galactosyltransferase. *Experimental Cell Research*, 1992; **201**: 330–334

Witter JP, Balish E, Gatley SJ. Origin of excess urinary nitrate in the rat. *Cancer Research*, 1982; **42**: 3654–3658

Yang CS, Wang ZY. Tea and cancer. *Journal of the National Cancer Institute*, 1993; **85**: 1038–1049

Zhang Y, Talalay P, Cho CG, Posner GH. A major inducer of anticarcinogenic protective enzymes from broccoli: isolation and elucidation of structure. *Proceedings of the National Academy of Sciences*, 1992; **89**: 2399–2403

Discussion

Hester H. Vorster

Department of Nutrition, Potchefstroom University, Republic of South Africa

The description of large bowel cancer by Bingham and Cummings typifies it as a chronic disease of lifestyle in which the presence of a combination of environmental risk factors over time will precipitate the disease in susceptible individuals with appropriate inherited or acquired genetic patterns and/or mutations. These authors suggest that the promoting dietary factors are total energy, fat and meat, while cereals, vegetables and fruits are protective. The roles of these foods and their constituents are supported by attractive and experimentally reasonably well substantiated biochemical and genetic mechanisms—at both molecular and cellular level.

Controversies

However, not all studies could identify these foods as risk factors. The prospective cohort study of 35 215 women in Iowa, USA (Bostick *et al*, 1994) showed sucrose and sucrose-containing foods (other than ice-cream and milk), height, Body Mass Index and number of live births, to be risk factors. This study raised questions regarding associations with accepted risk factors such as meat, fat and protein, as well as protecting factors such as parity and physical activity. Another dietary controversy is the role of calcium. Slattery *et al* (1994) showed that increased calcium intakes decreased risk in older men, possibly by binding intraluminal fatty acids and bile salts. However, Kampman and colleagues (1994) could not demonstrate a beneficial effect on large bowel cancer risk with increased intakes of dairy products and calcium.

There are many possible reasons for these discrepancies. Risk factors may differ in older and younger subjects (Slattery *et al*, 1994). Dietary factors may be influenced by existing microflora. Moore and Moore (1995) found high concentrations of *Bacteroides* and *Bifidobacterium* species in high-risk populations and more *Lactobacillus* species and lactic acid-producing *Eubacterium aerofaciens* in populations with a low risk of bowel cancer. Dietary factors may have different effects in the right and left colon. Yang and colleagues (1994) reported that dietary fat elevated risk for left colon cancer significantly but only slightly for the right colon. Interactions between and levels of different risk factors could also contribute to these discrepancies. Frentzel-Beyme and Chang-Claude (1994) suggest that the low large bowel cancer mortality in vegetarians is more related to other factors, such as health-conscious behaviour and healthy lifestyles, than to diet. It is of course possible that the strong genetic component of large bowel cancer (Fitzgerald et al, 1991) may be modified by dietary and other environmental factors. Swerdlow et al (1995) could not demonstrate differences in colon cancer rates in people born in England and Wales compared to New Zealand, with and without migration between the two countries.

Possible lessons from South Africa

Proposed risk factors should explain differences in large bowel cancer rates in different populations. Table 6.2 shows the age-standardised incidence rates (ASIR) of histologically diagnosed colon cancer in South African populations (Sitas and Pacella, 1994). Rates are much lower in blacks than in whites and also lower in blacks than in Indians and coloureds. Mortality from some chronic diseases of lifestyle such as hypertension, stroke and diabetes mellitus among South African blacks is high, but mortality from coronary heart disease (CHD) and colon cancer is still very low (Bradshaw et al, 1995). Could this mean that Africans have, perhaps through some sort of natural selection, a genetic protection against large bowel cancer? Or that CHD and large bowel cancer need a longer transition period in developing populations to emerge than hypertension, stroke and diabetes? Or that these diseases have different dietary determinants?

Table 6.2 Crude and age-standardised incidence rates (ASIR)[a] of histologically diagnosed colon cancer in 1989 in South African population groups

	Population group							
	Whites		Asians		Coloureds		Blacks	
Variable	F	M	F	M	F	M	F	M
Total: all cancers	10 155	12 451	494	368	1799	1745	9642	9276
Rank: colon cancer	7	8	6	6	7	11	19	22
Number of colon cancers (%)	378	390	17	18	55	46	83	102
	(3.72)	(3.13)	(3.44)	(4.89)	(3.09)	(2.64)	(0.86)	(1.10)
Crude	15.00	15.72	3.56	3.83	3.37	2.92	0.60	0.74
ASIR[a]	11.91	16.35	6.07	6.86	5.16	5.39	1.00	1.26
Cumulative	1.44	1.97	0.94	1.06	0.72	0.58	0.12	0.14
Risk[b]	69.44	50.76	106.38	94.34	138.89	172.41	833.33	714.29

Source: National Cancer Registry, Sitas and Pacella (1994)
[a] World standard, per 100 000
[b] Risk is expressed as one in x number of people. Also adjusted for age unknown

The American experience indicates that it is probably not a genetic protection. Although one large study with 75 266 patients showed a higher incidence of large bowel cancer in whites than in blacks (Cooper *et al*, 1995), others (Coates *et al*, 1995; Ji *et al*, 1994) reported higher rates for blacks. The study of Ji and colleagues (1994) also showed a higher urinary excretion of heterocyclic aromatic amines (produced by high-temperature cooking of protein foods) in blacks, supporting meat and protein as risk factors. Furthermore, Van't Hof *et al* (1995) found no ethnic difference in patterns of cell proliferation, suggesting that carcinogenic mechanisms in the colon both in whites and in blacks are the same.

South African blacks seem to have higher levels of faecal short-chain fatty acids than whites (Segal *et al*, 1995), indicating that differences in large bowel cancer rates may be related to the availability of fermentable substrates which in turn are related to the diet. Table 6.3 and Figure 6.4 illustrate mean macronutrient intakes of South Africans, obtained by a recent meta-analysis of the literature (Vorster *et al*, 1995). Blacks still have a lower fat intake (Table 6.3) and higher plant compared to animal protein intake (Figure 6.4) than the other groups. However, dietary fibre intakes of all groups, including urban blacks, were low. (The exception was a very high intake reported in one study for rural black women.) But Table 6.3 also shows that calculated starch intakes of the black groups were substantially higher than those of the other population groups. It is suspected that the staple, maize porridge, is often eaten cold in many poor households (Venter *et al*, 1996) providing substantial amounts of resistant starch that could be fermented in the colon, producing large amounts of butyrate with its protective effect against large bowel cancer (Macfarlane and Cummings, 1991).

The above observations in South Africans are compatible with the theory of Bingham and Cummings that animal protein (meat) and fat promote large bowel cancer while plant food sources, which can provide rich supplies of resistant starch, protect against large bowel disease.

References

Bostick RM, Potter JD, Kushi LH *et al.* Sugar, meat, and fat intake, and non-dietary risk factors for colon cancer incidence in Iowa women (United States). *Cancer Causes and Control*, 1994; **5**: 38–52

Bradshaw D, Bourne D, Schneider M, Sayed R. Mortality patterns of chronic diseases of lifestyle in South Africa. In: Fourie J, Steyn K, eds. *Chronic Diseases of Lifestyle in South Africa*. MRC Technical Report. Tygerberg: MRC, 1995: 5–32

Coates RJ, Greenberg RS, Liu MT *et al.* Anatomic site distribution of colon cancer by race and other colon cancer risk factors. *Diseases of the Colon and Rectum*, 1995; **38**: 42–50

Cooper GS, Yuan Z, Landefeld CS, Johanson JF, Rimm AA. A national population-based study of incidence of colorectal cancer and age. Implications for screening in older Americans. *Cancer*, 1995; **75**: 775–781

Fitzgerald GW, Cameron BH, Cox J. Hereditary site-specific colon cancer in a Canadian kindred. *Arctic Medical Research*, 1991; **Suppl**: 465–467

Table 6.3 Mean (SD) of macronutrient intakes of 2717 adult South Africans obtained with a 24-hour recall method

Nutrient	Whites	Urban blacks	Coloureds	Indians	Rural blacks
Men	$n = 259$	$n = 383$	$n = 288$	$n = 254$	
Energy (MJ)	10.6	8.5	9.2	8.2	–
	(3.8)	(3.7)	(3.6)	(3.1)	–
Total fat (g)	102.5	58.2	89.6	75.6	
	(42.8)	(39.9)	(46.0)	(39.9)	
Total protein (g)	97.4	78.1	82.1	69.5	–
	(39.6)	(43.5)	(35.6)	(38.2)	–
Total carbohydrate (g)	280	282	240	231	–
	(122)	(112)	(106)	(88)	–
Dietary fibre (g)	18.5	19.5	13.7	16.9	–
	(10.6)	(13.5)	(8.8)	(8.6)	–
Sugar (g)	89.3	50.8	78.4	72.8	
	(61.4)	(47.8)	(54.1)	(46.2)	
Starch (g) (calculated)	172.2	211.7	147.9	141.3	
Women	$n = 399$	$n = 481$	$n = 301$	$n = 257$	$n = 95$
Energy (MJ)	6.4	6.4	6.4	5.6	10.2
	(2.5)	(2.6)	(2.7)	(2.0)	(3.3)
Total fat (g)	60.8	46.3	63.6	75.6	46.0
	(27.9)	(28.9)	(34.4)	(53.3)	(28.0)
Total protein (g)	59.0	56.5	58.1	47.0	83.0
	(22.0)	(28.2)	(26.9)	(25.1)	(60.0)
Total carbohydrate (g)	183	222	177	164	409
	(85)	(89)	(79)	(62)	(122)
Dietary fibre (g)	13.7	14.6	10.7	13.1	37
	(7.8)	(8.8)	(6.4)	(6.6)	(16)
Sugar (g)	51.8	45.8	62.8	48.4	61.0
	(40.3)	(37.9)	(41.9)	(33.3)	(36.0)
Starch (g) (calculated)	117.5	161.6	103.5	102.5	311.0

Source: Meta-analysis of South African literature, Vorster *et al* (1995)

Frentzel-Beyme R, Chang-Claude J. Vegetarian diets and colon cancer: the German experience. *American Journal of Clinical Nutrition*, 1994; **59**: 1143S–1152S

Ji H, Yu MC, Stillwell WG *et al.* Urinary excretion of 2-amino-3,8-dimethylimidazo-[4,5-f] quinoxaline in white, black and Asian men in Los Angeles County. *Cancer Epidemiology Biomarkers and Prevention*, 1994; **3**: 407–411

Kampman E, Van't Veer P, Hiddink GJ, van Aken-Schneijder P, Kok FJ, Hermus RJ. Fermented dairy products, dietary calcium and colon cancer: a case-control study in The Netherlands. *International Journal of Cancer*, 1994; **59**: 170–176

Macfarlane GT, Cummings JH. The colonic flora, fermentation and large bowel digestive function. In: Phillips SF, Pemberton JH, Shorter RG, eds. *The Large Intestine: Physiology, Pathophysiology and Disease*. New York: Raven Press, 1991: 51–92

Moore WE, Moore LH. Intestinal floras of populations that have a high risk of colon cancer. *Applied Environmental Microbiology*, 1995; **61**: 3202–3207

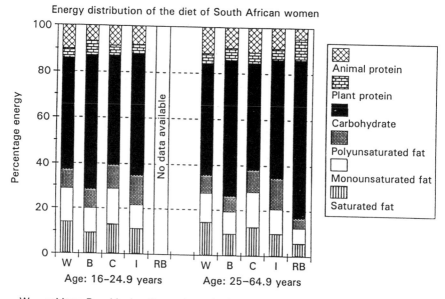

W = whites; B = blacks; C = coloureds; I = Indians (Asians); RB = rural blacks

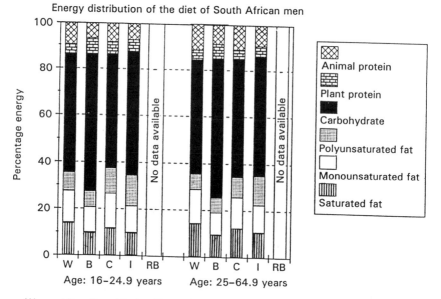

W = whites; B = blacks; C = coloureds; I = Indians (Asians); RB = rural blacks

Figure 6.4 Energy distribution of the diet of South African men and women

Segal I, Hassan H, Walker AR, Becker P, Braganza J. Fecal short chain fatty acids in South African urban Africans and whites. *Diseases of the Colon and Rectum*, 1995; **38**: 732–734

Sitas F, Pacella R. *National Cancer Registry of South Africa. Incidence and Geographical Distribution of Histologically Diagnosed Cancer in South Africa, 1989.* Johannesburg: South African Institute for Medical Research, 1994: 1–89

Slattery ML, Potter JD, Sorenson AW. Age and risk factors for colon cancer (United States and Australia): are there implications for understanding differences in case-control and cohort studies? *Cancer Causes Control*, 1994; **5**: 557–563

Swerdlow AJ, Cooke KR, Skegg DC, Wilkinson J. Cancer incidence in England and Wales and New Zealand and in migrants between the two countries. *British Journal of Cancer*, 1995; **72**: 236–243

Van't Hof A, Gilissen K, Cohen RJ *et al.* Colonic cell proliferation in two different ethnic groups with contrasting incidence of colon cancer: is there a difference in carcinogenesis? *Gut*, 1995; **36**: 691–695

Venter CS, Vorster HH, Van Rooyen A, Kruger-Locke MM, Silvis N. Comparison of the effects of maize porridge consumed at different temperatures on blood glucose, insulin and acetate levels in healthy volunteers. *South African Journal of Food Science and Nutrition*, 1996; **2**: 2–5

Vorster HH, Jerling JC, Oosthuizen W, Becker P, Wolmarans P. Nutrient intakes of South Africans: an analysis of the literature. Johannesburg: Roche Products, 1995: 1–41

Yang G, Gao Y, Ji B. Comparison of risk factors between left and right-sided colon cancer. *Chung Kuo I Hsueh Ko Hsueh Yuan Hsueh Pao*, 1994; **16**: 63–68

7
Interactions between diet and endogenous hormones: possible role in breast cancer

Elio Riboli and Rudolf Kaaks

International Agency for Research on Cancer, Lyon, France

Breast cancer is one of the most frequent cancers occurring in women, with an estimated total of 719 000 cases world-wide (Parkin *et al*, 1993). It has long been known that breast cancer incidence varies widely around the world. It is five to eight times more frequent in North America, Europe and Australia than in most Asian countries (Doll, 1967). Studies in migrants from low- to high-incidence areas have shown that breast cancer rates increase substantially in subsequent generations born in the country of immigration, generally equalling the incidence in the local population (McMichael and Giles, 1988; Kelsey and Horn-Ross, 1993). Since the early laboratory experiments of Tannenbaum (1942) much of the research into the causes of breast cancer has focused, on the one hand, on diet and, on the other hand, on factors related to sexual maturation, reproductive life and hormones. In recent years, many experimental animal studies and metabolic or observational studies on breast cancer risk in humans have investigated the links between endogenous sex hormones and diet, anthropometry and physical activity (Key and Pike, 1988; Goldin, 1994).

Diet and breast cancer

About 20 years ago it was reported that breast cancer incidence was high in countries where national *per capita* consumption of fat (Armstrong and Doll, 1975) and of refined sugar was also high. These findings stimulated further epidemiological studies on diet and cancer, initially numerous case-control

Diet, Nutrition and Chronic Disease: Lessons from Contrasting Worlds.
Edited by P. S. Shetty and K. McPherson © 1997 John Wiley & Sons, Ltd.

studies and later on a smaller number of large prospective cohort studies. Results from case-control studies conducted in the 1970s and 1980s were supportive of a weak positive association between high fat consumption and breast cancer risk. The pooled data analyses from 12 case-control studies (Howe et al, 1990) estimated that for a difference in fat intake of 100 g per day, there was a 35% increase in breast cancer risk (13% in premenopausal and 48% in post-menopausal women). A pooled analysis of seven cohort studies involving a total of 337 819 women, among whom 4980 breast cancer cases occurred during follow-up, found no increase in risk with high consumption of total, saturated, mono- or polyunsaturated fats (Hunter et al, 1996) compared to low consumption. While these results do not completely exclude the hypothesis that high fat intake in adult life may be associated with a small increase in breast cancer risk, they contradict the hypothesis that total fat intake in adult life is a major determinant of the aetiology of the disease.

In addition to fat, epidemiological studies have also investigated the possible role of other dietary components in breast cancer risk. In particular, several studies have suggested that a diet rich in plant foods may be associated with reduced risk. The geographical distribution of breast cancer is compatible with this hypothesis, since the disease is generally less frequent in populations with a diet rich in cereals, legumes, root and other vegetables, as is the case for most populations in South-East Asia and eastern and central Africa. In these populations, however, other known risk factors of breast cancer are also less frequent, such as obesity, early menarche, late first pregnancy and late meno-pause.

The results of case-control studies on breast cancer and vegetables were reviewed by Steinmetz and Potter (1991) and Block et al (1992). Three studies found that higher consumption of total vegetables (Katsouyanni et al, 1986), green vegetables (La Vecchia et al, 1987) or carrots (Hislop et al, 1988) was associated with a decrease in breast cancer risk of the order of 30–50%, compared to lower consumption. Two studies found lower breast cancer risk in subjects who had a diet high in fibre or beta-carotene or vitamin C, which are markers of consumption of vegetables, fruit and cereals (van't Veer et al, 1990; Graham et al, 1991). Finally, two early studies (Graham et al, 1982; Zemla et al, 1984) found no difference in breast cancer risk in relation to vegetable intake. In addition, two prospective studies undertaken in Canada (Rohan et al, 1993) and the US (Willett et al, 1992) reported results on dietary fibre, which can be assumed to be an indicator of total consumption of plant food, mainly in the form of vegetables, fruit and cereal products. The Canadian cohort (56 837 subjects, 519 incident breast cancer cases) found that women in the highest quintile of dietary fibre consumption (more than 25 g/day) had 30% lower breast cancer incidence. A similar reduction was observed for dietary intake of beta-carotene, suggesting that both were to some extent markers of vegetable and fruit consumption. The US Nurses' Health Study (Manson et al, 1990), in contrast, found no significant association between fibre intake and breast cancer incidence, although the confidence interval of the relative risk for fibre did not exclude a similar, modest reduction in risk.

Endogenous hormones

Sexual maturation, reproductive life, menopause and obesity are known risk factors for breast cancer. With few exceptions, most studies have found that breast cancer incidence was higher in women who had early menarche (before age 11 or 12), first child after the age of 30 or no child at all, and late menopause. In addition, overweight women are at higher risk after menopause, although before menopause they seem to have the same risk as normal weight women. Some studies even found that lean women had slightly higher breast cancer risk before menopause than overweight women. The association of all these factors with breast cancer risk is weak in terms of the magnitude of the effect, which is generally of the order of a 10–40% increase or reduction in risk. In fact, all these factors are thought to act by modifying steroid sex hormone patterns, which are believed to be a central endogenous factor in the development of breast cancer.

For its development, growth, differentiation and function, the mammary gland depends on circulating levels of oestrogens, androgens, progesterone and prolactin. However, the main hypothesis is that high endogenous oestrogen levels are the key hormonal factors acting on the mammary gland in the carcinogenic process. A theory has been put forward that a key role in breast cancer is played by the free fraction of circulating oestradiol, which is the very small portion of oestradiol (around 1–3%) which is not bound to the sex hormone binding globulin (SHBG) or other plasma proteins, and which is considered to be the most active fraction which binds to the cellular receptors of the target organs. Two major reviews published a few years apart (Key and Pike, 1988; Bernstein and Ross, 1993) concluded that overall higher exposure to endogenous as well as to exogenous oestrogens was associated with increased breast cancer risk, and that the evidence was stronger for postmenopausal than for premenopausal breast cancer.

More recently, the results of two large prospective cohort studies specifically designed to investigate breast cancer in relation to hormones and diet, brought substantial support for these early conclusions. The two studies are based in New York City (Toniolo et al, 1995) and Lombardy, Italy (Berrino et al, 1996). The main finding of the New York study was that risk of breast cancer was substantially increased in women who had higher levels of total oestradiol, free and albumin-bound oestradiol, and it was decreased in women who had a high proportion of oestradiol bound to SHBG. These results lend support to the biological hypothesis that breast cancer risk may be modulated by factors interfering not only with absolute oestrogen levels but with their biological availability to target tissues via regulation of the fraction bound to SHBG. The

Italian study found a five- to seven-fold increase in breast cancer risk in relation to high levels of total and free testosterone and total oestradiol (free oestradiol has not yet been measured). The marked effect of total and free testosterone found in this study is compatible with the main hypothesis that free oestradiol plays a central role in breast cancer. Androgens are important oestrogen precursors via aromatisation in adipose tissue, particularly after the menopause when the ovary stops producing oestradiol but continues to produce testosterone. In addition, testosterone has a higher affinity to SHBG, thus high testosterone levels lead to high free oestradiol levels.

Interactions of diet, nutritional status and steroid sex hormones

The best documented link is between overweight, SHBG levels, free oestradiol and testosterone. Quite an impressive number of metabolic studies have shown that obesity, in both women and men, is associated with higher levels of insulin, lower levels of SHBG and therefore higher free oestradiol levels. When over-weight subjects undergo a substantial weight loss, their SHBG levels increase, probably responding to decreased insulin levels (Kaaks, 1996). At the opposite end of the scale, girls affected by anorexia nervosa have low insulin levels, high SHBG levels and, in more advanced cases, amenorrhoea and anovulation. There is clinical evidence that improvements in their nutritional status is followed by a rise in insulin, a decrease in SHBG and, eventually, reactivation of the menstrual and ovulatory cycles. A complication to these schematic patterns is that amenorrhoea and anovulation are also found with a relatively higher frequency in obese than in normal weight women, and even more frequently in obese women with polycystic ovary syndrome.

   In addition to these fundamental and quite well demonstrated links, diet may contain substances which interact directly with hormonal patterns. The hypothesis that has attracted most attention in recent years concerns phyto-oestrogens (Adlercreutz, 1991). Phyto-oestrogens include a variety of compounds which share some stereochemical similarities with oestrogens and which are supposed to reduce the oestrogenic stimulation of target organs by real endogenous oestrogens. The most studied compounds are diphenols (ligneous and iso-flavones) which are found in several legumes at concentrations varying by one or two orders of magnitude. Phyto-oestrogens have been reported to compete with oestradiol for binding to oestrogen-binding sites. In addition, urinary excretion of phyto-oestrogens was found to be positively correlated to SHBG plasma levels (Adlercreutz et al, 1992).

Conclusions

The results of epidemiological studies conducted so far on diet and hormonal factors in relation to breast cancer risk suggest the following:

1. The association between breast cancer risk and dietary intake of major nutrients in adulthood, if any, is probably weak.
2. The link between steroid sex hormones and breast cancer risk is probably strong, particularly for bioavailable oestradiol and testosterone.
3. Changes in energy intake, diet composition and anthropometry can modify steroid hormone profile.
4. Non-nutrient food components, e.g. phyto-oestrogens, can modify steroid sex hormone levels in a direction favourable to a reduction of breast cancer risk.
5. One of the highest priorities for research into breast cancer prevention should be to identify achievable changes in diet, anthropometry and lifestyle which can favourably modify steroid sex hormone profile.

References

Adlercreutz H. Diet and sex hormone metabolism. In: Rowland IR, ed. *Nutrition, Toxicity and Cancer*. London: CRC Press, 1991: 237

Adlercreutz H, Mousavi Y, Clark J *et al*. Dietary phytoestrogens and cancer: in vitro and in vivo studies. *Journal of Steroid Biochemistry and Molecular Biology*, 1992; **41**: 331–337

Armstrong B, Doll R. Environmental factors and cancer incidence and mortality in different countries, with special reference to dietary practice. *International Journal of Cancer*, 1975; **15**: 617–631

Bernstein L, Ross RK. Endogenous hormones and breast cancer risk. *Epidemiological Reviews*, 1993; **15**: 48–65

Berrino F, Muti P, Micheli A *et al*. Serum sex hormone levels after menopause and subsequent breast cancer. *Journal of the National Cancer Institute*, 1996; **88**: 291–296

Block G, Patterson B, Subar A. Fruit, vegetables, and cancer prevention: a review of the epidemiological evidence. *Nutrition and Cancer*, 1992; **18**: 1–29

Doll R. *Prevention of Cancer: Pointers from Epidemiology*. London: The Nuffield Provincial Hospital Trusts, 1967

Goldin BR, Woods MN, Spiegelman DL *et al*. The effect of dietary fat and fiber on serum estrogen concentrations in premenopausal women under controlled dietary conditions. *Cancer*, 1994; **74**: 1125–1131

Graham S, Marshall J, Mettlin C, Rzepka T, Nemoto T, Byers T. Diet in the epidemiology of breast cancer. *American Journal of Epidemiology*, 1982; **116**: 68–75

Graham S, Hellmann R, Marshall J *et al*. Nutritional epidemiology of postmenopausal breast cancer in Western New York. *American Journal of Epidemiology*, 1991; **134**: 552–566

Hislop TG, Kan L, Coldman AJ, Band PR, Brauer G. Influence of estrogen receptor status on dietary risk factors for breast cancer. *Canadian Medical Association Journal*, 1988; **138**: 424–430

Howe GR, Hirohata T, Hislop TG *et al*. Dietary factors and risk of breast cancer: Combined analysis of 12 case-control studies. *Journal of the National Cancer Institute*, 1990; **82**: 561–569

Hunter DJ, Spiegelman D, Adami HO *et al*. Cohort studies of fat intake and the risk of breast cancer—a pooled analysis. *New England Journal of Medicine*, 1996; **334**: 356–361

Kaaks R. Nutrition, hormones, and breast cancer: Is insulin the missing link? *Cancer Causes & Control*, 1996; **7**: 605–625

Katsouyanni K, Trichopoulos D, Boyle P *et al*. Diet and breast cancer: a case-control study in Greece. *International Journal of Cancer*, 1986; **38**: 815–820

Kelsey JL, Horn-Ross PL. Breast cancer: magnitude of the problem and descriptive epidemiology. *Epidemiological Reviews*, 1993; **15**: 7–16

Key TJ, Pike MC. The role of estrogens and progestagens in the epidemiology and prevention of breast cancer. *European Journal of Cancer and Clinical Oncology*, 1988; **24**: 29–43

Key TJ, Roe L, Thorogood M, Moore JW, Clark GM, Wang DY. Testosterone, sex hormone-binding globulin, calculated free testosterone, and oestradiol in male vegans and omnivores. *British Journal of Nutrition*, 1990; **64**: 111–119

La Vecchia C, Decarli A, Franceschi S, Gentile A, Negri E, Parazzini F. Dietary factors and the risk of breast cancer. *Nutrition and Cancer*, 1987; **10**: 205–214

Manson JE, Colditz GA, Stampfer MJ *et al*. A prospective study of obesity and risk of coronary heart disease in women. *New England Journal of Medicine*, 1990; **322**: 882–889

McMichael AJ, Giles GG. Cancer in migrants to Australia; extending the descriptive epidemiological data. *Cancer Research*, 1988; **48**: 751–756

Parkin DM, Pisani P, Ferlay J. Estimates of the worldwide incidence of eighteen major cancers in 1985. *International Journal of Cancer*, 1993; **54**: 594–606

Rohan TE, Howe GR, Friedenreich CM, Jain M, Miller AB. Dietary fiber, vitamins A, C, and E, and risk of breast cancer: a cohort study. *Cancer Causes and Control*, 1993; **4**: 29–37

Steinmetz KA, Potter JD. Vegetables, fruit and cancer. I. Epidemiology. *Cancer Causes & Control*, 1991; **2**: 325–357

Tannenbaum A. The genesis and growth of tumors. III. Effects of a high-fat diet. *Cancer Research*, 1942; **2**: 468–475

Toniolo PG, Levitz M, Zeleniuch-Jacquotte A *et al*. A prospective study of endogenous estrogens and breast cancer in postmenopausal women. *Journal of National Cancer Institute*, 1995; **87**: 190–197

van't Veer P, Kolb CM, Verhoef P *et al*. Dietary fibre, beta-carotene and breast cancer: results from a case-control study. *International Journal of Cancer*, 1990; **45**: 825–828

Willett WC, Hunter DJ, Stampfer MJ *et al*. Dietary fat and fiber in relation to risk of breast cancer. An 8-year follow-up. *Journal of the American Medical Association*, 1992; **268**: 2037–2044

Zemla B. The role of selected dietary elements in breast cancer risk among native and migrant populations in Poland. *Nutrition and Cancer*, 1984; **6**: 187–195

Discussion

Timothy Key

Imperial Cancer Research Fund, Cancer Epidemiology Unit, University of Oxford, UK

The increases in breast cancer risk associated with early menarche and with late menopause indicate that risk is related to the duration of exposure of the breasts to the high levels of ovarian hormones characteristic of premenopausal women. The ovaries produce both oestradiol and progesterone, and although progesterone may play a role, the simplest hypothesis is that endogenous oestradiol is the most important hormone because it is the principal mitogen for the breast epithelial cells (Laidlaw *et al*, 1995). Epidemiological studies have not yet established whether the level of exposure to premenopausal oestradiol is important, but there is little information on this because studies need to collect blood several years before the diagnosis of cancer and, ideally, to collect several blood samples from each woman to characterise her oestradiol levels throughout a menstrual cycle.

The picture is becoming clearer for postmenopausal women, among whom three recent prospective studies have found that breast cancer risk is directly related to the serum concentration of oestradiol or to urinary oestrogen excretion (Toniolo *et al*, 1995; Berrino *et al*, 1996; Key *et al*, 1996). In the largest of these studies the risk for breast cancer was 2.6 times higher in women with the highest serum concentration of oestradiol than in women with the lowest concentration; the follow-up was only 5.5 years, but the relative risk was greater for women for whom serum was collected two or more years before diagnosis than for women diagnosed within two years of serum collection, suggesting that the increase in risk observed was not due to a preclinical effect of the disease on oestradiol metabolism (Toniolo *et al*, 1995). In both this study and that of Berrino *et al* (1996) there was also some evidence that risk is inversely related to the proportion of oestradiol bound to sex hormone binding globulin (SHBG) or to the serum concentration of SHBG. Obese postmenopausal women have an increased risk for breast cancer and have increased serum concentrations of oestradiol and reduced serum concentrations of SHBG.

Two of the well known risk factors for breast cancer, early menarche and postmenopausal obesity, are partly determined by nutritional factors, and these are the only links between nutrition and breast cancer that have been firmly established. The nature of the effect of nutrition on age at menarche is not completely understood, but a late menarche may be caused by a low energy intake and perhaps also by a low intake of meat or zinc and a high intake of dietary fibre (Kissinger and Sanchez, 1987; Meyer *et al*, 1990; de Ridder *et al*, 1991) as well as by increased physical activity (Merzenich *et al*, 1993). It is unlikely that dietary interventions to delay menarche deliberately would be acceptable, but it is possible that moderate dietary modifications could be used to delay the onset of regular ovulatory menstrual cycles, a possibility which has been demonstrated for moderate physical activity and which could cause an important reduction in breast cancer risk (Bernstein *et al*, 1987; 1994). Avoidance of obesity in postmenopausal women should cause a modest but worthwhile reduction in breast cancer risk.

A number of studies have investigated the effects of lowering fat intake or increasing fibre intake on plasma oestradiol concentrations in premenopausal and postmenopausal women. Among premenopausal women, diets very low in fat and high in fibre do appear to reduce oestradiol levels (Rose *et al*, 1991; Goldin *et al*, 1994; Bagga *et al*, 1995). Low-fat diets also appear to reduce oestradiol in postmenopausal women, probably partly due to the associated weight loss (Prentice *et al*, 1990).

There is currently great interest in phyto-oestrogens, a group of compounds with weak oestrogenic properties which occur in plants and which might alter endogenous oestradiol levels and breast cancer risk. Two recent small studies investigated the effect of soya phyto-oestrogens (isoflavones) on the menstrual cycle in premenopausal women. Cassidy *et al* (1994) used 45 mg per day of isoflavones and reported a 1.5 day increase in average cycle length due to an increase in the length of the follicular phase. Lu *et al* (1996) used 200 mg per day of isoflavones and reported a 3.5 day increase in average cycle length and large decreases in serum concentrations of both oestradiol and progesterone. More data from longer interventions are needed, but these studies suggest that phyto-oestrogens could have important effects in premenopausal women. The effects may be mediated through interference with the control of oestradiol production by feedback through the pituitary. This would not be expected to affect oestradiol production in postmenopausal women, and a recent large study using 165 mg per day of isoflavones did not find any clear evidence of hormonal effects in postmenopausal women (Baird *et al*, 1995). Two case-control studies have investigated whether soya may reduce the risk for breast cancer. In a relatively small study in Singapore, Lee *et al* (1991) reported a significant protective association in premenopausal women but not in postmenopausal women. However, a larger study in Shanghai and Tianjin found no protective association for soya among either premenopausal or postmenopausal women (Yuan *et al*, 1995).

The priorities for more research are (i) prospective studies of endogenous hormones and breast cancer risk, and (ii) the effects of nutritional factors, especially fibre and phyto-oestrogens, on hormonal patterns at menarche and in premenopausal and postmenopausal women.

References

Bagga D, Ashley JM, Geffrey SP *et al*. Effects of a very low fat, high fibre diet on serum hormones and menstrual function. *Cancer*, 1995; **76**: 2491–2496

Baird DD, Umbach DM, Lansdell L *et al*. Dietary intervention study to assess estrogenicity of dietary soya among postmenopausal women. *Journal of Clinical Endocrinology and Metabolism*, 1995; **80**: 1685–1690

Bernstein L, Ross RK, Lobo RA, Hanisch R, Krailo MD, Henderson BE. The effects of moderate physical activity on menstrual cycle patterns in adolescence: implications for breast cancer prevention. *British Journal of Cancer*, 1987; **55**: 681–685

Bernstein L, Henderson BE, Hanisch R, Sullivan-Halley J, Ross RK. Physical exercise and reduced risk of breast cancer in young women. *Journal of the National Cancer Institute*, 1994; **86**: 1403–1408

Berrino F, Muti P, Micheli A *et al*. Serum sex hormone levels after menopause and subsequent breast cancer. *Journal of the National Cancer Institute*, 1996; **88**: 291–296

Cassidy A, Bingham S, Setchell KDR. Biological effects of a diet of soy protein rich in isoflavones on the menstrual cycle of premenopausal women. *American Journal of Clinical Nutrition*, 1994; **60**: 333–340

de Ridder CM, Thijssen JHH, van't Veer P *et al*. Dietary habits, sexual maturation, and plasma hormones in pubertal girls: a longitudinal study. *American Journal of Clinical Nutrition*, 1991; **54**: 805–813

Goldin BR, Woods MN, Spiegelman DL *et al*. The effect of dietary fat and fibre on serum estrogen concentrations in premenopausal women under controlled dietary conditions. *Cancer*, 1994; **74**: 1125–1131

Key TJA, Wang DY, Brown JB *et al*. A prospective study of urinary oestrogen excretion and breast cancer risk. *British Journal of Cancer*, 1996; **73**: 1615–1619

Kissinger DG, Sanchez A. The association of dietary factors with the age of menarche. *Nutrition Research*, 1987; **7**: 471–479

Laidlaw IJ, Clarke RB, Howell A, Owen AW, Potten CS, Anderson E. The proliferation of normal human breast tissue implanted into athymic nude mice is stimulated by estrogen but not progesterone. *Endocrinology*, 1995; **136**: 164–171

Lee HP, Gourley L, Duffy SW, Esteve J, Lee J, Day NE. Dietary effects on breast-cancer risk in Singapore. *Lancet*, 1991; **337**: 1197–1200

Lu L-JW, Anderson KE, Grady JJ, Nagamani M. Effects of soya consumption for one month on steroid hormones in premenopausal women: implications for breast cancer risk reduction. *Cancer Epidemiology Biomarkers and Prevention*, 1996; **5**: 63–70

Merzenich H, Boeing H, Wahrendorf J. Dietary fat and sports activity as determinants for age at menarche. *American Journal of Epidemiology*, 1993; **138**: 217–224

Meyer F, Moisan J, Marcoux D, Bouchard C. Dietary and physical determinants of menarche. *Epidemiology*, 1990; **1**: 377–381

Prentice R, Thompson D, Clifford C, Gorbach S, Goldin B, Byar D. Dietary fat reduction and plasma estradiol concentration in healthy postmenopausal women. The Women's Health Trial Study Group. *Journal of the National Cancer Institute*, 1990; **82**: 129–134

Rose DP, Goldman M, Connolly JM, Strong LE. High-fiber diet reduces serum estrogen concentrations in premenopausal women. *American Journal of Clinical Nutrition*, 1991; **54**: 520–525

Toniolo PG, Levitz M, Zeleniuch-Jacquotte A *et al*. A prospective study of endogenous estrogens and breast cancer in postmenopausal women. *Journal of the National Cancer Institute*, 1995; **87**: 190–197

Yuan J-M, Wang Q-S, Ross RK, Henderson BE, Yu MC. Diet and breast cancer in Shanghai and Tianjin, China. *British Journal of Cancer*, 1995; **71**: 1353–1358

8
Assessing the net effect of alcohol consumption on mortality

Klim McPherson

Health Promotion Sciences Unit, London School of Hygiene & Tropical Medicine, London, UK

The dominant current health message for sensible consumption of alcohol is perceived as being entirely negative, because it discourages consumption (Paton, 1994). Its intent is to reduce the adverse consequences of excessive drinking, binge drinking and alcohol dependence. These consequences include, in particular, the attributable morbidity and mortality associated with accidents, abuse, anti-social behaviours, mouth and digestive cancers and cirrhosis. The attributable risks associated with breast cancer among women are also increasingly being cited.

The epidemiological literature on the question of alcohol-related deaths often gives rise to estimates of many thousands of deaths attributable to alcohol consumption. These estimates arise by limiting the consideration to those causes of death positively associated with alcohol consumption. This approach simply ignores relative risks less than unity (e.g. Anderson *et al*, 1988) and ignores diseases for which any protective effects, real or otherwise, are demonstrated (Sutocky *et al*, 1993). Thus, the apparent effects of alcohol consumption on mortality have an entirely predictable direction and considerable size.

The epidemiology of alcohol-related morbidity and mortality is more complicated, however, and new evidence does now need to be accommodated in any serious review of sensible drinking messages. The complications arise from three important aspects of the epidemiology:

- a possible important protective effect of moderate alcohol consumption on coronary heart disease (CHD), which is real rather than an artefact of selection;

Diet, Nutrition and Chronic Disease: Lessons from Contrasting Worlds.
Edited by P. S. Shetty and K. McPherson © 1997 John Wiley & Sons, Ltd.

- the poorly understood modifications of the relationship of alcohol consumption and disease with age and gender; and
- the possibility of important differences in the attributable effect of different kinds of alcoholic beverage and different methods of consumption, for example binge drinking.

Of course, these three are interrelated in a complicated way. For example, CHD is much more common among males than females, and among older people, and drinking patterns themselves vary importantly with age and gender. As we will show, however, the complications arise particularly from the possibility that alcohol consumption could have a net beneficial effect on the health of some groups in our society. This review concentrates on the first of these complications. It raises the poorly explored consequence of drinking messages which might seek to increase the consumption among some groups while attempting to reduce the consumption among others.

Research into health education methods which have such seemingly conflicting messages is immature. In the context of sensible advice about alcohol consumption, it typically assumes the often cited strong association between the average level of a population attribute and the prevalence of 'excess' levels (Rose and Day, 1990). This is used to indicate that health education messages can only invoke change in a single direction because, it is argued, the average level determines the proportion of those exposed to excess levels. Since the latter is to be reduced, the message must therefore unequivocally aim to reduce the average consumption in order to be effective. However, the original observation comes from comparisons between groups, and not from observing changes within groups. The relationship between mean level and the proportion consuming excess levels may well then be very different.

Furthermore, there is a danger that results for individuals on alcohol-related mortality will be inappropriately used to make recommendations regarding optimum consumption levels for populations (Skog, 1992). This would apparently tell us that, because of a J-shaped risk curve, it is likely that the *per capita* consumption of alcohol in most industrialised countries is three to five times higher than would be required for optimal population benefit (Anderson, 1995). These calculations make unduly strong assumptions about the nature of the data, i.e. requiring both a polynomial relationship and a constant coefficient of variation of the consumption distribution, as the mean level changes. The often observed notion that the standard deviation of a distribution is proportional to the mean is frequently assumed in analytical modelling, but represents nothing more than an empirical observation which has no intrinsic merit. In particular, the distribution of human behaviours as complicated as alcohol consumption may be expected to have no such basic relationship between mean and variance. It is precisely this which is poorly explored in health education research, and to assume *a priori* the nature of this relationship is to deny some possibly significant health advantage.

This brief review will summarise the importance of some of these questions by resorting to basic epidemiological modelling to illustrate the kind of dilemma facing policy-makers. People do not, of course, drink primarily for its health benefits, nor do they not drink largely because of long-term health consequences. Moderate alcohol consumption, it must be remembered, may entail a major advantage in poorly measured, but important, aspects of quality of life (Ritter, 1988). However, this will necessarily be ignored in the analyses which follow. Public policy on alcohol consumption is determined largely by the harder long-term health considerations and hence must be informed by the plausible consequences of alcohol consumption. The work reported below seeks to summarise the epidemiology of alcohol-related mortality. We investigate the mortality in England and Wales which can be attributable to current drinking patterns using the risks derived from published epidemiological studies. We will subsequently seek to model that alcohol-attributable mortality on likely changes which might arise, were the prevalence of drinking in various amounts to change. This work concentrates on mortality simply because cause-specific data are routinely available, by age and gender, for mortality but not for morbidity.

Methods

We have taken the relative risks of alcohol-related cause-specific mortality from four cohort studies. These studies were chosen because the possible selection effects of including people as abstainers who were in fact ex-drinkers, possibly rendered ill by their habit, have been attended to as far as is reasonably possible. Clearly it is not possible to eliminate the possible effect of biases such as this, without a randomised trial, but the aggregate evidence at the moment suggests that moderate drinking is causally associated with a reduced mortality, but others continue to dispute it (Shaper, 1995) as they have every right to do, somewhat in contradiction to the gathering consensus. The extent of any causative relationship is thus inadequately estimated at present, but could be large. There are perfectly clear biological mechanisms for such an effect, which are automatically accepted as strong evidence in other circumstances, for example hormone replacement therapy to prevent heart disease (McPherson, 1994).

Using these relative risks, we have applied them to the current age- and sex-specific drinking prevalences and calculated the percentage of current mortality attributed to alcohol consumption at different ages and genders. This process assumes that the relative risks represent causal associations, and hence to change the drinking patterns will change the risks of death accordingly. The purpose of this methodology is simply to provide a crude method of balancing the possible benefits with possible harm. We have assumed gender-specific relative risks, but have not generally modified the estimated relative risks according to age. This is because the data on which such modification would be based are sparse (Rehm and Sempos, 1995), but it is possible to undertake sensitivity analysis to investigate the likely effects. This has been done here.

In general, however, in what follows, the relative risks reported are assumed to apply to all ages for each disease equally. This may be an unreasonable assumption, but one commonly, if implicitly, assumed in epidemiology. However, for instance, in the recent report from the British Doctors study, Doll *et al* (1994) quote relative risks applicable to men recruited into a cohort study in 1951 and who had replied to a questionnaire about their drinking habits in 1978. At this time these men were on average 62 years old, and hence whatever is observed about their mortality, might well not apply to younger men, let alone women. While we might assume constant relative risks for changing ages, nowhere do we assume constant relative risks across genders.

Data

We have derived our estimates of relative risks from four large cohort studies. The first is the Kaiser Permanente study reported by Klatsky *et al* (1992). They report cause-specific relative risks in their cohort of around 129 000 individuals followed from 1978 to 1988. These risks are relative to lifetime abstainers. Secondly, the data from the American Cancer Society (ACS) cohort of 581 000 women and 277 000 men followed from 1959 for 12 years are used (Garfinkel *et al*, 1988; Boffetta and Garfinkel, 1990). The risks were adjusted for smoking and age, and no evidence for a selection effect among abstainers was found. Thirdly, the recent work in Copenhagen (Gronbaek *et al*, 1994) is used to estimate the overall percentage of attributable mortalities. Lastly, for comparison purposes the recent observations of Richard Doll and colleagues on the 13-year follow-up on males from the British Doctors study are used (Doll *et al*, 1994).

We have taken the estimates of current alcohol consumption from the General Household Survey (GHS) and mortality for the population of England and Wales for 1992 (Table 8.1). In 1992 the *Health of the Nation* target indicated that drinking less than 21 units per week for men and 14 units by women was unlikely to damage health. In late 1995 the Report of an Inter-Departmental Working Group (GB Department of Health, 1995) advised that for men, maximum health advantage is obtained by consuming between one and two units per day while regular consumption of between three and four units a day by men of all ages will not accrue significant health risk. Similar comments for women advocate between one and two units a day for maximum health advantage, but warn against consistently drinking more than three or more units a day because of the progressive health risk of increasing consumption. Thus, broadly speaking, safe drinking limits for men and women respectively were specified as 21 and 14 units per week, and are now 28 and 21 units. Note that the new limits are specified as daily amounts, and hence seek to spread the weekly consumption more uniformly throughout the week. However, according

Table 8.1   Alcohol consumption in England and Wales (1992)

		Age groups (%)			
	Units/week	16–24	25–44	45–64	65+
Males					
None	0	7	4	6	12
Moderate	1–20	61	64	69	74
High	22–50	23	24	19	12
Very high	51+	9	8	6	2
Females					
None	0	11	8	11	22
Moderate	1–14	72	78	78	73
High	15–35	13	12	10	5
Very high	36+	4	2	1	0

to the GHS categorisation above, these new levels are designated unambiguously as 'high'.

The methods of calculating attributable risks are standard epidemiological methodology and take account of the observed relative risks and the observed prevalence of drinking in several categories. Thus the attributable risk from a particular cause of death is the proportion of all deaths from that cause which can be attributed to alcohol consumption at current levels, that is to say, the proportion by which the mortality would be *reduced* if everybody was a lifetime abstainer from alcohol. Note that with a protective effect of alcohol the attributable risk will be the increase as percentage of the total that would result if everybody became an abstainer.

As an index of the magnitude of this metric, the proportion of lung cancer attributable to cigarette smoking is around 90% while the proportion attributable to passive smoking is around 4%. Thus, while passive smoking is common, the relative risk is low, but cigarette smoking remains common and carries a massive risk, relative to lifetime non-smokers, for lung cancer. Within the limits of epidemiological measurement, therefore, some 94% of lung cancer is attributable to cigarettes. In contrast, approximately a mere 15% of CHD is attributable to elevated cholesterol and another 15% to lack of exercise, given fairly arbitrary cut-off levels.

The attributable risk for all-cause mortality can be calculated from the component causes when the relative risk for each cause is known, but generally the risk is directly measured by simply aggregating all deaths. Thus all-cause mortality is taken as the aggregate statistic and in what follows the attributable risk percentages for particular causes are expressed as a percentage of all-cause mortality. Thus both the size of the relationship with alcohol and mortality from that cause are reflected, as well as how common is that cause. It is worth noting that in the British Doctors study (Doll *et al*, 1994), there were 230 deaths observed from alcohol-augmented causes and 1230 from ischaemic heart disease, thus illustrating the relative impact that any protective effect of alcohol consumption may have among such a group.

These calculations are done to enable the risks to be expressed on a single scale. Thus the relative risks of alcohol are high for cirrhosis, but low for CHD. Therefore almost all cirrhosis is attributable to alcohol, and only a small proportion of CHD is putatively prevented by alcohol. But obviously CHD is much more common than cirrhosis and hence such an effect could in principle swamp the cirrhosis effect in terms of numbers of deaths. The extent to which this is true, including all relevant causes, is essentially the question addressed by this analysis. Table 8.2 shows the proportion of deaths under age 65 by cause and also the number of years of life lost in England and Wales in 1990, given current mortality patterns. It can be easily seen that common diseases give rise to the greatest burden of death and that circulatory disease and breast cancer among women represent the commonest causes of death, while accidents and suicide become important as contributors to years of life lost, since they predominantly occur among young people.

Results—attributable mortality

Taking the risks associated with all-cause mortality first, the overall results are shown in Figure 8.1, which indicates the percentage increase or decrease in total mortality attributable to current levels of alcohol consumption. As discussed above, these data assume constancy of relative risk for all ages, which will not be

Table 8.2   Deaths in England and Wales by selected causes (1990)

	% deaths from all causes age <65		Working years of life lost 15–64	
	Males	Females	Males	Females
All cancers	29	45	179	196
Digestive organs	8	8	46	29
Breast cancer	–	13	–	59
Liver disease (inc. cirrhosis)	1	1	10	3
Circulatory	37	24	212	76
IHD	28	14	152	35
CVD	7	6	27	23
Accidents	8	4	159	46
RTA	4	2	97	26
Suicide	5	2	65	15
Total (all causes)	100	100	984	575

NB Total costs do not add to 100% because some causes, not related to alcohol consumption, are omitted

STUDY

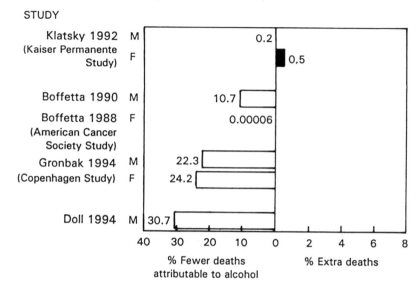

Figure 8.1   Four recent studies of alcohol and all-cause mortality—relative risks applied to population of England and Wales, 1992

accurate. However, it can be seen that, at the very least, the most reliable data on the epidemiology of alcohol-related deaths give rise to aggregated evidence which suggests that for men the overall effect is zero or beneficial and for women essentially zero. There is at the same time evidence from some studies to suggest that drinking alcohol may be causing fewer deaths in aggregate.

If we look at Figures 8.2–8.4, where the relative risks from the ACS study (Boffetta and Garfinkel, 1990) are used to make the aggregated estimates, the possible effects at different ages can be investigated. In the youngest age group, accidents have the largest effect but even they do not cause a net increase in mortality, if we assume (possibly wrongly) that relative risks for all causes apply as much to them. However, the numbers in this age group are very small. After that age CHD deaths quickly dominate the aggregate picture. Thus it does seem that for men, at current drinking patterns, as a first approximation, alcohol is responsible for a net reduction in mortality at all ages, which is particularly important at older ages.

For women, the situation is different because CHD is less common than in men, and breast cancer is much more common (Figures 8.5–8.7). Not until the 45–64-year age group does CHD protection begin to make a positive impact on the attributable mortality, and only after age 65 does the balance of mortality effects begin to equal out.

Clearly, these data suggest a precision which is not commensurate with the epidemiology. In particular, the effect on the balance between CHD and breast

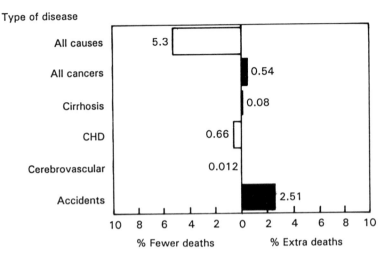

Figure 8.2   Percentage of all-cause mortality attributable to alcohol in males aged 16–24 years in England and Wales, applying ACS relative risk

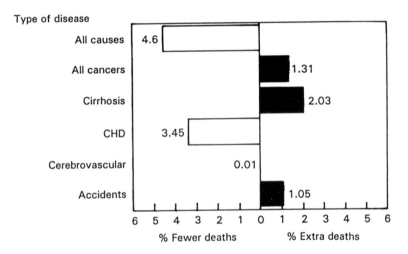

Figure 8.3   Percentage of all-cause mortality attributable to alcohol in males aged 25–44 years in England and Wales, applying ACS relative risk

cancer in women depends crucially on which estimates of relative risk are used. At one extreme the balance can be made to favour alcohol by taking the best protective estimates of alcohol on CHD and the least potent effect on breast cancer (Howe *et al*, 1991) (Figure 8.8) or at the other (Figure 8.9) by taking the results from the ACS study, which estimates a low protective effect on CHD, and another overview on breast cancer which estimates a strong dose-related effect

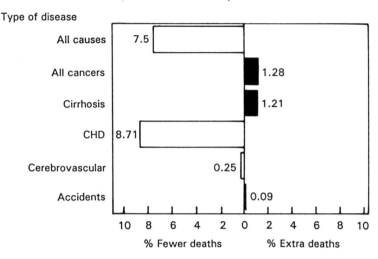

Figure 8.4   Percentage of all-cause mortality attributable to alcohol in males aged 45–64 years in England and Wales, applying ACS relative risk

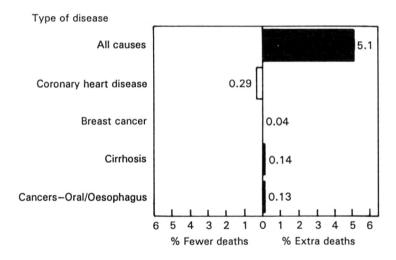

Figure 8.5   Percentage of all-cause mortality attributable to alcohol in females aged 16–24 years in England and Wales, applying ACS relative risk

for alcohol (Longnecker *et al*, 1988). Clearly, the truth could be between these estimates or, just possibly, even not included by them. It is quite possible, for instance, that the apparent effect of alcohol on breast cancer is entirely an artefact of confounding with other dietary constituents (for example, fat consumption), and that in reality women changing alcohol intake would have no effect at all on

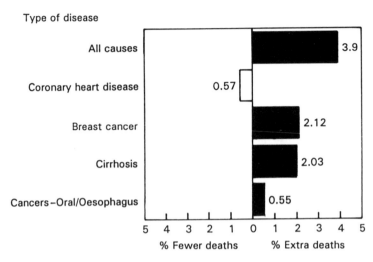

Figure 8.6 Percentage of all-cause mortality attributable to alcohol in females aged 25–44 years in England and Wales, applying ACS relative risk

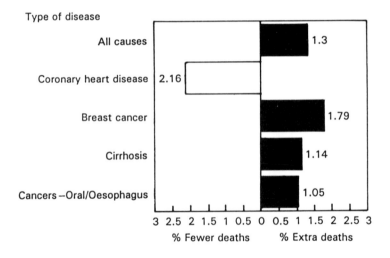

Figure 8.7 Percentage of all-cause mortality attributable to alcohol in females aged 45–64 years in England and Wales, applying ACS relative risk

breast cancer risk (McPherson *et al*, 1993). In the case of women particularly, these uncertainties are massively important because, as we have seen, the aggregated effect of alcohol on mortality is obviously strongly determined by its

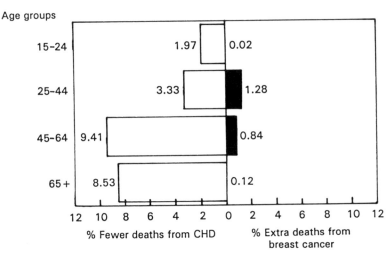

Figure 8.8 High protective effect on CHD vs low (40 g/day threshold) risk for breast cancer applying RRs for CHD from Nurses' Health Study

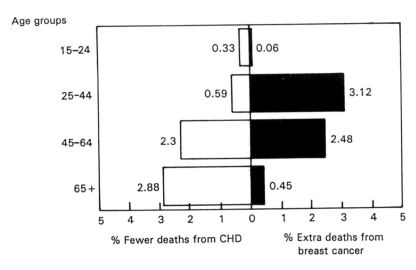

Figure 8.9 Low protective effect on CHD vs high (dose-response) risk for breast cancer applying RRs for CHD from American Cancer Society Study

effect, assumed to be causative, on breast cancer. The relative risks for breast cancer are shown in Figure 8.10 and for CHD in Figure 8.11.

Drinks per day	Low risk (ACS)	Higher risk (KPS)
0	1	1
0-5	1	1.1
5-10	1.1	1.2
10-21	1	1.3
21-32	1	1.5
32+	1.7	1.7

Figure 8.10 Relative risks for breast cancer to be applied to the female population of England and Wales

Units alcohol per week	American Cancer study	Kaiser Permanente study	Nurses' Health study
0	1.0	1.0	1.0
>0-0.5	0.85	0.9	0.8
>0.5-10	0.85	0.5	0.6
>10-21	1.01	0.7	0.6
>21-32	0.89	0.7	0.6
>32	1.1	1.2	0.4

Figure 8.11 Relative risks for CHD by alcohol consumption to be applied to the female population of England and Wales. ACSS: age-adjusted; KPS: adjusted for age and smoking; NHS, adjusted for several possible confounders

Conclusions

It does seem highly likely that moderate consumption of alcohol is causatively associated with a reduction in overall mortality rates. This will largely be as a consequence of the beneficial effects on CHD, mediated most plausibly via an elevation of HDL cholesterol and possibly anti-thrombotic effects, which might explain the low apparent dose threshold of protection and the protection among older people (Rankin, 1994). This very crude investigation into the aggregate mortality associated with alcohol consumption leads to conclusions from which no simple message emerges.

This work attempts to balance the benefits against the risks of current levels of consumption in a manner by which net effects can be demonstrated. Within the bounds of epidemiological error (and probably invoking some assumptions which are too bold) the argument is finely balanced. The implications on policy are complicated. Clearly any reductions from excessive levels is always a sound option. But if this means encouraging some of those who drink a little to abstain altogether then the health consequences could be quite serious and possibly deleterious on balance.

The future research endeavour will require greater sophistication in the modelling process and greater reliability in the estimates of risk, if this is to inform policy more usefully. It will further require a stronger understanding of the effects of complicated (seemingly conflicting) messages on the behaviour of populations. It does not seem obvious to us that the observed strong association, across cultures, of the average level of alcohol consumption with prevalence of excess levels, applies necessarily to changing levels in a single culture. These same cross-cultural comparisons yield very strong negative associations of aggregated consumption with CHD mortality rates (Criqui and Ringel, 1994), which are also important.

For the moment this work simply points to the possibility that the risks attributable to abstention could be as, or more, important, in public health terms, as the risks attributable to current levels of reported excessive drinking. In older men this seems most likely, and possibly among women too, if the observed association with breast cancer is not itself causative. Alcohol, unlike hormone replacement therapy (Studd, 1992) and other similar interventions whose prophylactic potential is essentially a side-effect, has to overcome an implicit, if not overt, hostility from the medical and other influential professions. A long historic association with drinking problems (Edwards, 1989) and their health effects, whose seriousness should certainly not be dismissed, tends to colour the overall picture (Edwards *et al*, 1994).

However, we do need to know more about the exact nature of any protective effects and to have more reliable age-specific estimates of risk (Anderson *et al*, 1993). It is also important to have a more coherent and reliable picture of the differences that both type of beverage and type of consumption have on risk. A recent review has concluded that in the absence of more adequate scientific knowledge and informed community debate, it is unethical to promote low alcohol intake as a preventive health measure (Holman and English, 1996). Both of those preconditions clearly deserve much effort and encouragement.

We certainly have much further to go before there is any serious danger of anyone, other than the alcohol industry of course (Casswell, 1993), actually promoting low alcohol intake among non-drinkers. It remains perfectly possible that for some groups, particularly the young, and especially if they are female, such promotion would be seriously misleading. But the risks even then which might be associated with moderate drinking, so long as it is divorced from driving and other independently dangerous activities, are small and might give rise to an ultimately healthy, life-enhancing and convivial habit.

References

Anderson P. Excess mortality associated with alcohol consumption. *British Medical Journal*, 1988; **297**: 824–826

Anderson P. Alcohol consumption and all cause mortality. *Addiction*, 1995; **90**: 481–484

Anderson P, Cremona A, Paton A, Turner C, Wallace P. The risk of alcohol. *Addiction*, 1993; **88**: 1493–1508

Boffetta P, Garfinkel L. Alcohol drinking and mortality among men enrolled in an American Cancer Society prospective study. *Epidemiology*, 1990; **1**: 342–348

Caswell S. Public discourse on the benefits of moderation: implications for alcohol policy development. *Addiction*, 1993; **88**: 459–465

Criqui MH, Ringel BL. Does diet or alcohol explain the French paradox? *Lancet*, 1994; **344**: 1719–1723

Doll R, Peto R, Wheatley K, Gray R, Sutherland I. Mortality in relation to consumption of alcohol: 13 years' observations on male British doctors. *British Medical Journal*, 1994; **309**: 911–917

Edwards G. As the years go rolling by. Drinking problems in the time dimension. *British Journal of Psychiatry*, 1989; **154**: 18-26

Edwards G, Anderson P, Barbour TF. *Alcohol Policy and the Public Good*. Oxford: Oxford University Press, 1994

Garfinkel L, Boffetta P, Stellman SD. Alcohol and breast cancer: a cohort study. *Preventive Medicine*, 1988; **17**: 686–693

Great Britain Department of Health. *Sensible Drinking. Report of an Interdepartmental Working Group*. London, 1995

Gronbaek M, Deis A, Sorensen TI et al. Influence of sex, age, body mass index, and smoking on alcohol intake and mortality. *British Medical Journal*, 1994; **308**: 302–306

Holman CDJ, English DR. Ought low alcohol intake to be promoted for health reasons? *Journal of the Royal Society of Medicine*, 1996; **89**: 123–129

Howe G, Rohan T, Decarli A et al. The association between alcohol and breast cancer risk: evidence from the combined analysis of six dietary case-control studies. *International Journal of Cancer*, 1991; **47**: 707–710

Klatsky AL, Armstrong MA, Friedman GD. Alcohol and mortality. *Annals of Internal Medicine*, 1992; **117**: 646–654

Longnecker MP, Berlin JA, Orza MJ, Chalmers TC. A meta-analysis of alcohol consumption in relation to breast cancer. *Journal of the American Medical Association*, 1988; **260**: 652–656

McPherson K. The policy implications of HRT: is there a case for preventive intervention? In: Sharp I, ed. *Coronary Heart Disease: Are Women Special?* London: National Forum for Coronary Heart Disease Prevention, 1994: 141–152

McPherson K, Englesman E, Conning D. Breast cancer. In: Verschuren PM, ed. *Health Issues Related to Alcohol Consumption*. ILSI Europe, 1993

Paton A, ed. *ABC of Alcohol*. London: BMJ Publishing Group, 1994

Rankin JG. Biological mechanisms at moderate levels of alcohol consumption that may affect the development, course and/or outcome of coronary heart disease. *Contemporary Drug Problems*, 1994; **21**: 45–57

Rehm J, Sempos CT. Alcohol consumption and all cause mortality. *Addiction*, 1995; **90**: 471–480

Ritter C. Social supports, social networks and health behaviours. In: Gochman DS, ed. *Health Behaviour, Emerging Research Perspectives*. New York: Plenum Press, 1988

Rose G, Day S. The population mean predicts the number of deviant individuals. *British Medical Journal*, 1990; **301**: 1031–1034

Shaper AG. The 'unhealthy abstainers' question is still important. *Addiction*, 1995; **90**: 488–490

Skog OJ. Epidemiological and biostatistical aspects of alcohol use, alcoholism and their complications. In: Erickson PG, Kalant H, eds. *Windows on Science*. Toronto: Addiction Research Foundation, 1992

Studd J. Complications of hormone replacement therapy in post-menopausal women. *Journal of the Royal Society of Medicine*, 1992; **85**: 376–378

Sutocky J, Shultz JM, Kizer KW. Alcohol related mortality in California 1980–1989. *American Journal of Public Health*, 1993; **83**: 817–823

Acknowledgement

ILSI Europe Alcohol Task Force is thanked for their support for this work.

Discussion

A. Gerald Shaper

Royal Free Hospital School of Medicine, London, UK

The overall message of this review is that for middle-aged men and possibly for women as well, moderate drinking is a healthy and life-enhancing habit—do not abstain.

Five major studies are used by Professor McPherson to derive estimates of relative risk which are then applied to the England/Wales population using a method with many assumptions, and in particular assuming that the relative risks reported apply to all ages equally, which is clearly not the case. The relative risks for four of these studies use as baseline non-drinkers in middle age, i.e. ex-drinkers and lifelong teetotallers combined, and in the fifth study, lifelong teetotallers. The subjects range from people in a health insurance scheme, to volunteers recruited in an unspecified way, to British doctors, in whom alcohol intake was recorded 27 years after recruitment in the surviving one-third of the cohort. However, all these studies show a protective effect of alcohol, although only one provides a description of the characteristics of the non-drinkers who constitute the baseline. These studies were chosen because the 'possible selection effects of including people as abstainers who were in fact ex-drinkers, possibly rendered ill by their habit, have been attended to'. This summary dismissal ignores major issues concerning the characteristics of non-drinkers and of those who change their habits over time (Shaper, 1990).

Among middle-aged British men, two-thirds of the non-drinkers are ex-drinkers who have many characteristics likely to increase their morbidity and mortality. With increasing age, there is a steady downward drift from heavy to moderate drinking and towards abstinence, under the influence of accumulating ill-health not necessarily related to alcohol intake. In the British Regional Heart Study (Shaper *et al*, 1994), heavy drinkers at screening who were no longer heavy drinkers five years later were at least twice as likely to have acquired a new diagnosis of coronary heart disease (CHD) or to have gone onto new regular medication, compared with those who remained heavy drinkers. Despite these phenomena which increase the risk of cardiovascular events and total mortality in non-drinkers, there does appear to be a small protective effect of alcohol on CHD, and there are sound biological mechanisms that could account for such benefit. There is, however, no dose–response relationship. Despite the benefit to CHD, there is little or no reduction in total mortality. The approach of most concern is that which actually encourages those who do not drink to do so for the sake of their coronary arteries and their life expectancy. Professor McPherson, the Copenhagen workers, Sir Richard Doll and his colleagues, the BMA and the Government Inter-Departmental Working Group all state, in one way or another, that abstinence from alcohol might seriously damage your health. Based as it is on the increased risk in non-drinkers compared with drinkers, this claim goes beyond the evidence available, and should not be made (Wannamethee and Shaper, 1988).

In conclusion, mortality statistics are an inappropriate measure for determining policy on alcohol. The small protective effect of alcohol on CHD has been exaggerated and extrapolated beyond the evidence on total morbidity and mortality.

References

Shaper AG. Alcohol and mortality: a review of prospective studies. *British Journal of Addiction*, 1990; **85**: 837–847

Shaper AG, Wannamethee G, Walker M. Alcohol and coronary heart disease: a perspective from the British Regional Heart Study. *International Journal of Epidemiology*, 1994; **23**: 482–494

Wannamethee G, Shaper AG. Men who do not drink: a report from the British Regional Heart Study. *International Journal of Epidemiology*, 1988; **17**: 307–316

9
The public health impact of globalisation of food trade

Tim Lang

Centre for Food Policy, Wolfson School of Health Sciences, Thames Valley University, London, UK

On 15 April 1994, world trade leaders initialled a new General Agreement on Tariffs and Trade (GATT) deal. The tortuous eight-year Uruguay Round negotiation had come to an end. Within two years, 130 or so countries had ratified the agreement, few with any extensive national public debate; India and the USA were exceptions. The vast majority of world trade is now subject to GATT rules. Agriculture, for the first time, had been drawn under the GATT umbrella and the proponents of the idea that trade liberalisation is the means to deliver greater economic good had achieved a momentous victory. The GATT was driven by the theory of economic liberalisation, replacing the post-war Keynesian consensus which had accorded the state the right to intervene in markets (Cockett, 1994). Not only was the contentious policy area of agriculture included in the new system, now overseen by the newly created World Trade Organization, but areas of potential dissent such as biotechnology patents were also covered under the agreement on Intellectual Property Rights. This chapter argues that the era of trade liberalisation symbolised by this agreement has considerable implications for a number of goals espoused by world bodies and public health practitioners. These include food security, consumer information and choice and environmental protection.

Food security is a goal of the Food and Agriculture Organization. Its Committee on World Food Security states:

> 'Food security' means that food is available at all times, that all persons have means of access to it, that it is nutritionally adequate in terms of quantity, quality and variety, and that it is acceptable within the given culture. Only when all these conditions are in place can a population be considered 'food secure'. We aim to achieve lasting

Diet, Nutrition and Chronic Disease: Lessons from Contrasting Worlds.
Edited by P. S. Shetty and K. McPherson © 1997 John Wiley & Sons, Ltd.

self-reliance at the national and household levels. In order to succeed, our initiatives must be founded on principles of economic viability, equity, broad participation, and the sustainable use of natural resources. (Committee on World Food Security, 1996: para. 4)

The World Bank defines food security as 'access by all people at all times to enough food for an active and healthy life' (World Bank, 1986). The GATT agreement is based on an entirely different model—that cheaper commodities should not be impeded from having access to hitherto protected markets. Even before the final GATT agreement, critics from both developing and developed economies were arguing that the free trade model which the GATT enshrined was based upon an inappropriate understanding of the food challenges ahead (Raghavan, 1990; Watkins, 1991; Coote, 1992). A variety of arguments were rehearsed: that free trade is fine for televisions or motor cars, but not for food; that free trade is a misnomer and that, in practice, it is a set of rules which generally suit the powerful (Watkins, 1992); that, while affluent consumers would benefit from cheaper goods, as would companies who could (threaten to) switch production to where labour costs are low, the poorest nations and the poorest within nations would lose out (Watkins, 1989; Lang and Hines, 1993); that affluent companies would have access to previously communally owned seeds and plants (Shiva and Holla-Bhar, 1993). Whatever their foci, the critics agreed that the new regime would be especially hard for sub-Saharan Africa, a fact acknowledged by proponents of trade liberalisation such as the Organisation for Economic Cooperation and Development and the World Bank (Goldin et al, 1993).

These arguments with regard to the GATT—for, against and mosaics of both—can be seen to have drawn upon most discourses in world affairs and the human sciences, but public health was barely a consideration. The exception was some concern about the role of food health standards—mainly in relation to contaminants and technical standards. These were covered by the creation of a new global system for setting minimum standards, the Sanitary and Phytosanitary Standards (SPS) and Technical Barriers to Trade (TBT) agreements within the GATT. 'Influence' was handed to the Codex Alimentarius Commission. This process for setting standards leaves much to be desired. Although a meeting of governments, this vast system of 20 committees, with a total of 2758 participants in a two-year cycle of meetings, was found to have a quarter of its participants from large international companies (Avery et al, 1993). This imbalance is at odds with the spirit of much recent community health thinking which stresses local participation, empowerment and transparency (e.g. WHO, 1985; 1987; Baum and Sanders, 1995; Lupton, 1995).

The study of Codex (Avery et al, 1993), with its committees covering issues such as pesticides, veterinary drug residues and food contaminants, found that:

• 104 countries participated, as did over 100 of the largest multinational food and agrochemical companies.

- The vast majority (96%) of non-governmental participants represented industry.
- There were 26 representatives from public interest groups compared with 662 industry representatives.
- Nestlé, the largest food company in the world, sent over 30 representatives to all Codex committee meetings, in total more than most countries.
- Most representation came from rich, Northern countries. Over 60% came from Europe and North America, with the poor countries of the South dramatically underrepresented: only 7% from Africa and 10% from Latin America.
- Of the participants on the working group on standards for food additives and contaminants, 39% represented transnational corporations or industry federations, including 61 representatives from the largest food and agrochemical companies in the world.
- Of the 374 participants on the committee on pesticide residue levels, 75 represented multinational agrochemical and food corporations, and 34 of these were from the world's top 20 agrochemical companies; only 80 participants represented the interests of developing countries.
- The USA sent more representatives to Codex than any other country (50% of them representing industry) and almost twice as many as the entire continent of Africa.

Globalisation: new and old

While the GATT cannot be blamed for public health problems or trends underway long before it, GATT's restructuring of world affairs has profound implications for public health in that it celebrates a school of economics which professes the triumph of individualism over 'society', of markets over social care, and the virtues of privatised, rather than community, responsibility. Needs are defined as that to which the market can respond. Citizenship is reduced to consumerism (Gabriel and Lang, 1995). Competing in the global marketplace becomes a managerial *mantra* to encourage people, North and South, to work harder and longer.

Much has been written about the meaning of globalisation (e.g. Hirst and Thompson, 1996), but in the case of food, we should be wary about equating the changes in the world food economy with those of personal computers or cars. Computers are a modern invention. Cars began to be subject to global forces of production and design at the beginning of the 20th century. But food was subject to global trends, tastes and demands centuries ago, as historians of spices, grains, salt and sugars remind us (Mintz, 1985; Rowling, 1987; Adshead, 1992). Nevertheless, there is a qualitative and quantitative gearing up in the present wave of globalisation. The selling of a Northern (American) diet to the world is an example. As the North learns, from epidemiologists, the doubtful joys of consuming a highly processed diet, replete with saturated fats and lower than desirable in antioxidants, this diet is being exported globally, with governments and public health agencies relatively powerless to do anything to halt the process.

Indeed, in a long-term strategy document, the US Department of Agriculture positively revels in the new opportunities to sell 'high-value, consumer food products' to countries in the Asia Pacific rim which have hitherto provided epidemiological evidence about the value of low-fat diets (USDA, 1995). This same strategy document concludes that there is a 'great outlook for processed foods' from the 'growth in fast food and family-style restaurants' and 'growth in Western-style supermarkets'. This is to accompany the decline of agriculture in Asia and a rapid urbanisation which will be a 'benefit... to US exporters' who will be able to target consumers who 'are now more localised and easier to reach with market promotion activities'. This picture reinforces that painted by others for food in the 1950s and 1960s (Friedmann and McMichael, 1989) and for the grain trades (Morgan, 1979). The export of Northern diets to the South is also reminiscent of the process whereby tobacco sales were encouraged in the South once sales were being constrained in the North due to concerted public health measures, health education campaigns and fiscal measures.

Public health agencies are easily lampooned as 'killjoys' and 'health missiona-ries' if they try to temper the kind of food products heavily advertised in these global marketing initiatives. Consumers are said to be able to 'look after themselves', when the evidence from societies where advertising is subject to few constraints shows that their knowledge is fragmented and, from an early age, affected. Like the ancient English King Canute who tried to halt the rise of the sea's unstoppable tide, dietary burgerisation is presented as driven by youthful demand, when it is in fact brilliantly and ruthlessly marketed (Lobstein, 1988). The burger has become a symbol of modernity and the triumph of an American mode of eating, a metaphor for how rational, bureaucratic society orders production of any good and the fulfilment of any need (Ritzer, 1993). But who, in the world's financial media or elected assemblies, makes the policy connections with the alarming rise in obesity in the USA (Surgeon General of the United States, 1988)? And who comments on the doubtful health, not to say ethics, of subsidising exports of wheat grain and meat consumption to food cultures where wheat is foreign and meat a rare luxury (Rifkin, 1992; Carruthers, 1995)? Who, too, spoke for the billions of small farmers, the world's majority of rural dwellers or for the case that if everyone emulated the energy- and fat-rich Northern diet, the planet would be put under gross strain (McMichael, 1993; Ritchie, 1996)? Is it beyond the realm of possibility that, over the next decades, we shall witness a spread of so-called 'western diseases of affluence' such as coronary heart disease and some of the food-related cancers?

Pending medical cures for these diseases or technical fixes in the form of new 'functional' foods or pharmaceutical drugs, the epidemiological evidence suggests that dietary habits can be changed (WHO, 1990). But this requires policy priority to be given to nurturing the role of food within culture (Mennell *et al*, 1992) rather than bowing to a narrow conception of the market. This requires governments to govern, or at least to right the imbalance between corporate power and individual consumers.

Fragmentation of food culture

Some people benefit, of course, from the globalisation package of deregulation, the imposition of narrow criteria of economic efficiency, international competitiveness, and a dogmatic reliance on the market. Before the GATT's ink was dry, the large farmers, the traders and the big food companies were arguing that they could compete in the tough climate. In the sphere of consumption, as Durning (1992) has argued, the world is already fragmenting into three discernible consuming classes, for which diet is a key indicator (Table 9.1).

Consumer culture, not just in food, is driven by the ecologically overconsuming classes. Although icons such as McDonald's tend to hog the headlines, it is important to recognise that a long and powerful transformation of society is underway. Ritzer (1993) has called it 'McDonaldization'. Aspirations for a lifestyle are translated into dietary form; they may be driven by the affluent but copied by the less well-off. 'Peasant' becomes a term of abuse, synonymous with the past.

Similarities of lifestyle bond the rich of North and South, as well as the poor (Gabriel and Lang, 1995; Watkins, 1995). The rich, Durning's consumers, can choose from up to 20 000 items on the hypermarket shelves, drawn from around the world in a brilliant, efficiently run system of production and distribution (Raven and Lang, 1995). This delivers fresh green beans to the UK in mid-winter, flown in from Kenya or The Gambia. Biodiversity on the shelves is not necessarily reflected in the contract fields (whence this abundance comes) which are drawn into a cash-cropping, intensive monoculture (Jenkins, 1992). Contracting and year-round production in the South is distributed to affluent consumers in the North (Feder, 1977; Thrupp, 1995). Case studies by Oxfam have indicated that countries such as the Philippines and Mexico are already finding their grain markets, maize in particular, being seriously undermined by

Table 9.1 World consumption classes, 1992

Category of consumption (Population)	Consumers 1.1 billion	Middle 3.3 billion	Poor 1.1 billion
Diet	Meat, packaged food, soft drinks	Grain, clean water	Insufficient grain, unsafe water
Transport	Private cars	Bicycles, bus	Walking
Materials	Throwaways	Durables	Local biomass

Source: Durning, 1992

an influx of highly (and unfairly) subsidised US and European Union grains (Watkins, 1996).

Even before the new GATT, Southern agricultural investment was rapidly becoming export-led to pay national debts (Oxfam International, 1996; UNDP, 1995). In The Gambia, roads have been installed radiating from the airport, in order to get fresh foods to Northern Europe faster (Barrett and Browne, 1994). This sets The Gambia in competition with Kenya, a competition from which only the trader and the distant consumer benefit. In the short term, this may yield advantages, but it sets up a pattern of development, which, as is suggested by the experience of Chile and Brazil, both huge net exporters of fruit, exacerbates inequalities at home and creates a new dependency culture. Raikes has memorably termed this process 'modernising hunger' (Raikes, 1988).

Proponents of globalisation argue that, without trade liberalisation, the poor will starve. This argument is disarming, but erroneous. There are *already* worrying levels of nutritional inadequacy. The United Nations estimates that one in five persons in the developing world suffers from chronic hunger—800 million people in Africa, Asia and Latin America—and that 'over 2 billion people subsist on diets deficient in the vitamins and minerals essential for normal growth and development, and for preventing premature death and such disabilities as blindness and mental retardation' (UNICEF, 1993). There is also strong evidence of the effect of low income on diet in affluent countries (e.g. Dowler and Rushton, 1994; Low Income Project Team, 1996); these remind us of what happens when social policies bend to economic philosophy. The range of foods that people on low incomes can 'choose' from is itself a meaningful nutrition indicator (Dowler, 1995). Inequality within and between nations is itself a potent health indicator (Wilkinson, 1992: Brunner, this volume, Chapter 4).

Thirty years ago, the combined incomes of the richest fifth of the world's people were 30 times greater than those of the poorest fifth. Today their incomes are over 60 times greater. The number of dollar billionaires has been estimated to be 358 in 1994 (Broad and Cavanagh, 1995). This relatively tiny number of people was calculated to be collectively worth some US$762 billion, which is approximately equivalent to the combined income of the world's poorest 2.5 billion citizens, just under a half of humanity. This sharp fissure through the globalisation process manifests itself in consumer food culture and reflects the rapid concentration of national and international economies everywhere.

The assets of the largest 300 firms in the world are now worth approximately a quarter of the productive assets in the world (*The Economist*, 1993). Transnational corporations (TNCs) now account for 70% of total world trade (i.e. in all goods, not just food). Of those TNCs, the top 350 now account for around 40% (Daly and Goodland, 1992). In food, such power is common, according to research by the United Nations Centre on Transnational Corporations (UNCTC, 1981) and high levels of concentration are common in the food system

(Tansey and Worsley, 1995). Cargill, a family-owned commodity trader, has 60% of world cereal trade (Lang and Hines, 1993). The biggest five corporations control 77% of the cereals trade, the biggest three have 80% of the banana market, the biggest three have 83% of cocoa and the biggest three have 85% of the tea trade (Madden, 1992).

Even in affluent Europe, small, craft and local food producers and traders are under pressure. Between 1980 and 1990, according to UK government census figures, 11% of UK farmers and 34% of farm workers stopped farming, continuing a process begun with industrialisation, but accelerated by the European Union's Common Agricultural Policy (CAP) (SAFE, 1993). Nevertheless, the fiscal impact of CAP is considerable. For instance, 80% of farm support that actually gets to farmers (as opposed to traders or stores) goes to the largest 20% of farms (Great Britain House of Lords, 1992).

Dietary clash of cultures?

To public health specialists, a key contemporary cultural indicator is not the number or plight of farmers and growers, but fruit and vegetable consumption. Generally, in the westernisation of diet, there has been a shift from fresh items (unprocessed, uncooked materials) to frozen or pre-cooked foods. Variations occur even within affluent regions. The British eat fewer vegetables than any other European country, at least half the amount of France, Spain and Italy. This is a significant factor in the UK's lamentable record of food-related ill-health (GB COMA, 1994). Vegetables (and fruits) contain many of the protective factors for coronary heart disease and some cancers (WHO, 1990) which are Britain's main sources of premature death. A government study of the Scottish diet, for instance, found that Scottish children's diets were 'the worst in the western world' (Scottish Office Home and Health Department, 1993). A high proportion of children eat neither green vegetables nor fruit. If this is the picture today, in 1960 it was even more marked, with Scotland eating 60% less vegetables, for instance, than the national average (GB MAFF, 1991).

While UK fruit consumption has increased significantly since the mid-1970s, this is largely accounted for by the very sharp rise in purchases of fruit juice. This raises potential conflict between nutrition and ecology. From the nutritional perspective, source of nutrients is perhaps irrelevant; to the environmental perspective it is not. Northern fruit juice consumption is increasingly of juices from long-distant fruit, notably oranges from Brazil. A study by the Wupperthal Institute in Germany calculated that 80% of Brazilian orange production is consumed in Europe. Annual German consumption occupied 370 000 acres of Brazilian productive land, three times the land down to fruit production in Germany. If this level of German orange juice consumption was replicated world-wide, 32 million acres would be needed just for orange production (Kranendonk and Bringezau, 1994). The increasing range of fruit available throughout the year also contributes to this rise in consumption. A rare attempt to address this conflict was pioneered by the North Karelia project. This set up a scheme to increase fruit and vegetable consumption in this region of Finland from locally grown and processed berries and fruits, while simultaneously meeting employment and environmental objectives (Kuusipalo *et al*, 1988).

Saturated markets, not just saturated fats

The epidemiological evidence on the impact of diet on human health is reasonably clear (WHO, 1990; Cannon, 1992), and echoes the work on the Mediterranean Diet by Ancel Keys and colleagues (1970; 1980), which first provided evidence for the failure of the 'advanced' diet. The message about variations of diet even within populations fits the overall picture, and was reinforced by the huge Chinese dietary survey (Chen Junshi *et al*, 1990).

Today, as food styles are exported, consumers world-wide are encouraged to think of food and drink as coming not from farmers or the earth but from giant corporations. A study in China, for instance, found that 65% of people in China recognise the brand name of Coca-Cola; 42% recognise Pepsi, 40% recognise Nestlé (Gallup, 1995). The global reach of large food corporations is now a major 'driver' behind dietary change (Barnet and Cavanagh, 1995). Brand marketing is facilitated by revolutions in distribution and production. The arrival of this so-called post-Fordist economy, marked by 'flexible specialisation' systems of production, renders the distributor rather than the consumer sovereign (Raven and Lang, 1995), yet much of the orientation of health promotion is centred on educating and informing the consumer. It is likely that this strategy will have to change in coming years (Gabriel and Lang, 1995; Caraher *et al*, 1996). In most markets subject to global trade liberalisation, concentration is rapid, and in many national markets, one or two manufacturers now dominate. The main concern of these giants is not saturated fats, but saturated markets. The tendency for technology-driven modern food systems to yield increases in labour and land productivity simultaneously creates a tendency to over-produce and to 're-fashion nature' in a global assembly line (Goodman and Redclift, 1991). The biotechnology revolution is an extension of this process.

In the food sector, no one has been more significant in revolutionising global food economies than the food retailers (Thrupp, 1995; Raven and Lang, 1995). UK data suggest that the same amount of food merely travels further, up and down the motorways, thereby externalising costs (mainly energy costs) to the environment. These costs are not reflected in the 'cheaper' food prices, as no one actually pays, but every citizen experiences them, and some receive ill-health from them, for example from pollution from increased traffic (Public Health Alliance, 1991). A German study of strawberry yoghurt found ecological absurdities in the system of processing, packaging and distribution, such that a theoretical truckload of 150 g yoghurts would travel 1005 km (Boege, 1993; Paxton, 1994).

The strawberries came from Poland, yoghurt from North Germany, corn and wheat flour from the Netherlands, jam from West Germany and sugar beet from East Germany. The aluminium for use on the cover travelled 300 km. Only the milk and glass jar were local to Stuttgart, where the yoghurt theoretically 'came from'. To produce one truckload of strawberry yoghurt, 10 000 litres of diesel fuel had been burned. In Britain, the distance that food is transported has gone up by nearly 50% between 1976 and 1992. The growth of long-distance food in the UK has been the single greatest cause of increasing road freight distance travel (Hillman, 1994).

Independent small retailers tend to source their food more locally, whereas giant stores want the regularity of supply that can only be given by large factories, large contracts, large growers and all-year-round sources (Feder, 1977). The process also sets developing country producers against each other in the race to feed the affluent, for instance Kenya against The Gambia in vegetable production (Barrett and Browne, 1994). This also has the effect of institutionalising reliance upon distant lands, the 'ghost acres' phenomenon, where the supposed efficiency of Northern farming is in fact subsidised by cheap inputs from abroad, notably in the form of animal feeds (Paxton, 1994; van Brakel and Zagema, 1994). Just under half of European animal feed is imported, 20% of it soya. In 1989, 77% of Brazil's soya bean exports went to Europe. In 1970, 1.4 million hectares in Brazil were down to soya. By 1988, it was 10.5 million (Smith, 1993). Brazil had, until recently, one of the world's worst child malnutrition rates. The Netherlands now needs to export animal manure; its soils cannot cope with absorbing the by-products of this intensification, and it now exports dung to other European states, and even to India. Cheap fossil fuel energy makes agriculture and long-distance transport economically viable. The damage is externalised onto the environment.

A theoretical 'average' European weekend shopping trolley contains goods that have already travelled 4000 km before the shopper takes them home (Griffiths, 1993). The European Commission's Taskforce on the Environment calculated that there would be a 30–50% increase in trans-frontier lorry traffic from 1993 following the opening of national borders within the Single European Market (European Commission, 1992). Total lorry traffic is expected to double between 1989 and 2010. The reality of hypermarket shopping is that people have to use their cars to get food, thereby severing a connection between health-enhancing exercise and their daily lives. Expending energy then becomes an additional lifestyle burden: the financial and emotional cost of a gym or sport. According to the UK government's National Travel Survey, the number of shopping trips in Britain rose by 28% between 1975/6 and 1989/91 and the total distance travelled increased by 60% over the same period (Whitelegg, 1995). The number of car-dependent trips and the distance travelled have gone up rapidly. In 1985 62% of people used their car for their main shopping; by 1993 this had risen to 73% (Henley Centre, 1994). This change in distribution not only gives retailers power over the entire food system, but also affects what the farmer grows and how she or he grows it, by the use of contracts and specifications, and also affects poor consumers. They have to pay for transport that they can ill afford. Needless to say, the specifications stipulate that food is unblemished, of a certain size, uniformity, and so on, which only a narrow form of farming can produce. Shops sell vegetables from all over the world, that can be grown, and often used to be grown, locally.

The impact on food culture and public health

In theory, under the GATT agreement, subsidies are to be phased down, but serious doubts have been expressed as to whether that is happening. Oxfam is not alone in doubting the morality of US and European Union policies towards developing nations (Watkins, 1995; 1996). The European Union's own Liaison Committee of Development Non Government Organisations (NGOs) of the European Union has argued:

> Reliance on trade to achieve national food security is not usually an appropriate policy for developing countries: dependence on food imports creates vulnerability to world markets and prices. In reality trade flows are controlled more by powerful corporations than by governments. We urge a greater degree of self-reliance in food production, at national or regional level.
> (Liaison Committee of Development NGOs to the European Communities, 1994)

Any country that participates in a deregulated global food system is likely to find its potential to create a sustainable local food system weakened by a reliance upon foreign suppliers. An export orientation imposed on its farmers means a dislocation in food culture: produce is sold which is not consumed locally, and products are consumed which are produced elsewhere. This new economic regime undermines the policies of those developing countries which were previously committed to policies of national food self-reliance, such as Mexico and the Philippines (Watkins, 1996).

GATT's supporters claim that the least developed countries are exempt from having to remove their agricultural import barriers and that, in the case of staple foods, no developing country has to follow GATT tariff regulations designed to reduce import barriers. But this ignores the fact that the International Monetary Fund structural adjustment programmes require exactly this condition, thus rendering the GATT exemption virtually meaningless. The reasons that developing countries agreed to this was that they hoped that the GATT agreement would reduce the dumping of surplus Northern food and offer the possibility of more access for developing countries' produce to the markets of the North.

Proponents of the trade liberalisation model of development make much of the GATT's 21% reduction in the volume of subsidised exports, glossing over the fact that this still leaves about 80% still in place. The EU CAP's subsidies for grain are to be reduced by 30%, but already development agencies and trade analysts have expressed dissatisfaction with the deal, saying this will not end the disastrous dumping of exports on developing countries. The EU has swapped one form of subsidy for another, taking away the direct support of markets and replacing it with direct subsidies to the farmer (Gardner, 1994).

The GATT vision for agriculture is for it to be more export-focused, and to emulate the Northern model of industrialised efficiency. National barriers to protect local production are to be dismantled. Self-reliance is out, trade is in. As a result, regional food security is being eroded and urbanisation accelerated. The United Nations Population Fund (UNFPA) already warns that developing countries will face huge new internal migration from rural to urban areas as people look for work. On current trends, which should be treated with caution, world population will grow by 2.6 billion by the year 2025 (CWFS, 1996). Some 1.3 billion will be added to the workforces of Asia, Africa and Latin America in the next decade. Cities will contain half the world's population by 2020 (UNFPA, 1994).

At present around 3 billion of the world's 5.5 billion people live in rural areas (UN, 1991). If the rural–urban spread of population of some of the richest 'efficient' agricultural systems like Canada, Australia or the UK were to be applied to the world, 1.9 billion of those rural dwellers would live in towns. To do what? Fed by whom? On current trends, these new urban dwellers will be cheap urban labour, if they are lucky. No wonder agricultural policy experts are once more rehearsing the argument that restraints on US and EU overproduction should be reversed. Now the argument is that the North should feed the South (Carruthers, 1995; Ritchie, 1996). The goal of food security could be evaporating in the face of new commercial reality benefiting the North's intensive farmers. One does not have to be a Malthusian to view this scenario with some trepidation. Where is employment to come from? The GATT voices fall silent at this point.

For all its complexity, the globalisation process, driven by Northern tastes and marketed everywhere in the name of Northern culture and capital, offers formidable challenges to food and public health thinking. When governments argue that they can do little but bow to market pressure and facilitate its mechanisms, the very notion of public health intervention may be troublesome. This is an ideological issue rather than a real barrier to action (Hirst and Thompson, 1996). The world actually needs a shift away from cheap export-led food policies to more local production for local use everywhere. This requires more people on the land, not throwing people off to make the economic audit of farming look more 'efficient'. The goal should be to build a better quality of life in the country, not to drive people into towns; to reduce inequalities; and to make public and environmental health part of economics, not a bolt-on extra. As part of this re-invention of the public health function, new indices will be needed to integrate environmental, consumer and health considerations. For example, the promotion of variety of species—hitherto a concern of ecologists—may provide a pointer. Diversity from farm to plate, too, is measurable, as is the distance that food travels—the so-called 'food miles/kilometres' indicator.

References

Adshead SAM. *Salt and Civilisation*. London: Macmillan, 1992

Avery N, Drake M, Lang T. *Cracking the Codex: Report for 50 Consumer NGOs*. London: National Food Alliance, 1993

Barnet R, Cavanagh J. *Global Dreams*. New York: Simon & Schuster, 1995

Barrett H, Browne A. *The internationalisation of vegetable production: the incorporation of sub-Saharan Africa with particular reference to The Gambia*. Unpublished paper. Coventry University, School of Natural and Environmental Sciences, Geography Division, 1994

Baum F, Sanders D. Can health promotion and primary health care achieve health for all without a return to their more radical agenda? *Health Promotion International*, 1995; **10**: 149–160

Boege S. *Road Transport of Goods and the Effects on the Spatial Environment*. Wupperthal: Wupperthal Institute, 1993

Broad R, Cavanagh J. Don't neglect the impoverished South. *Foreign Policy*, 1995; **101**: 18-35

Cannon G. *Food and Health: The Experts Agree*. London: Consumers' Association, 1992

Caraher M, Dixon P, Lang T. *Buying, eating and cooking food: A review of a national data set on food attitudes, skills and behavioural change*. Report to the Health Education Authority, January 1996

Carruthers ID. *2020 Vision for World Food Supply*. Paper for British Association meeting, 1995. Wye: Department of Economics, 1995

Chen Junshi T, Campbell C, Li Junyao, Peto R. *Diet, Lifestyle and Mortality in China*. Oxford: Oxford University Press, 1990

Cockett R. *Thinking the Unthinkable: Think-tanks and the Economic Counter-Revolution 1931–1983*. London: HarperCollins, 1994

Committee on World Food Security (CWFS). *Towards Universal Food Security*. Draft policy statement and plan of action. 21st Session. Item III. Rome: Food and Agriculture Organisation. 29 January–2 February 1996

Coote B. *The Trade Trap: Poverty and the Global Commodity Markets*. Oxford: Oxfam, 1992

Daly H, Goodland R. *An Ecological-Economic Assessment of Deregulation of International Commerce under GATT*. Washington, DC: World Bank Environment Department, September 1992

Dowler E. Looking for 'fresh' food: Diet and lone parents. *Proceedings of the Nutrition Society*, 1995; **54**, 759–769

Dowler E, Rushton C. *Diet and Poverty in the UK*. London: Department of Public Health and Policy, publication 11, London School of Hygiene & Tropical Medicine, 1994

Durning AT. *How Much is Enough?: The Consumer Society and the Future of the Earth*. London: Earthscan, 1992

The Economist. *Survey of Multinationals*, 27 March 1993

European Commission. *1992: The Environmental Dimension. Taskforce Report on the Environment and the Internal Market*. Brussels: European Commission, 1992

Feder E. *Strawberry Imperialism*. The Hague: Institute of Social Studies, 1977

Friedmann H, McMichael P. Agriculture and the state system: rise and decline of agricultures, 1870–present. *Sociologica Ruralis*, 1989; **29**: 2

Gabriel Y, Lang T. *The Unmanageable Consumer: Contemporary Consumption and its Fragmentation*. London: Sage, 1995

Gallup. *Financial Times Exporter*, Summer 1995

Gardner B. EU dumping to continue. In CIIR, ed. *The GATT Agreement on Agriculture: Will it Help Developing Countries?* London: Catholic Institute for International Relations, 1994

Goldin I, Knudsen O, van der Mensbrugghe D. *Trade Liberalisation: Global Economic Implications*. Paris: OECD, 1993

Goodman D, Redclift M. *Refashioning Nature: Food, Ecology and Culture*. London: Routledge, 1991

Great Britain Committee on Medical Aspects of Food Policy (GB COMA). Cardiovascular Review Group. *Nutritional Aspects of Cardiovascular Disease*. London: HMSO, 1994

Great Britain House of Lords Select Committee Report on the European Communities. *Development and the Future of the Common Agricultural Policy*. HL Paper 791, London: HMSO, 1992

Great Britain Ministry of Agriculture, Fisheries and Food (GB MAFF). *Household Food Consumption and Expenditure 1990, with a Study of Trends over the Period 1940-90. Annual Report of the National Food Survey Committee*. London: HMSO, 1991

Griffiths J. A freer flow of goods. *Financial Times*, 12 March 1993

Henley Centre. *Planning for Social Change*. London: Henley Centre for Forecasting, 1994

Hillman M. *Changing Patterns of Shopping, Drawn from National Travel Surveys 1975/76 to 1989/91*. London: Policy Studies Institute, 1994

Hirst PQ, Thompson, G. *Globalization in Question: The International Economy and the Possibilities of Governance*. Cambridge: Polity Press, 1996

Jenkins R. *Bringing Rio Home: Biodiversity and Farming*. London: Sustainable Agriculture, Food and Environment Alliance, 1992

Keys A, ed. Coronary heart disease in seven countries. American Heart Association Monograph No. 29. *Circulation*, 1970; **41** (suppl 1), 1–211

Keys A. *Seven Countries: A Multivariate Analysis of Death and Coronary Heart Disease*. Cambridge, MA: Harvard University Press, 1980

Kranendonk S, Bringezau B. *Major Material Flows Associated with Orange Juice Consumption in Germany*. Wupperthal: Wupperthal Institute, 1994

Kuusipalo J, Mikkola M, Moisio S, Puska P. Two years of the East Finland Berry and Vegetable Project: an offshoot of the North Karelia Project. *Health Promotion International*, 1988; **3**, 313–317

Lang T, Hines C. *The New Protectionism: Protecting the Future against Free Trade*. London: Earthscan, 1993

Liaison Committee of Development NGOs to the European Communities. *Food Security Beyond 2000*. Brussels, January 1994

Low Income Project Team (LIPT). *Low Income, Food, Nutrition and Health: Strategies for Improvement. Report of the Low Income Project Team of the Nutrition Taskforce*. London: Department of Health, 1996

Lobstein T. *Fast Food Facts*. London: Camden Press, 1988

Lupton D. *The Imperative of Health: Public Health and the Regulated Body*. London: Sage, 1995

Madden P. *A Raw Deal: Trade and the World's Poor*. London: Christian Aid, 1992

McMichael AJ. *Planetary Overload: Global Environmental Change and the Health of the Human Species*. Cambridge: Cambridge University Press, 1993

Mennell S, Murcott A, van Otterloo AH. *The Sociology of Food: Eating, Diet and Culture*. London: Sage, 1992

Mintz SW. *Sweetness and Power: The Place of Sugar in Modern History*. New York: Viking, 1985

Morgan D. *Merchants of Grain*. London: Weidenfeld and Nicolson, 1979

Oxfam International. *Multilateral Debt: The Human Costs*. Oxford: Oxfam, 1996

Paxton A. *The Food Miles Report*. London: Sustainable Agriculture, Food and Environment (SAFE) Alliance, 1994

Public Health Alliance. *Health on the Move: Policies for Health-Promoting Transport: The Policy Statement of the Transport and Health Study Group*. Birmingham: Public Health Alliance, 1991

Raghavan C. *Recolonization: GATT, the Uruguay Round and the Third World*. London: Zed Press, 1990

Raikes P. *Modernising hunger: famine, food surplus and farm policy in the EEC and Africa*. London: Catholic Institute for International Relations /James Currey, 1988

Raven H, Lang T. *Off our Trolleys?: Food Retailing and the Hypermarket Economy*. London: Institute for Public Policy Research, 1995

Rifkin J. *Beyond Beef: The Rise and Fall of the Cattle Culture*. New York: Dutton, 1992

Ritchie M. *World Food Shortages and the Threat to Sustainable Farming: the Paradox of Higher World Market Prices for Grains*. Minneapolis: Institute for Agriculture and Trade Policy, 1996

Ritzer G. *The McDonaldization of Society: An Investigation into the Changing Character of Contemporary Social Life*. Thousand Oaks, CA: Pine Forge Press, 1993

Rowling N. *Commodities: How the World was Taken to Market*. London: Free Association Books, 1987

SAFE. *What future?* London: Sustainable Agriculture, Food and Environment Alliance, 1993

Scottish Office Home and Health Department. *The Scottish Diet. Report of the James Committee*. Edinburgh: Scottish Office, 1993

Shiva V, Holla-Bhar R. Intellectual piracy and the neem tree. *The Ecologist*, 1993; **23**: 223–227

Smith, A. The world of soya. *Food Matters Worldwide*, 1993; **19**

Surgeon General of the United States. *The Surgeon General's Report on Nutrition and Health*. Washington, DC: US Department of Health and Human Services, 1988

Tansey G, Worsley T. *The Food System: A Guide*. London: Earthscan, 1995

Thrupp LA. *Bittersweet Harvest for Global Supermarkets: Challenges in Latin America's Agricultural Export Boom*. Washington, DC: World Resources Institute, 1995

United Nations. *World Urbanisation Prospects 1990*. New York: Oxford University Press for the United Nations, 1991

United Nations Centre on Transnational Corporations (UNCTC). *Transnational Corporations in Food and Beverage Processing*. New York: UNCTC, 1981

United Nations Children's Fund (UNICEF). *Food, Health and Care: The UNICEF Vision and Strategy for a World Free from Hunger and Malnutrition*. New York: UNICEF, 1993

United Nations Development Programme (UNDP). *Human Development Report 1995*. New York: UNDP, 1995

United Nations Fund for Population Activities (UNFPA). *State of the World Population 1994*. New York: UNPFA, 1994

United States Department of Agriculture (USDA). *Long-term Agricultural Trade Strategy FY 1996*. Washington, DC, 1995

van Brakel M, Zagema B. *Sustainable Netherlands*. Amsterdam: Friends of the Earth International, 1994

Watkins K. *Agriculture and Farm Trade in the GATT*. CAP Briefing no. 20. London: Catholic Institute for International Relations, March 1989

Watkins K. Agriculture and food security in the GATT Uruguay Round. *Review of African Political Economy*, 1991; **50**: 38–50

Watkins K. *Fixing the Rules*. London: Catholic Institute for International Relations, 1992

Watkins K. *The Oxfam Poverty Report*. Oxford: Oxfam, 1995

Watkins K. *Creating Dependence: the Impact of Northern Food Systems on the South*. Southeast Asian NGO Conference on Food Security and Fair Trade, Quezon City, Philippines, 13–16 February 1996

Whitelegg J. *Driven to Shop*. London: SAFE Alliance/Lancaster: Eco-logica, 1995

Wilkinson RG. National Mortality Rates: The Impact of Inequality? *American Journal of Public Health*, 1992; **82**: 1082–1084

World Bank. *Poverty and Hunger: Issues and Options for Food Security in Developing Countries*. Washington, DC: World Bank, 1986

World Health Organization (WHO). *Health for All by the Year 2000*. Copenhagen: World Health Organization, 1985

World Health Organization (WHO). *The Ottawa Charter for Health Promotion*. Copenhagen: World Health Organization, 1987

World Health Organization (WHO). *Diet, Nutrition and the Prevention of Chronic Diseases*, Technical Series no. 797. Geneva: World Health Organization, 1990

Discussion

Anthony J. McMichael

Epidemiology Unit, London School of Hygiene & Tropical Medicine, UK

Tim Lang has presented an admirable compilation and critique of many facets of this complex topic. Nevertheless, there are three aspects that warrant further exploration:

1. The need to see contemporary globalisation as part of a longer narrative of economic restructuring of the modern world; to distinguish it from the preceding era of politically coordinated national economic management; and to note its potentially transitional nature as we move to an uncertain, perhaps unsustainable, future.
2. The need to give balanced consideration to the *full* spectrum of public health consequences of globalisation of food trade—that is, both the direct consequences of over-nutrition and under-nutrition and the more diffuse consequences from the social and ecological disruptions attendant upon that globalisation.
3. Related to the second point, we need to recognise the ecological nature of this

topic. Too many of our policy-makers—and scientists—still think of food-and-health in technical single-issue terms, directed at ensuring adequate intakes of specified nutrients, minimising exposure to potentially toxic contaminants, and ensuring microbiological safety. Meanwhile, our international food trade degrades productive land, diminishes biodiversity, creates monoculture vulnerability, and dismantles historically evolved sustainable patterns of land-use.

Human societies have traded food throughout recorded history, whether it be spices entering Renaissance Europe or salt and iodine-rich coastal foods carried up the mountain slopes in Papua New Guinea and South America. Such regional and international trade is traditionally transacted on a bilateral basis, often subject to local constraints, customs and conventions. At the height of the Roman Empire, 1000 tons of wheat were imported daily to Rome from North Africa. Providing bread and circuses for an urban population of approximately one million was a constant struggle. Many tons of imported elephants, bears, lions and Christians were also required.

Globalisation is different. It is something more than the world-wide expansion of trade. It seeks to reshape and integrate the world according to the prevailing Western models of economic development and consumption. Its most obvious goals are enhanced economic activity, efficiency and profitability. It must therefore inculcate preferences in an ever-expanding consumer market. We see it with cigarettes, motor cars and food. As the barriers of Communism erode, as transnational companies accrue more power and freedom, as deregulation and privatisation proceed apace, and as national governments are increasingly confined to a minimalist role of economic management, so public health considerations have come under siege on a wide front.

Lang has argued that the new era of global trade liberalisation, embodied in the 1994 GATT agreement, will greatly affect agriculture and the distribution of food. It will result in an escalation of existing trends in food production and processing practices—including a consolidation of monopoly control, in the diversion and dismantling of local food production and culture, in the prolongation of the gap between rich and poor and the 'modernising of hunger' (Raikes, 1988), and in the manipulation of urban consumer food preferences. In turn, he argues, this will cause the spread of the chronic degenerative diseases of nutritional 'affluence' in those targeted consumer populations. He describes a globalised world in which attention to the public health consequences of dis-nutrition is usurped by the economic manager's mantra of successful competition in the new global marketplace. Thus, food is no longer to be seen principally as *nutrition*—as it has long been implicitly understood within human culture; nor is food even to be seen as *basic energy*—as it is often measured by FAO and others concerned to avert frank hunger. Instead, food becomes a tradeable *commodity*; it becomes an instrument of economic management, political leverage, and commercial profit.

Lang describes the US Department of Agriculture salivating over the prospects of selling value-added energy-dense consumer foods to increasingly accessible, media-impressionable, Asian countries, indifferent to considerations of the near-certain adverse public health consequences. This is global 'dietary burgerisation'. Something about that sounds eerily familiar. In this country we are currently gripped by the socially damaging consequences of a Ministry of Agriculture, Fisheries and Food that similarly acts as the *de facto* advocate of producer interests; it therefore supports cheap, profitable, mass-produced food, while appearing indifferent to consumer health.

There is manifestly great public health portent in the macroscopic processes that Lang describes. But I suggest that we cannot easily make sense of the so-called 'globalisation' of food trade unless we know a little about its history. The modern human species has been foraging for food for 150 000 years, farming it for 10 000 years, and industrially processing it for 100 years. For a brief 40 years we have been seeking a coordinated international strategy to feed the world's rapidly expanding, newly decolonised, populations. In the 1950s and 1960s, the Fordist–Keynesian form of Western national capitalism—i.e. the politically managed model of mass production that brought postwar national prosperity to the First World—was diffused across the expanding array of nation-states. Economic development strategists assumed that this idealised model, based on the US political economy, was the way forward to self-sufficiency. A gradual internationalisation of food production and distribution followed, including the beginnings of the Green Revolution, the marketing of unprecedented food surpluses and the unsubtle competition for client states during the Cold War.

Subsequently in the 1970s, instability of trade and exchange rates occurred, coupled with the oil crisis and a flood of Euro-dollars. This, plus the collapse of various commodity prices and the resultant debt crisis in the 1980s, unleashed new forces of internationalisation. Nation-states were adrift on a turbulent ocean of newly mobilised, deregulated, capital. Meanwhile, Western-based transnational companies were gaining in size and influence. The Green Revolution, which had produced some spectacular gains in agricultural yields over two to three decades, began to lose momentum. Clearly, the international Development Project was faltering, and debt repayments were seriously jeopardised. Accordingly, the IMF moved to restructure precarious Third World national economies, and a new round (the Uruguay Round) of GATT negotiations was initiated in the mid-1980s. This, as Lang points out, included agriculture for the first time.

So, here we are in the 1990s, living through a transitional era in a rapidly changing world. The more general question has been asked: 'Are these restructuring processes presaging a new order—or simply rearranging the old order, now in crisis?' (McMichael, 1994). Global capital markets and transnational firms are integrating and transforming local food systems. New and internationally standardised 'social diets', divergent from traditional diets, are emerging. Meanwhile, a carefully managed specialty production and niche marketing of profitable foods has arisen—exotic fruits, fragrant coffee beans, *légumes fines*, and cut flowers. Thus, First World luxuries displace Third World necessities.

If this globalised configuration is indeed part of a new economic order, then its implications for public health may go well beyond those discussed by Lang. However, there is lively debate about the nature and extent of this globalisation process (Sklair, 1991). Is it a process or an outcome? The sheer scale of the modern operation of transnational companies, the freedoms they increasingly enjoy in a deregulated world, and the evolving and empathetic policies of the Western-dominated multilateral finance institutions all make globalisation *seem* real enough.

Meanwhile, ranged against globalisation are some countervailing forces. Humans are fundamentally tribal—as, tragically, we keep reminding ourselves with disastrous conflicts. Our cultures are surprisingly resilient. Various new social movements have arisen in response to the threats posed by globalised economic activities to local environments, societies and culture. These groups, now linking up around the world, draw increasing attention to the various adverse environmental and social impacts of the economic development agenda. Finally, deep-seated local and national concerns over food security ensure that access to food—that is, its social *use* value as opposed to its *exchange* value in the marketplace—remains a powerful criterion of political legitimacy.

So, the globalisation of food trade is recognisably a *new* stage in the longer historical process of the transformation and appropriation, by international capital, of the production and distribution of food. We should also note, however, that the food trade has been less amenable to capital-intensive industrialising processes than are the production and distribution of non-biological commodities. So, the food story is more complex than are those, say, for clothing, cars and electronic goods. There is an irreducible *biological* basis to the production of food, via plants and animals, and to its consumption by ingesting and digesting humans. Those biological realities limit the possibilities for industrial transformation and appropriation of food production, processing and distribution (Goodman and Redclift, 1991).

Lang is properly concerned about the impact of globalisation upon local food security and public health. Globalisation, in its quest for international integration of production and marketing, substantially articulated between subsidiary firms *within* powerful diversified transnational corporations, tends to cause *dis*-integration at the national and local levels. In the same way that hypermarket chains, with their standardised routines and products across and between countries, cause disorganisation and weakening of local shopping centres that are well attuned to local needs, so globalisation is, by definition, indifferent to localised impacts.

Now, there is some good, along with all of this actual or potential bad! For example, globalisation *has* increased the year-round availability of fresh fruit and vegetables (FFV)—at least for privileged urban populations (Friedland, 1994).

Before this century, FFV were seasonal. Then we saw the emergence of Latin American 'banana republics' as that durable tropical fruit became an export crop. Subsequently, First World supermarkets have increasingly demanded year-round supplies of FFV, such that by the 1980s Western consumers could depend on: (i) an extended growing season—achieved via new plant-breeding, horticultural techniques, and international diversity of production sites, and (ii) an increased range of FFV—especially tropical exotic fruits and vegetables.

But the good news is eclipsed by the bad news. We can envisage four main types of public health impact consequent upon the globalisation of world food trade. They are:

1. *The inculcation of imbalanced and calorically excessive Western diets in non-Western populations.* The pattern of ensuing chronic disease burdens is now extensively chronicled (WHO, 1990).
2. *The dietary deprivation of poor rural populations, whose local agricultural resources have been diverted into export agriculture*—and who, by remaining or becoming impoverished, are unable to purchase adequate replacement food.
3. *The health consequences of community disintegration, population displacement, unemployment, and seasonal farm-labouring on foreign-owned cash-crop plantations.* The studies of René Loewenson (1988), in Zimbabwe, attest to the adverse maternal and child health consequences that have resulted from the insecure seasonal employment of local women. The competitive pressures that Lang describes, between Kenya and The Gambia, in the scramble to supply cheap fresh vegetables to Europe would have similar health consequences for those source communities. Other examples abound in the literature—for example, the displacement to the remote Amazon of thousands of peasants from south-eastern Brazil because of agribusiness acquisition of land for the export-production of soybeans; or the displacement of forest-dwelling and agrarian groups in Central America because of the need for new pastoral land to produce burger meat for the USA (McMichael PD, 1996).
4. *The probable future public health consequences of the systemic environmental damage that results from the huge 'ecological footprints' of the globalised agro-food industry.* The problem is not just that the mix of food products urged upon urban consumers may be unhealthy—it is that the production of much of this food is wasteful of energy and resources, and is *not* the basis for an ecologically sustainable diet for 10 billion people in the next century. This issue extends now to the massive and growing contributions of fossil fuel combustion, flatulent cows and irrigated agriculture to greenhouse gas accumulation. Increasingly, we understand and foresee the adverse public health consequences that will result from living in a climatically altered world (McMichael AJ *et al*, 1996).

Lang emphasises the first of these four categories of health impact. He mentions the second, and refers to the modernisation of hunger. However, he has not explicitly addressed the last two categories of impact—although he does note each of the underlying problems.

The burgeoning distances that the prospective contents of a cup of yoghurt now travel in a trade-liberalised Europe, as described by Lang, are matched by countless other environmentally damaging absurdities. I pay little more for a bottle of Australian wine in London than I did in Adelaide; however, someone somewhere must eventually pay for the externalised environmental 'costs' of that bottle's energy-intensive transport half way around the world. Likewise, I presume that The Netherlands' exportation of their unmanageable excess of domestic cattle dung to India is not via magic carpet; that transportation too incurs large environmental costs. Thus, much about our increasingly globalised food trade depends on sleight-of-hand accounting. Payment of those accounts cannot be deferred indefinitely.

This leads me to my third main point—the need to perceive, and to communicate, the essentially ecological dimensions of this topic. It is clear from much that Lang has said, from considering the wider messages from the BSE episode about the consequences of unnatural and intensive methods of food production, and from several of the arguments that I have presented here that we depend on the long-term productivity of complex ecological systems for our food supplies. Food is *not* like dishwashers, cars and radios.

A ready reminder of the ecological complexity underlying food production and health comes from a recently identified nutritional problem faced by poor populations in underdeveloped countries. A review by the Washington-based International Food Policy Research Institute concludes that the Green Revolution, while achieving widespread caloric success, has led to increases in maternal anaemia and in childhood deficiencies in iron, zinc and beta-carotene (Seymour, 1996). The higher-yielding strains of wheat and rice, replete with more energy-rich macronutrients, do not achieve comparable increases in these micronutrients. Again, the message is that, as we tinker with natural food-producing processes and systems, so we risk unforeseen adverse ecological outcomes. The recent fate of the Grand Banks cod fishery reminds us that some such heavy-handed mismanagement can lead to serious, sometimes irreversible, consequences.

In conclusion, as Lang has argued, the real problems with the globalisation of food production and distribution are that, first, economic control has moved from national governments to largely unaccountable (or at least deregulated) transnational capital, and, second, the underlying ethic has moved from seeking coordinated national social gain—however inadequately or unevenly—to seeking private profit. As long as the marketplace eclipses the legislative chamber, the prospect for public health is bleak. We must dare to hope that globalisation, as we are currently coming to know it, will in turn be replaced by an ethic of ecologically sustainable development.

That would be good for public health.

References

Friedland WH. The global fresh fruit and vegetable system: An industrial organization analysis. In: McMichael PD (ed), *The Global Restructuring of Agro-Food Systems.* Ithaca: Cornell University Press, 1994, 173–189

Goodman D, Redclift M. *Refashioning Nature. Food, Ecology and Culture.* London: Routledge, 1991

Loewenson R. Labour insecurity and health: an epidemiological study in Zimbabwe. *Social Science and Medicine,* 1988; **27**: 733–741

McMichael AJ, Andro M, Carcavallo R *et al.* Population health impacts. In: Watson RT, Zinyowera MC, Moss RH (eds), *Climate Change 1995: Impacts, Adaptations and Mitigation of Climate Change: Scientific-Technical Analyses.* Contribution of Working Group II to the Second Assessment Report of the Intergovernmental Panel on Climate Change. Cambridge and New York: Cambridge University Press, 1996

McMichael PD. Introduction: Agro-food system restructuring—unity in diversity. In: McMichael PD (ed), *The Global Restructuring of Agro-Food Systems.* Ithaca: Cornell University Press, 1994, 1–17

McMichael PD. *Development and Social Change: A Global Perspective.* Thousand Oaks, CA: Pine Forge Press, 1996

Raikes P. *Modernising Hunger: Famine, Food Surplus and Farm Policy in the EEC and Africa.* London: Catholic Institute for International Relations/James Currey, 1988

Seymour J. Hungry for a new revolution. *New Scientist,* 30 March 1996, 32–37

Sklair L. *Sociology of the Global System.* Hemel Hempstead: Harvester Wheatsheaf, 1991

World Health Organization. *Diet, Nutrition and the Prevention of Chronic Diseases.* Technical Report Series, No. 797. Geneva: WHO, 1990

10
Some aspects of Norwegian nutrition and food policy

Kaare R. Norum

Institute for Nutrition Research, University of Oslo, and National Nutrition Council, Oslo, Norway

In 1946 when Norway instituted the National Nutrition Council (NNC), the main nutritional problem was that little food was available in a post-war situation. Hence, until around 1950, the main challenges for the Norwegian nutrition and food policy were to ensure enough and varied food for the population. After 1950, however, the dietary problems changed in character, with overnutrition and unbalanced diet becoming more prevalent. There was a substantial increase in mortality from coronary heart diseases (CHD) (Norwegian Central Bureau of Statistics, 1987), an increase which was most probably associated with changes in food habits and lifestyle. The General Director of Health set up an expert committee which led to an official Norwegian report on the relationship between diet and cardiovascular diseases. The experts recommended a decrease in the fat content of the national diet to 30% of the dietary energy, mainly by reducing the intake of saturated fat (Nicolaysen *et al*, 1963) and the report formed a basis for the subsequent developments related to Norwegian nutrition and food policy. However, it took some time before an official nutrition and food policy was formulated.

As the relationship between diet and CHD gradually gained acceptance, the NNC made several attempts to influence government policy goals in line with the new knowledge. Simultaneously, consumer interest in and concern with food and health were growing, which brought nutritional issues to the attention, not only of politicians, but also of the media and the general public. These efforts resulted in considerable attention to the issues of nutrition, health and agriculture. Yet they were not adequate to create actual changes at policy level. Until 1973, the Ministry of Social Affairs and the Directorate of Health, who were responsible for

Diet, Nutrition and Chronic Disease: Lessons from Contrasting Worlds.
Edited by P. S. Shetty and K. McPherson © 1997 John Wiley & Sons, Ltd.

nutrition policy, played a passive role, and made no explicit effort to bring about policy changes.

The first White Paper on nutrition and food policy

At the FAO/WHO World Food Conference in Rome in 1974, it was stated that each nation should have a nutrition and food policy. The Norwegian delegation at the Conference was headed by the Minister of Agriculture, who took the initiative to formulate a nutrition and food policy, and presented a White Paper on *Norwegian nutrition and food policy* to the Parliament (Norwegian Ministry of Agriculture, 1975). The main goals were:

- the encouragement of healthy dietary habits;
- the formulation of a nutrition and food policy in accordance with the recommendations of the World Food Conference;
- the increased production and consumption of domestic food and strengthening of the ability to increase rapidly the degree of self-sufficiency in the food supply; and, as the highest priority;
- utilisation of the food production resources in the economically weaker areas.

The policy document stated that the Government would prepare a policy which would contribute to the following:

> The beneficial aspects of the diet are to be preserved. Conditions will be arranged so that the diet is better adapted to nutritional requirements, while general demands for taste, variety and diversity are stressed. The different nutritional requirements of special groups such as children and young people, pregnant and breastfeeding mothers, the elderly, must also be taken into consideration.
>
> In order to obtain a better adaptation of the diet to nutritional requirements it is especially important to curtail the proportion of fat in the energy supply. An objective should be to reduce the proportion of fat to 35% of the energy supply through a gradual alteration of the diet.
>
> The decrease in the supply of fat should be replaced by foods containing starch—primarily cereals and potatoes. There should be an attempt to limit the proportion of sugar in the energy supply.
>
> The proportion of polyunsaturated fatty acids in the total fat intake should be increased.

The goal for the average fat consumption in the policy document was 35% energy, whereas the experts had advocated for 30% energy (Nicolaysen *et al*, 1963). The official goal was a compromise between the NNC and the agricultural lobby who feared that a lower fat target would lead to a reduced consumption of meat and dairy products.

In this first White Paper on nutrition policy it was pointed out that the central question was the *means* to be used to influence the production and consumption of food products in accordance with the objectives of the policy. Emphasis was put on collaboration between the public sector; organisations, enterprises and employees in the relevant economic sectors; voluntary organisations; and various categories of households. In particular, the information, education and training measures were emphasised, aiming at motivating people to adopt better dietary habits, ensuring a broad general knowledge of the main principles of a nutritionally healthy diet, and providing for the possibility of acquiring necessary skills.

To achieve this, a wide range of measures have been used, including:

- public and professional education and information;
- setting of consumer and producer price and income subsidies jointly in nutritionally justifiable ways;
- the adjustment of absolute and relative consumer food price subsidies;
- ensuring low prices for food grain, skimmed and low-fat milk, vegetables and potatoes;
- the avoidance of low prices for sugar, butter and margarine;
- the marking of regulations to promote provision of healthy foods by retail stores, street vendors and institutions; and
- the regulation of food processing and labelling.

One of the successes of the Norwegian food and nutrition policy was the information and public education organised by the NNC, especially through the use of programmes on the national public television channel, and nationwide, long-lasting nutrition campaigns. Higher training or education at university level was also important. The Nordic School of Nutrition at the University of Oslo has trained nutritionists since 1965, and by 1990 almost 500 nutritionists from the Nordic Countries had graduated. More than two-thirds of this group are Norwegian, of whom about 70 specialised in clinical nutrition (Oshaug, 1994).

There is now significant development of nutrition education within the Medical Faculty of the University of Oslo, which was virtually non-existent in the early 1970s. Nutrition as a subject developed first as an elective, and later as a compulsory, course where students were exposed to nutrition as an area of applied biochemistry and physiology with lectures including diet, clinical nutrition and nutrition policy. In 1990, the teachers running the course also produced a tailor-made textbook of nutrition intended for medical students (Bjørneboe et al, 1990).

Two other projects in the health sector were of great importance for implementation of the nutrition policy. First, the 'Oslo Study', a randomised prospective study which showed that a change in diet reduced CHD in middle-aged men who had high blood cholesterol levels (Hjermann et al, 1981). The men in the treatment group reduced their saturated fat intake, which led to a 10% reduction in their blood cholesterol level, whereas the control group did not get any dietary advice, and their blood cholesterol level remained unchanged. After five years the CHD incidence in the treatment group was only half that in the control group. The results of the Oslo Study convinced both the population and the politicians of the importance of changing to a leaner diet. Secondly, the National Health Screening Service (NHSS) has been and still is conducting health surveys in all parts of Norway (Bjartveit *et al*, 1979). All inhabitants aged 40 are offered a health examination including measurement of blood lipids, blood pressure and chest X-ray. Those with high risk factors for CHD are referred to the local health authorities for follow-up. The health surveys have given valuable information on CHD risk factors, and have documented changes in these parameters during the period when the country has had an active nutrition policy (Bjartveit *et al*, 1991).

The Norwegian Government encouraged farmers to increase production of food grain, potatoes, vegetables and low-fat milk. Measures were introduced to stabilise milk and meat production to avoid over-production. In collaboration with farmers' organisations, an attempt was made to produce more grass-fed than grain-fed beef. In addition, the pork produced was less fatty than before.

In 1982 the Government presented a White Paper *On the Follow-Up of Norwegian Nutrition Policy* prepared by the Norwegian Ministry of Health and Social Affairs (1982). In 1993 the Nutrition and Food Policy was integrated in *Challenges in Health Promotion and Prevention Strategies* (Norwegian Ministry of Health and Social Affairs, 1993), which brought nutrition even closer to public health.

Resistance to the Nutrition and Food Policy

Progress in implementing the nutrition policy was slow in the first years after its approval by the Parliament in 1976. Two main reasons were that the dairy and meat industry were against the policy, and that the NNC had little power and political influence. The dairy industry tried to counteract the policy by producing foreign experts who claimed that milk, butter and other dairy products had no influence on risk factors for CHD, and that therefore the Norwegian nutrition policy was built on false premises. This led to a survey among leading scientists in the field of atherosclerosis and lipid metabolism (Norum, 1978). The survey clearly showed that the Norwegian nutrition policy was built on a solid scientific foundation. The NNC tried to get the dairy industry to produce a low-fat milk for the Norwegian market, but this met with resistance. However, after the NNC had organised a successful consumer-based campaign for the consumption of skimmed milk instead of whole milk, the dairy industry gave in, and in collaboration with NNC a low-fat milk was introduced in 1984, which has since been the main choice of consumers in Norway.

The Norwegian Nutrition and Food Policy has also had internal conflicts. For example, the objective of increasing local food production led to more Norwegian wheat for human consumption. However, Norwegian grain was more expensive than wheat on the international market, and simultaneously with an official campaign to eat more cereals, bread became more expensive!

Some results of the Norwegian Nutrition and Food Policy

Surveys have revealed that knowledge of diet and health has increased in the Norwegian population in the past 15 years, and that attitudes concerning healthy dietary habits have become more positive. These changes in knowledge and attitude are reflected in a change in the diet of the population (Tables 10.1 and 10.2).

Dietary data are obtained from the annual reports of the NNC, presenting food consumption data based on wholesale figures, and from the household consumption surveys published by the Norwegian National Bureau of Statistics.

The main changes in the Norwegian diet during the period 1975–1993 have been a reduction of fat, mainly due to a reduction in saturated fat, and an increase in the consumption of vegetables, fruits and cereals. Concomitant with these changes the surveys done by the Norwegian NHSS have shown that blood cholesterol has decreased by about 10% in the general population (Bjartveit *et al*, 1991; Johansson *et al*, 1996). These changes are reflected in a large reduction in the mortality due to CHD among middle-aged Norwegian men and women (Figure 10.1).

Table 10.1   Food consumption at wholesale level (kg per person per year)

	1970	1975	1980	1985	1990	1995
Cereals	71	75	80	75	79	81
Potatoes, unrefined[a]	79	71	60	63	51	48
Potatoes, refined[b]	7	8	12	17	19	23
Vegetables	40	37	51	47	55	58
Fruits	67	74	75	85	72	81
Meat	43	52	55	54	54	59
Eggs	10	10	11	13	11	11
Fish, approximate[c]	30	35	–	–	40	40
Whole milk (3.8%)	172	169	164	124	56	50
Low-fat milk (1.5%)	–	–	–	28	84	85
Skimmed milk (0.1%)	14	26	28	30	31	29
Cheese	9	10	12	13	13	14
Cream	6.7	6.7	7.1	6.7	6.8	6.7
Butter	5.4	4.7	5.6	4.8	3.3	3.1
Margarine, total	19	18	16	14	13	14
Low-fat margarine	–	–	–	0.2	2.4	2.7
Oil and other fats[d]	4.4	4.2	4.7	4.1	4.0	3.9
Sugar, syrup, honey, etc.	42	32	43	42	41	43

[a] Potatoes not for industrial use
[b] Potatoes used to produce potato products
[c] Figures for fish consumption are only approximate
[d] Includes cooking oils, cooking fats, and fat used in food manufacturing for mayonnaise, salads, chocolate, biscuits, etc.
Source: Norwegian Nutrition Council (1995)

Table 10.2 Dietary energy and energy-providing nutrients at wholesale level (per person per day)

	1970	1975	1980	1985	1990	1993
Energy (kcal)	2860	2900	3170	3020	2910	2980
Protein (g)	85	86	94	94	94	96
Fat (g)	126	129	135	122	111	112
Carbohydrate (total)	352	345	390	378	377	392
Starch (g)	185	174	185	174	177	185
Sugar (g)	115	91	120	118	118	122
Dietary fibre (g)	–	21	23	24	22	23
Percentage distribution of energy						
Protein	12	12	12	13	13	13
Fat	39	40	38	35	35	34
Carbohydrate[a]	49(16)	48(13)	50(15)	51(16)	52(16)	53(17)

[a]Values in parentheses are percentage energy from sugar
Source: Norwegian Nutrition Council (1995)

The nutrition policy in Norway from 1975 to 1990 was to a large extent aimed at a reduction in premature CHD. This goal has to some extent been attained, and the current nutrition policy has therefore somewhat changed in comparison with what was formulated in 1975.

The Nutrition and Food Policy in Norway today

In the report Challenges in Health Promotion and Prevention Strategies (Norwegian Ministry of Health and Social Affairs, 1993) the Nutrition and Food Policy is integrated into the Health policy, and is based on the experience gained following the earlier parliamentary White Papers. The current Norwegian Nutrition and Food Policy has four main goals:

To reduce the prevalence of dietary-related diseases and damage to health in the population

To ensure such a reduction the Government intends to implement a policy that will support the following main objectives:

- A national diet in line with the recommendations of the NNC.
- Breast-feeding of babies should continue at a high level.
- The nutrition-related differences in health status in the population should be reduced.
- Dietary treatment should be integrated in primary and secondary prevention of diet-related diseases within the health services.

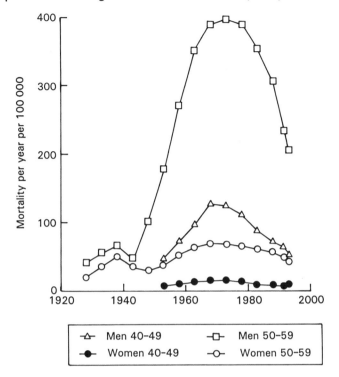

Figure 10.1 Mortality from coronary heart disease in Norway (data provided by the Norwegian National Bureau of Statistics)

The goals deal with both the national diet, including that of infants, the present inequality in health, especially with regard to cardiovascular diseases, and ways to change approaches within the health services. Special emphasis is placed on changes in food consumption so that it fulfils the recommendations of the NNC:

- Reducing the proportion of energy derived from fat in the diet to 30%, by lowering the proportion of saturated fat.
- The fibre content of the diet should be increased to 25 g per person per day by increasing the consumption of cereals, potatoes, vegetables and fruit.
- Sugar should contribute no more than 10% of energy.
- Salt intake should be reduced to 5 g per person per day.
- Consumption of fish should increase.
- Consumption of dairy products, meat and meat products with lower fat content should be encouraged.
- Consumption of butter, hard margarine, high-fat potato products and snacks should be reduced.
- Frequent intake of grilled, fried, smoked or salted foods should be avoided.

To ensure food safety

The policy requires:

- that foods are free from infectious agents and do not contain approved food additives in quantities which are a risk to health; and
- that consumer demands for food quality, safety and security are met. Special emphasis should be placed on improving the mapping, monitoring and warning systems for food-borne diseases. Included in this part of the policy is ensuring that the water supply satisfies the quality requirements laid down by the Norwegian authorities.

To strengthen consumers' influence on the Nutrition and Food Policy

The government will ensure that consumers have the opportunity to sustain a healthy diet. A consumer policy will be implemented, which promotes a healthy diet through differential prices, food availability, food labelling/claims and information and marketing, in order to achieve this.

To contribute to safe production, distribution and marketing of food products and to safe consumption patterns in terms of health, the environment and appropriate use of resources

Food production shall satisfy society's requirements for safe and ethically acceptable norms and allow for protection of animals and plants, genetic resources and environmental resources. This aspect of the nutrition and food policy is an adjustment to sustainable development, meaning that production should be ecologically sustainable on a long-term perspective. This links the modern nutrition and food policy to international work for environmental protection and human rights for food and health. In this respect, it is appropriate to quote the following recommendations regarding food production from The Brundtland Commission (World Commission on Environment and Development, 1987):

> The industrialized countries must reduce overproduction of agricultural products, so that world market prices will reflect the real production costs. In the short term this implies higher costs for food-importing from developing countries. But it will mean a real stimulus to increase production in developing countries.

Governmental implementation bodies

At ministerial level, the National Nutrition Council (NNC), and the National Food Control Authority (NFCA) are responsible for coordination of the implementation of the Nutrition and Food Policy.

The NNC was established in 1937, reorganised in 1946, and is today an expert body consisting of 23 members, with competence in nutritional biology, clinical nutrition, epidemiology, agricultural economy, community nutrition and nutrition policy, working in close cooperation with research institutions. The mandate for the NNC is:

- to be an advisory body to Ministries and others in matters concerning food supply and nutrition;
- to describe and evaluate the nutritional situation in Norway;
- to propose new strategies and measures in order to reach nutritional goals;
- to give assistance and suggestions to research councils and research institutions;
- to contribute to the promotion and coordination of professional work on diet and nutrition, nationally and internationally;
- to be actively engaged in nutrition education and ensure that public information on nutrition meets its recommendations.

One important task for the Council is formulation of the Norwegian dietary guidelines. These guidelines, first published in 1954, have been the theoretical basis for nutrition-related health promotion, and were incorporated as the scientific foundation in the Nutrition and Food Policy. The last version of the guidelines, revised in 1989, was prepared in cooperation with the other Nordic countries (Standing Nordic Committee on Food, 1989).

During the past few years the administration of the Nutrition Council has been strengthened from being a small secretariat to an efficient administrative body with broad nutritional knowledge, operating in close contact both with the Ministry of Health and with the Nutrition Council and its members. This has been very important in enabling the NNC to implement and coordinate nutrition-related activities in many different sectors of society. An intersectoral approach is one of the most important elements in Norwegian nutrition and food policy.

The NFCA was established in 1988 in order to administer legislation related to food. It is responsible for coordinating and guiding the executive control system, which consists of 82 Local Food Control Authorities covering all the municipalities in Norway. These local food control offices are responsible for inspecting the production, import, storage and transport of food. During the past few years, the work of some Local Food Control Authorities has been strengthened and has been involved in broader nutritional work in collaboration with the local health services.

Conclusion

The official Nutrition and Food Policy White Papers (Norwegian Ministry of Agriculture, 1975; Norwegian Ministry of Health and Social Affairs, 1982; 1993) have been very useful strategic documents in the effort to improve public health in

Norway over the past 20 years. The NNC has played an important role in the implementation by formulating a consistent and scientific basis for the policy.

A great deal has been learned about the formulation and execution of a nutrition and food policy at national level.

- It takes time to get politicians interested in the issue. In order to get a comprehensive policy, the Government needs to develop a policy which has broad political support and is not susceptible to changes linked to specific governments in power.
- A nutrition and food policy must address problems related both to inequality and lack of food (malnutrition), as well as to cardiovascular diseases and other health problems related to too much food and changes in lifestyle (overnutrition).
- The nutrition message to the public must be scientifically based, consistent, credible and relevant for the target groups of the population. It must be practical and easy to understand.
- An effective administrative body (e.g. a Nutrition Council) and a strong secretariat are needed so that it is clear who has the daily responsibility for implementing the policy.
- The Nutrition Council must report to the responsible Ministry and to the Parliament at regular intervals.
- The members of the Nutrition Council should be independent experts in nutrition, diet and health with broad experience.
- Cooperation between the Nutrition Council, NGOs, the food industry and other key players is important.

Today, we can see several changes in Norwegian eating habits. The consumption of cereals, vegetables, fruit and low-fat milk has increased. Furthermore, there has been a reduction in the intake of margarine, butter and whole milk. This has led to a reduction of total fat from 40% to 34% of the food energy, mainly by a reduction of saturated fat. Concomitant with the changes in diet, there has been a reduction in the level of plasma cholesterol in the population, and a reduction in death from CHD. This reduction is nearly 50% in men aged 40-49 years old, and also substantial in other age groups and among women. It is likely that the Norwegian Nutrition and Food Policy has played an important role in changing dietary habits and thus contributed to the decline in heart disease.

However, there are some warning signals for the future. The rules and regulations of CEC and GATT, which Norway has to respect, make it difficult to subsidise and price according to health preference. There is a tendency to rapid changes in eating and meal patterns, especially among young people. This, combined with aggressive marketing from companies producing fast food and 'junk food', make it very important to have a Nutrition Council with standing and ability to provide scientifically based information on the important relationship of diet, nutrition and public health.

References

Bjartveit K, Foss OP, Gjervig T, Lund-Larsen P. The cardiovascular disease study in Norwegian counties. Background and organization. *Acta Medica Scandinavica*, 1979; **634** (supplement): 1-70

Bjartveit K, Stensvold I, Lund-Larsen PG, Gjervig T, Krüger Ø, Urdal P. Hjerte- og karundersøkelser i norske fylker. Bakgrunn og gjennomføring. Status 1986-90 for isikomønster blant 40-42 åringer i 14 fylker [Cardiovascular screenings in Norwegian counties. Background and implementation.] Status of risk pattern during the period 1986-90 among persons aged 40-42 years in 14 counties. *Tidsskrift for den Norske Lægeforening*, 1991; **111**: 2063-2072

Bjørneboe GE, Drevon CA, Norum KR (eds). *Mat og medisin. Generell og klinisk ernæring* (*Food and Medicine. General and Clinical Nutrition*). Oslo: Universitetsforlaget, 1994: 1-391

Hjermann I, Velve Byre K, Holme I, Leren P. Effect of diet and smoking intervention on the incidence of coronary heart disease. Report from the Oslo Study Group of a randomized trial in healthy men. *Lancet*, 1981; **ii**: 1303-1310

Johansson L, Drevon CA, Bjørneboe GE. The Norwegian diet during the last hundred years in relation to coronary heart disease. *European Journal of Clinical Nutrition*, 1996; **50**: 277-283

Nicolaysen R, Eeg-Larsen N, Jervell A *et al. Betenkning om forholdet mellom fett og hjerte-kar-sykdommer* (*Fat and Coronary Heart Disease*). Oslo: Nasjonalforeningen for folkehelsen/Det Norske råd for hjerte- og karsykdommer, 1963

Norum KR. Some present concepts concerning diet and prevention of coronary heart disease. *Nutrition and Metabolism*, 1978; **22**: 1-7

Norwegian Central Bureau of Statistics. *Health Statistics 1987*. Oslo: Central Bureau of Statistics, 1987

Norwegian Ministry of Agriculture. *Norwegian Nutrition and Food Policy*. Report No. 32 to the Storting (1975-76). Oslo: Royal Norwegian Ministry of Agriculture, 1975

Norwegian Ministry of Health and Social Affairs. *On the Follow-up of Norwegian Nutrition Policy*. Report No. 11 to the Storting (1981-82). Oslo: Royal Norwegian Ministry of Health and Social Affairs, 1982

Norwegian Ministry of Health and Social Affairs. *Utfordringer i helsefremmende og forebyggende arbeid* (*Challenges in Health Promotion and Prevention Strategies*). Report No. 37 to the Storting (1992-93). Oslo: Royal Norwegian Ministry of Health and Social Affairs, 1993

Norwegian Nutrition Council. *Annual Report, 1995*. Oslo: Norwegian Nutrition Council, 1995

Oshaug A. Nutrition security in Norway? A situation analysis. *Scandinavian Journal of Nutrition*, 1994; **38**: 1-68

Standing Nordic Committee on Food. *Nordic Nutrition Recommendations*. Uppsala: National Food Administration, 1989

World Commission on Environment and Development (The Brundtland Commission). *Our Common Future*. Oxford: Oxford University Press, 1987

Discussion

Pekka Puska

National Public Health Institute, Helsinki, Finland

Non-communicable diseases, and especially cardiovascular diseases, represent the major health burden in industrialised countries, and a rapidly growing problem in developing countries. At the same time this is an area in which major health gains can be achieved. In most of the developed world about half of deaths are due to cardiovascular diseases.

Extensive medical research has been carried out during the past few decades to learn about the causes and mechanisms of atherosclerotic cardiovascular diseases. Research has involved large epidemiological studies within and between populations, basic biochemical and animal studies, intervention trials and large-scale community-based preventive studies. Although undoubtedly there is still a great deal to discover, much has already been learnt to aid prevention. In fact, so much is known that it can be argued that the main question for chronic disease prevention is not 'what to do', but 'how to do it'. The key question is: how can the existing knowledge best be applied for effective prevention in real life?

Elevated blood cholesterol is a major nutritional risk factor for atherosclerotic cardiovascular disease, and especially for its most common fatal outcome, coronary heart disease (CHD). It is strongly and consistently related to CHD in prospective studies, in population comparisons, in animal studies, and in preventive trials. Considering the totality of the evidence, it is very likely that the association is a causal one. Furthermore, it may be argued that elevated blood cholesterol is a basic risk factor, giving individuals and populations the basic susceptibility to atherosclerotic diseases, upon which other factors act.

Over the past two decades, a great number of international and national recommendations have been made concerning the dietary changes needed for the prevention of CHD. Although the details of the recommendations vary, the main trends are remarkably similar. The recommended dietary changes are:

- reduction in saturated fat intake;
- partial substitution of saturated fat for unsaturated fat;
- reduction in dietary cholesterol intake;
- increase in fibre intake;
- avoidance of being overweight.

Successful change: From research to public policy

Since elevated blood cholesterol is a major risk factor for a significant public health problem, action to change the situation is badly needed. Because blood cholesterol levels relate closely to the general dietary pattern of the population, this action cannot be a simple one; instead, comprehensive measures are needed. Dietary habits of any population are deeply rooted in cultural and economic features of the country, which is why successful long-term changes in dietary habits can hardly take place without changes in public policy as well. But usually, before such changes take place, a long period of development is needed. This chain is illustrated in Figure 10.2. Research, basic and applied, has shown the important role that LDL-cholesterol plays in the atherosclerotic process and how blood cholesterol levels are influenced by diet. Demonstration projects in communities and other settings show how relevant changes can be implemented in real life.

Once convinced that evidence exists, expert groups and governmental commit-tees have gradually made recommendations to the general public about a healthy diet. The first to respond to the new medical knowledge are often active health organisations, such as heart associations. In many countries, a variety of campaigns have been launched, to make people aware of the links between diet and heart disease and how they should act on this knowledge. Gradually more sectors of the community/society, such as NGOs, health services and schools, have responded, and started to participate in the action. The action includes various types of health education, screening programmes, patient consulting, etc. With increased public (that is, consumer) interest, the food industry starts to respond. Industry sees that there is a market for cholesterol-lowering food (and drug) items; the influence of strong health arguments has thus increased.

Usually at a rather late stage of this development, public policy, plans,

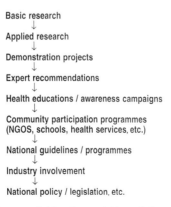

Basic research
↓
Applied research
↓
Demonstration projects
↓
Expert recommendations
↓
Health educations / awareness campaigns
↓
Community participation programmes
(NGOS, schools, health services, etc.)
↓
National guidelines / programmes
↓
Industry involvement
↓
National policy / legislation, etc.

Figure 10.2   The process of successful implementation of change: from research to public policy

decisions and legislation come into the picture. Because of conflicting interests, public administration usually works slowly and major decisions are made only when the change process has gone some way. Political decision-makers are not so much influenced by expert statements as they are by feedback from their constituencies. Although Figure 10.2 is drawn to show a temporal sequence of events, the order of events is not in fact so clear and much overlap occurs.

The following are particularly important aspects in a successful public policy:

- Intersectoral collaboration
- The presence of a responsible agency, national focal point
- Nutrition education programmes
- Support for voluntary organisations
- Food labelling policies
- Food pricing policies
- Research and demonstration
- International collaboration.

The Finnish example

Finland, in the 1960s and early 1970s, had extremely high mortality rates from CHD, and other atherosclerotic cardiovascular diseases. The rates for men were the highest in the world. Against this background it is understandable that Finland—its scientists, health experts and decision-makers—have been proactive to change the situation. The process that has taken place in Finland during the past 20–30 years gives a good example of the development from research to public policy described above—for lowering the high cholesterol levels through general dietary changes, in order to cut down the heart disease rates (Pietinen *et al*, 1996). This process has generally been a very positive one, but many difficulties and constraints have been encountered and lessons learned.

The North Karelia Project was started in 1972 as a response to growing public concern, and to build on the previous research results. When elevated serum cholesterol, related to diet, was suspected to be a major risk factor in Finland, a logical step was to start a demonstration project, to develop and study methods to change the situation. The province of North Karelia, with the highest rates of mortality due to CHD in Finland, was chosen as the pilot area. After the good results and experiences of the initial five-year period, the project actively started to contribute to the national development, while demonstration work in North Karelia continued (Puska *et al*, 1995).

Generally very large and favourable dietary changes have taken place in Finland in accordance with the recommendations. Figure 10.3 shows the respective and substantial changes in mean serum cholesterol level of Finnish men. The changes among women were even greater. Figure 10.4 shows the dramatic decrease in CHD mortality of Finnish men during the past 20 years (and in North Karelia, particularly in the 1970s). A separate analysis has indicated that

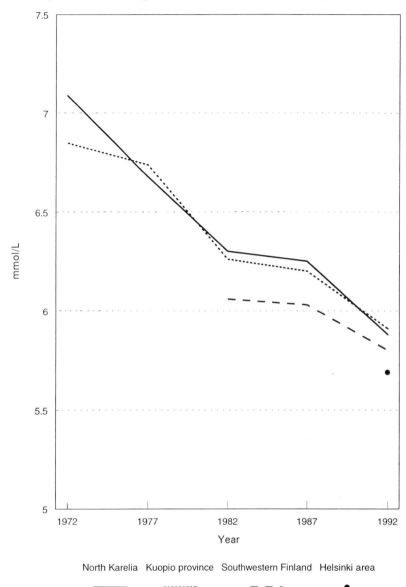

Figure 10.3 Mean serum total cholesterol levels in the different areas of Finland 1972–1992 (FINRISK Surveys, men 30–59 years)

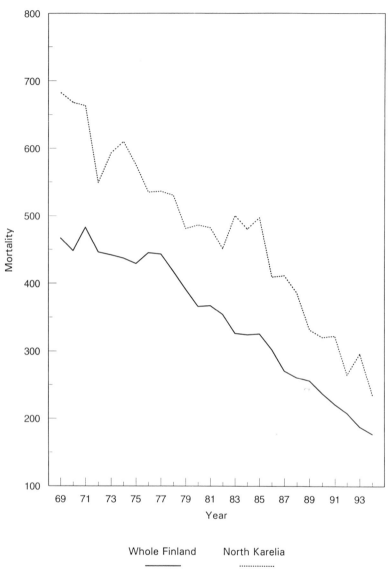

Figure 10.4 Age adjusted coronary heart disease mortality in North Karelia and in all of
Finland 1965–1994 (35–64 years, men)

reduction in the population cholesterol level has been responsible for about half the decline in coronary mortality (Vartiainen et al, 1994).

Conclusion

Successful dietary interventions need simultaneously to provide people with the necessary skills and support for the change, and to ensure that feasible nutritional changes are adopted as public policy. Interventions should at the same time apply the relevant findings of medical/nutritional research and appropriate principles of social and behavioural sciences. In addition, sufficient resources and commitment are needed. In order to influence public policy, health programmes should mobilise people and communities for change, and demand support from political decision-makers. With growing consumer interest, a healthy food industry contributes to the change and also influences public policy.

References

Pietinen P, Vartiainen E, Seppänen R, Aro A, Puska P. Changes in diet in Finland from 1972 to 1992. Impact on coronary heart disease risk. *Preventive Medicine*, 1996; **25**: 243–250

Puska P, Tuomilehto J, Nissinen A, Vartiainen E, eds. *The North Karelia Project. 20 Year Results and Experiences*. Helsinki: University Press, 1995

Vartiainen E, Puska P, Pekkanen J, Tuomilehto J, Jousilahti P. Changes in risk factors explain changes in mortality from ischaemic heart disease in Finland. *British Medical Journal*, 1994; **309**: 23–27

11
Symposium: The burgeoning global burden of obesity

11.1 The problem of obesity world-wide

Prakash S. Shetty and Alison E. Tedstone

Human Nutrition Unit, London School of Hygiene & Tropical Medicine, UK

Obesity is becoming an increasingly important public health problem. It is now estimated that world-wide, about 100 million people are obese. Obesity is associated with an increased likelihood of non-insulin-dependent diabetes mellitus (NIDDM), hypertension, hyperlipidaemia and cardiovascular disease. It is also associated with increased rates of breast, colorectal and uterine cancer. Obesity is thus an important factor in the increasing morbidity and mortality due to chronic, non-communicable diseases.

The practical and clinical definition of obesity is based on the Body Mass Index (BMI; weight in kg/(height in m)^2) (WHO, 1995). It is generally agreed that a BMI of greater than 30 is indicative of clinical obesity while a BMI of 25.0–29.9 is suggestive of overweight in an individual. The recommended cut-offs are appropriate for the identification of the extent of overweight or obesity in individuals and population groups. The WHO Expert Committee in its Report (WHO, 1995) concluded that weight gain and overweight/obesity are associated with increased morbidity and mortality and that weight cycling, that is, cycles of weight loss followed by weight regain, may also be associated with increased morbidity and mortality. The Committee was of the opinion that weight loss in obesity is difficult to sustain, is of uncertain benefit to health in the long term and

Diet, Nutrition and Chronic Disease: Lessons from Contrasting Worlds.
Edited by P. S. Shetty and K. McPherson © 1997 John Wiley & Sons, Ltd.

may lead to weight cycling, and hence the primary prevention of obesity must be our main concern.

Obesity is a major public health issue since it is increasingly common in most industrialised societies and is increasing even in many of the less affluent, developing countries. Prevalence of obesity is high in the USA and in Europe, particularly in Eastern Europe and Mediterranean countries. High rates of prevalence are seen among the American Indians, Hispanics and the Pacific and Indian Ocean islanders, such as the Melanesians, Micronesians and Polynesians (Hodge et al, 1995). The prevalence of obesity is much lower in African and Asian countries.

Obesity in developed countries

Table 11.1 summarises some of the available recent data on the prevalence of obesity among adults in industrialised and developed countries. The prevalence of obesity is high in the USA, even allowing for the fact that surveys in the USA have used a BMI cut-off of 27.8 for males and 27.3 for females to define obesity (US Department of Health and Human Services, 1994). It is higher among US blacks than whites, and also among the indigenous population of American Indians and also the Hispanic Americans (Kumanika, 1993). Obesity is relatively common in Europe especially among women, and in Southern and Eastern Europe in particular (Seidell, 1995). Apart from The Netherlands, where the prevalence of obesity has remained stable between 1974 and 1986 (Blokstra and Kromhout, 1991), in most other countries of Europe the trends are indicative of an increase in obesity among the adult population. For instance, the prevalence in the adult population doubled from 6% and 8% in 1980 to 13% and 15% in 1991 in England (UK Department of Health, 1993). Increases in the prevalence of obesity are also seen in most countries of Europe over the past decade.

Table 11.1   Prevalence of obesity in developed countries

Country	Year	Obesity definition (BMI cut-off point)	Age range (years)	Males (%)	Females (%)
Australia	1989	30	25–69	11.1	12.7
Netherlands	1993	30	20–59	8.0	10.0
Germany	1990	30	25–69	17.2	19.3
Sweden	1988/89	30($\male$); 28.6($\female$)	16–84	5.3	9.1
Canada	1991	27	25–64	30	20
Israel	1986	30	50–84	15.9	32.7
UK					
England	1993	30	16–64	13.0	16.0
USA					
Whites	1988/91	27.8($\male$); 7.3($\female$)	20–74	32.0	33.5
Blacks	1988/91	27.8($\male$); 27.3($\female$)	20–74	31.8	49.2

Table 11.2 Proportion of adults with overweight/obesity in some countries of Africa, Asia and Latin America

| Country | Year | Proportion (%) of population | |
		BMI = 25–29.9	BMI > 30
Africa			
Congo (women)	1986/87	11.8	3.4
Ghana	1987/88	17.1	0.9
Mali	1991	6.4	0.8
Morocco	1984/85	18.7	5.2
Tunisia	1990	28.6	8.6
Asia			
China	1982	7.2	1.0
India	1988/90	3.0	0.5
Latin America			
Brazil	1989	25.1	8.6
Cuba	1982	26.9	9.5
Peru	1975/76	24.8	9.0

Source: Adapted from Shetty and James, 1994

Obesity in developing countries

The problem of obesity among adults is not confined to the industrialised, developed world. The prevalence of obesity in several countries of the developing world is high, and in some of them high rates of obesity are already evident in children as well as adults. The present prevalence of obesity is highly variable between developing countries and within populations of a country, although in general the prevalence of obesity is higher in women than in men. Table 11.2 shows the problem of adult obesity in some countries of Africa, Asia and Latin America.

There is an alarming trend, suggestive of a burgeoning problem of obesity, which will contribute to increases in other chronic, non-communicable diseases and present a huge health burden for the less affluent countries. These changes reflect the presence of newly acquired risks relating to diet and lifestyle changes associated with rapid urbanisation accompanying the economic development of the country. With life expectancy increasing in developing countries and the consequent changes in the demographic profile of the population, obesity and the concurrent morbidity due to other chronic diseases are only likely to increase further.

References

Blokstra A, Kromhout D. Trends in obesity in young adults in The Netherlands from 1974–1986. *International Journal of Obesity*, 1991; **15**: 513–521
US Department of Health and Human Services, United States. Washington DC: US Department of Health and Human Services, 1994

Hodge AM, Dowse GK, Zimmer PZ *et al.* Prevalence and secular trends in obesity in Pacific and Indian Ocean island populations. *Obesity Research*, 1995; **3** (Suppl 2): 77–87

Kumanyika SK. Special issues regarding obesity in minority populations. *Annals of Internal Medicine*, 1993; **119**: 650–654

Seidell JC. Obesity in Europe: scaling an epidemic. *International Journal of Obesity*, 1995; **19** (Suppl 3): S1–S4

Shetty PS, James WPT. *Body Mass Index: A Measure of Chronic Energy Deficiency in Adults.* Food and Nutrition Paper No. 56. Rome: Food and Agricultural Organisation, 1994

UK Department of Health. *The Health of the Nation: One Year On . . . A Report on the Progress of the Health of the Nation.* London: HMSO, 1993

WHO Expert Committee Report. *Physical Status: The Use and Interpretation of Anthropometry.* WHO Technical Report Series 854. Geneva: World Health Organization, 1995

11.2 Appetite, food intake and human obesity

Andrew M. Prentice

MRC Dunn Clinical Nutrition Centre, Cambridge, UK

In the past two decades there has been a radical shift towards the view that most forms of obesity are caused by a defective regulation of appetite causing overconsumption of energy. This has not always been the view. Examination of the 1983 Royal College of Physicians' report on obesity (Royal College of Physicians, 1983) reveals multiple chapters covering potential defects in energy expenditure, and only one on food intake. The reason for the dominance of research into brown fat, diet-induced thermogenesis, futile cycles and other putative differences in metabolic efficiency between lean and obese individuals hitherto, was largely the result of the belief in data from the results of food records which indicated that obese people did not necessarily overeat. If this were the case then, it was reasoned, they had to be remarkably efficient in their utilisation of energy, thus creating a surplus to be stored as fat even when the obese consumed a normal diet.

The development in the mid-1980s of the doubly labelled water (DLW) technique for accurately measuring free-living energy expenditure in humans provided the first means of cross-validating food records. The new method has repeatedly proved that obese people must be hyperphagic (Prentice *et al*, 1986; Bandini *et al*, 1990; Prentice *et al*, 1996) and hence has refocused attention on the importance of appetite regulation in the aetiology of obesity (Prentice *et al*, 1989). This paper briefly reviews the evidence to support the above statement, and then

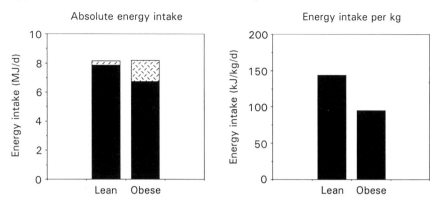

Figure 11.1 Typical estimates of food intake in lean and obese women. The hatched area indicates correction for energy mobilised from body fat during measurement period. Data from Prentice *et al* (1986)

discusses the latest research into the regulation of appetite ranging from molecular genetics to country-wide epidemiological studies.

Evidence implicating hyperphagia in the causation of obesity

When estimating the habitual food intake of humans as they live their normal lives, scientists are forced to rely on the subjects themselves to record their own consumption patterns. As we now know, this seemingly trivial task is fraught with

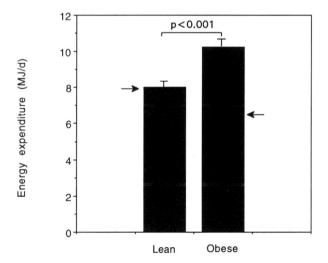

Figure 11.2 Total free-living energy expenditure of lean and obese women. Measurements made using the doubly labelled water method. Arrows indicate self-recorded food intake. Data from the same women as in Figure 11.1 (Prentice *et al*, 1986)

difficulties, especially in affluent countries where there are deep and complex psychoses regarding food and body image. Figure 11.1 illustrates some of our own measurements of food intake in groups of lean and obese women in Cambridge. The data were collected using the 'gold standard' seven-day weighed intake method, and were examined by a very experienced dietitian who discarded all obviously implausible data (Prentice et al, 1986). These results seem to suggest that the obese women were eating no more than the lean ones in spite of their 50% greater bodyweight, and appeared to survive on a much lower energy ration.

Figure 11.2 illustrates DLW estimates of energy expenditure in the same women and shows that this was not the case (Prentice et al, 1986). The obese women expended significantly more energy, and since they had been weight-stable for some months they must also have been consuming more energy to support this greater expenditure. Figure 11.2 shows the excellent agreement between intake and expenditure in the lean women, while the obese women under-recorded their food intake by over 3.5 MJ/d (over 800 kcal/d). The extent of individual biases in recording food intake in obese and weight-conscious (post-obese) women can be extreme, with some of the errors exceeding 50% even after a dietitian has screened the records (Black et al, 1993). Many other studies using metabolic balance procedures, DLW estimates, or calculations based on the physiological principles governing energy needs, have subsequently endorsed the contention that overweight and obese people usually under-record their food intake (Schoeller, 1990; Schoeller et al, 1990; Black et al, 1991; Goldberg et al, 1991; Lichtman et al, 1992; Mertz, 1992). Although it does not prove that simple overeating is the initial cause of obesity, it at least allows for this as a strong possibility.

Energy needs to develop and support obesity

It is well recognised that there only needs to be a very small positive error in the regulation of energy balance for obesity to develop (Jéquier, 1992). Even the fattest man in the world who recently died weighing 73 stone (465 kg) only required a daily energy excess equivalent to a small bar of chocolate in order to become so fat. It is futile to try to detect such discrepancies because the measurement techniques are not precise enough, and there is so much behavioural noise in day-to-day changes in energy intake and expenditure. However, a consideration of the energy that is needed to support an obese person can yield some critical insights into eating behaviour.

Figure 11.3 shows data from a recent compilation of all the available DLW measurements of energy expenditure in overweight and obese men and women (Prentice et al, 1996). Note that the average very obese man requires ~ 18 MJ/d (~ 4500 kcal/d) and the average very obese woman requires ~ 13 MJ/d (~ 3000 kcal/d) just to remain weight-stable. At these intakes the people concerned would not be gluttonous; they would simply be consuming what was required to support their increased mass. We know from other studies that at this level of obesity

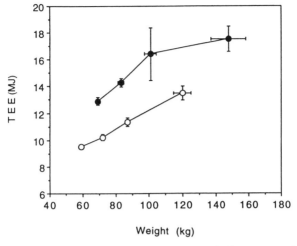

Figure 11.3 Total free-living energy expenditure (TEE) in lean, overweight and obese men and women. Data compiled from all available published results (Prentice *et al*, 1996). Subjects divided into Body Mass Index categories: <25.0, 25.0–29.9, 30.0–35.0 and >35 kg/m². Key: male, •; female, o

many physiological processes are trying to re-establish a lower body fat mass: energy expenditure is high; fat oxidation rates are elevated; peripheral tissues are resistant to insulin; and so on. In spite of this, the drive to eat is so powerful as to overcome all of these autoregulatory processes, and food intakes remain very high. Such is the public opprobrium attached to obesity that very obese patients often resort to elaborate cover-up procedures, and frequently claim to be eating very little, and are never seen eating in public.

Obesity as an eating disorder

The above illustrations of how difficult it is to discover the truth about human feeding behaviour are described in order to emphasise the critical role that behavioural psychologists can play in the diagnosis and treatment of disordered eating as a cause of certain obesities. There has been important progress in this field in recent years, assisted by the adoption in 1994 of research criteria for the definition of Binge Eating Disorder (BED) as a recognised syndrome related to bulimia, but without the purging, and hence resulting in obesity (American Psychiatric Association, 1994). It has been estimated that about 30% of patients in specialist obesity clinics satisfy the stringent criteria for BED (Jebb and Prentice, 1995). These include: recurrent episodes of bingeing an amount of food which is definitely larger than most people would eat; a sense of a lack of control over eating; eating when not physically hungry; eating alone; subsequent guilt; and marked internal distress over binge eating (American Psychiatric Association, 1994).

Epidemic obesity at the population level: gluttony or sloth?

In many affluent countries the prevalence of obesity is increasing at a disturbing rate. In the UK over half the adult population is overweight and the proportion with clinical obesity (Body Mass Index > 30 kg/m^2) doubled between national surveys in 1980 and 1991 (GB Department of Health, 1995). Clearly this is caused by an excess of energy intake, but can it be contributed to gluttony, sloth or both? Analysis of secular changes as assessed by the British National Food Survey (NFS) (GB MAFF, 1940–1994) indicates that the *per capita* energy intake has been declining by up to 20% since 1970, while obesity rates have been escalating (Prentice and Jebb, 1995). There are some concerns over the exact validity of the NFS data since, until recently, it has only made a *pro rata* adjustment for meals eaten outside the home. However, it seems certain that energy intake has not risen over this period. The implication of this finding is that levels of physical activity must have declined at an even greater rate than the fall in energy intake. Elsewhere we have provided an analysis of the secular and social class trends in physical activity and argued that these are more closely related to the prevalence of obesity than are changes in dietary variables (Prentice and Jebb, 1995). None the less, it must be the case that the British population is, on average, consuming excess energy in relation to their lowered energy requirements created by a sedentary lifestyle, and it is useful to examine why our physiological systems fail to recognise these reduced requirements and to downregulate food intake accordingly.

Passive overconsumption induced by high-fat diets

A key factor in the failure of energy regulation appears to be the high fat content of modern diets. Figure 11.4 illustrates the profound change in the proportion of dietary energy derived from fat in the British diet over the past 50 years. In the 1940s each kilojoule of carbohydrate was associated with 0.6 kJ of fat, in the 1990s with 0.9 kJ of fat—an increase of 50%. There is considerable evidence, both at the individual and the population level, that obesity is associated with the consumption of a high-fat diet. Analysis of time trend data and of international variations in obesity rates usually implicates a high fat intake as a likely causative factor (Lissner and Heitmann, 1995). The chief exceptions seem to be the former Eastern block nations where obesity levels are high in spite of apparent low fat intakes. Cross-sectional studies within populations also reveal significant associations between obesity and the percentage of energy that an individual derives from fat (Dreon *et al*, 1988; Gazzaniga and Burns, 1991; Tremblay *et al*, 1991; Bolton-Smith and Woodward, 1994; Gibney, 1995; Hill and Prentice, 1995). Such studies are virtually unanimous in this respect and are probably robust even in spite of some concerns about macronutrient-specific under-reporting (Heitmann and Lissner, 1995).

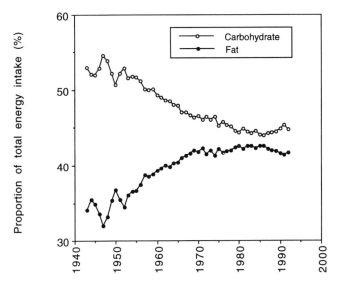

Figure 11.4 Secular changes in the fat-to-carbohydrate ratio of the British diet between the 1940s and the 1990s. Data from National Food Survey (GB MAFF, 1940–1994)

The arguments that dietary fat is not causally related to obesity, presented elsewhere in this book (Willett, this volume, Chapter 5), are based solely on the results of long-term low-fat intervention trials and on the fact that obesity rates are escalating in the US at a time when the fat content of the diet appears to be declining very slightly. The first of these observations is likely to be influenced by progressive non-compliance with the low-fat diet, especially since Lissner and Heitmann (1995) have shown good rates of spontaneous weight loss in short-term low-fat, but energy-unrestricted, diets. The second observation fails to account for the fact that obesity evolves over decades and will require decades to resolve. There is bound to be a considerable time-lag between the onset of causal (or curative) events and the final outcome. It is thus premature to make judgements about long-term secular trends in response to any decrease in fat intake which may be slowly occurring.

The reasons that people select a high-fat diet are, as yet, poorly understood. They range from macro-economic factors which are permissive of the production and purchase of diets with a high level of animal protein and fat, to individual food choices which may be governed by an inherent physiological preference for fat (Drewnowski, 1993) or simply by familial entrainment. In this field there is currently an active debate as to whether the development of fat substitutes will be able to overcome our modern preference for fatty foods without the individual having to exert their own cognitive control (Rolls, 1994).

Physiological mechanisms underlying high-fat hyperphagia

The phenomenon of excess energy intake induced by fatty diets in both human and animal experiments is so strong that it is routinely described as high-fat hyperphagia. A series of experiments done by us graphically illustrate how easily energy balance can be perturbed by alterations in the fat content of the diet (Stubbs *et al*, 1995a, b).

In the first study lean men were allowed to eat freely during three seven-day periods in a whole-body calorimeter which permitted the accurate measurement of changes in their fat balance. The diets appeared to be identical and were matched for palatability. However, the fat content was covertly manipulated to 20, 40 or 60% of energy for the separate runs. On the 20% fat diet the men spontaneously lost around 200 g of fat over seven days. On the 60% fat diet they gained almost 700 g of fat. The remarkable feature of these changes is that the men were selected as being constitutionally lean (and hence as good regulators in normal life), that they had no idea that they had lost or gained fat when it was subsequently revealed to them, and that even after seven days there appeared to be no autoregulatory adjustment in food intake.

In the second study the same treatments were imposed on free-living men. This time fat balance could not be measured outside the calorimeter, but energy balance was measured using the DLW method. The results are illustrated in Figure 11.5 alongside the first experiment. There was a virtually identical treatment effect (indicated by the slope across the three diets), but it occurred at a different absolute level, indicating an important interaction with physical

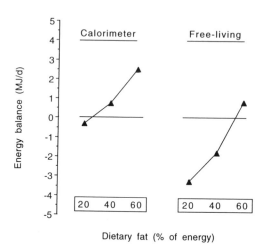

Figure 11.5   Effect of covert manipulation of the fat content of diets on energy balance in lean men. Left-hand figures show data from seven days in a whole-body calorimeter. Right-hand figures show data from 14 days free-living. Data from Stubbs *et al* (1995a, b)

activity. Outside the confines of the whole-body calorimeter the subjects were able to tolerate a 40% diet without gaining fat, but when physically inactive inside the chamber the 40% diet induced rapid fat deposition of 100 g per day. Other workers have found similar effects when the fat content of diets is covertly manipulated (Lissner *et al*, 1987; Kendall *et al*, 1991). The reason that subjects gained and lost fat in these experiments is that they continued to eat the same bulk of food (presumably due to previous conditioning effects whereby they had learnt to assess appropriate amounts of food for their requirements) and made no adjustment for the altered energy density. This is typical of the effects of high-fat diets (Stubbs, 1995; Poppitt and Prentice, 1996) and has been described as 'passive overconsumption' because it occurs unintentionally without the consumption of excess bulk (Blundell *et al*, 1995). The same phenomenon is partly responsible for the cafeteria-feeding effect in laboratory rodents.

A third experiment used the same manipulations of fat content but the changes were acheived at a constant energy density (Stubbs and Prentice, 1993). This eliminated the high-fat hyperphagia, thus suggesting that much of the effect of fat is mediated simply through its extra energy density. The only other similar experiment to have been performed in humans found similar results using liquid formula diets (van Stratum *et al*, 1978).

Short-term experiments using classic pre-load and test-meal paradigms also tend to confirm that fat has a low satiety effect (Cotton *et al*, 1993; Cotton and Blundell, 1994; Blundell *et al*, 1995), particularly in certain obese subjects and restrained eaters (Lawton *et al*, 1993; Rolls *et al*, 1994).

Recent advances in the molecular biology of appetite control

In the past year there have been rapid and exciting developments in studies of the molecular genetics of obesity. These originated from the publication in late 1994 of the sequence of the *ob* gene responsible for obesity in *ob/ob* mice which have a defective copy (Zhang *et al*, 1994). It was demonstrated that the gene was only expressed in adipose tissue, and that humans possess a similar gene showing close homology. The *ob* gene codes for a hormone now named 'leptin' which is widely assumed to act primarily as a satiety factor which sends feedback signals determined by the size of, or energy flux through, the adipocyte (Rink, 1994). These findings have reawakened a long-standing interest in the concept of an 'adipostat' which could provide a long-term modulator of energy balance determined by the size of the fat stores (Kennedy, 1953). Studies with synthetic leptin have already shown that it causes profound appetite suppression and weight loss in *ob/ob* mice, and has a lesser effect in wild-type mice (Halaas *et al*, 1995). It has no effect in *db/db* obese mice or *fa/fa* rats where the obesity is caused by a receptor defect (Halaas *et al*, 1995). Most recently, receptors for leptin have been identified in the choroid plexus (Tartaglia *et al*, 1995), and have been shown to be identical to the *db* receptor in mice and the *fa* receptor in rats (Chua *et al*,

1996). Defects of both of these have been known for years to cause obesity. The mode of action of leptin in the hypothalamus may be to balance the activity of appetite suppressing (GLP-1) and stimulatory (neuropeptide-Y) neurotransmitters (Scott, 1996). As far as humans are concerned it already seems clear that most obese people have high levels of circulating leptin (Hamilton *et al*, 1995; Lonnqvist *et al*, 1995) and as yet no examples of a defective gene have been found. It is being speculated that certain obese patients might possess defective receptors which make them leptin-resistant, and it is already known that the human homologue of the receptor gene is likely to reside on chromosome 1p31 (Chua *et al*, 1996).

In assessing the implications of these developments it is necessary to be both cautious and optimistic—cautious because it is evident that the developing epidemic of obesity must be caused by social, behavioural and environmental changes since it is occurring within a relatively constant gene pool; optimistic because, at the very least, the elucidation of the biology of leptin will greatly enhance our understanding of how energy balance is regulated. At best it might lead to therapeutic advances for affected patients. A further reason for optimism is that it is already helping to build integrated approaches to obesity research from molecular biology, through cellular metabolism and whole-body physiology, to epidemiology. These seem likely to yield early dividends in understanding and hence tackling the burgeoning problem of obesity.

References

American Psychiatric Association. *Diagnostic and Statistical Manual of the American Psychiatric Association*. 3rd edn. Washington, DC: American Psychiatric Association, 1994

Bandini LG, Schoeller DA, Dietz WH. Energy expenditure in obese and nonobese adolescents. *Pediatric Research*, 1990; **27**: 198–203

Black AE, Goldberg GR, Jebb SA, Livingstone MB, Cole TJ, Prentice AM. Critical evaluation of energy intake data using fundamental principles of energy physiology. 2. Evaluating the results of published surveys. *European Journal of Clinical Nutrition*, 1991; **45**: 583–599

Black AE, Prentice AM, Goldberg GR *et al*. Measurements of total energy expenditure provide insights into the validity of dietary measurements of energy intake. *Journal of the American Dietetic Association*, 1993; **93**: 572–579

Blundell JE, Cotton JR, Delargy H *et al*. The fat paradox: fat-induced satiety signals versus high fat overconsumption. *International Journal of Obesity*, 1995; **19**: 832–835

Bolton-Smith C, Woodward M. Dietary composition and fat to sugar ratios in relation to obesity. *International Journal of Obesity*, 1994; **18**: 820–828

Chua SC, Chung WK, Wu-Peng XS *et al*. Phenotypes of mouse diabetes and rat fatty due to mutations in the OB (leptin) receptor. *Science*, 1996; **271**: 994–996

Cotton JR, Blundell JE. Dietary fat, food habits and appetite. *Nutrition and Food Science*, 1994; **6**: 4–9

Cotton JR, Burley VJ, Blundell JE. High fat foods and hyperphagia: No feedback for the control of appetite. *International Journal of Obesity*, 1993; **17**: 409–416

Dreon DM, Frey-Hewitt B, Ellsworth N, Williams PT, Terry RB, Wood PT. Dietary fat:carbohydrate ratio and obesity in middle-aged men. *American Journal of Clinical Nutrition*, 1988; **47**: 995–1000

Drewnowski A. Human preferences for sugar and fat. In: Fernstrom JD, Miller GD, eds. *Appetite and Body Weight Regulation: Sugar, Fat and Macronutrient Substitutions.* Boca Raton, FL: CRC Press, 1993: 137–148

Gazzaniga JM, Burns TL. The relationship between diet composition and body fatness in preadolescent children. *Journal of the American Dietetic Society (suppl)*, 1991; **91**: A-63

Gibney MJ. Epidemiology of obesity in relation to nutrient intake. *International Journal of Obesity*, 1995; **19**: 51–53

Goldberg GR, Black AE, Jebb SA et al. Critical evaluation of energy intake data using fundamental principles of energy physiology. 1. Derivation of cut-off limits to identify under-recording. *European Journal of Clinical Nutrition*, 1991; **45**: 569–581

Great Britain (GB) Department of Health. *Obesity: Reversing the Increasing Problem of Obesity in England.* London: Department of Health, 1995

Great Britain Ministry of Agriculture, Fisheries and Food (GB MAFF). *Household Food Consumption and Expenditure (Annual reports, 1940–1994).* London: HMSO, 1940–1994

Halaas JL, Gajiwala KS, Maffei M et al. Weight-reducing effects of the plasma protein encoded by the obese gene. *Science*, 1995; **269**: 543–546

Hamilton BS, Paglia D, Kwan AY, Deitel M. Increased obese mRNA expression in omental fat cells from massively obese humans. *Nature Medicine*, 1995; **1**: 953–956

Heitmann BL, Lissner L. Dietary underreporting by obese individuals—is it specific or non-specific? *British Medical Journal*, 1995; **311**: 986–989

Hill JO, Prentice AM. Sugar and body weight regulation. *American Journal of Clinical Nutrition*, 1995; **62**: 264S–274S

Jebb SA, Prentice AM. Is obesity an eating disorder? *Proceedings of the Nutrition Society*, 1995; **54**: 721–728

Jéquier E. Caloric balance versus nutrient balance. In: Kinney JM, Tucker HN, eds. *Energy Metabolism: Tissue Determinants and Cellular Corollaries.* New York: Raven Press, 1992: 123–136

Kendall A, Levitsky DA, Strupp BJ, Lissner L. Weight loss on a low-fat diet: consequence of the imprecision of the control of food intake in humans. *American Journal of Clinical Nutrition*, 1991; **53**: 1124–1129

Kennedy GC. Role of depot fat in hypothalamic control of food intake in rat. *Proceedings of the Royal Society, London B*, 1953; **140**: 578–592

Lawton CL, Burley VJ, Wales JK. Blundell JE. Dietary fat and appetite control in obese subjects: weak effects on satiation and satiety. *International Journal of Obesity*, 1993; **17**: 409–416

Lichtman SW, Pisarska K, Berman ER et al. Discrepancy between self-reported and actual caloric intake and exercise in obese subjects. *New England Journal of Medicine*, 1992; **327**: 1893–1898

Lissner L, Heitmann BL. Dietary fat and obesity: evidence from epidemiology. *European Journal of Clinical Nutrition*, 1995; **49**: 79–90

Lissner L, Levitsky DA, Strupp BJ, Kalkwarf HJ, Roe DA. Dietary fat and the regulation of energy intake in human subjects. *American Journal of Clinical Nutrition*, 1987; **46**: 886–892

Lonnqvist F, Arner P, Nordfors L, Schalling M. Overexpression of the obese (ob) gene in adipose tissue of human obese subjects. *Nature Medicine*, 1995; **1**: 950–953

Mertz W. Food intake measurements: is there a 'gold standard'? *Journal of the American Dietetic Association*, 1992; **92**: 1463–1465

Poppitt SD, Prentice AM. Energy density and its role in the control of food intake: evidence from metabolic and community studies. *Appetite*, 1996; **26**: 153–174

Prentice AM, Black AE, Coward WA *et al.* High levels of energy expenditure in obese women. *British Medical Journal*, 1986; **292**: 983–987

Prentice AM, Black AE, Murgatroyd PR, Goldberg GR, Coward WA. Metabolism or appetite: questions of energy balance with particular reference to obesity. *Journal of Human Nutrition and Dietetics*, 1989; **2**: 95–103

Prentice AM, Jebb SA. Obesity in Britain: Gluttony or sloth? *British Medical Journal*, 1995; **311**: 437–439

Prentice AM, Black AE, Coward WA, Cole TJ. Energy expenditure in overweight and obese adults in affluent societies: an analysis of 319 doubly-labelled water measurements. *European Journal of Clinical Nutrition*, 1996; **50**: 92–97

Rink TJ. In search of a satiety factor. *Nature*, 1994; **372**: 406–407

Rolls B. Changing the preferences for fat in foods. *Nutrition Reviews*, 1994; **52**: 21–23

Rolls BJ, Kim-Harris S, Fischman MW, Foltin RW, Moran TH, Stoner SA. Satiety after preloads with different amounts of fat and carbohydrate: implications for obesity. *American Journal of Clinical Nutrition*, 1994; **60**: 476–487

Royal College of Physicians. Obesity. A report of the Royal College of Physicians. *Journal of the Royal College of Physicians, London*, 1983; **17**: 3–65

Schoeller DA. How accurate is self-reported dietary energy intake? *Nutrition Reviews*, 1990; **48**: 373–379

Schoeller DA, Bandini LG, Dietz WH. Inaccuracies in self-reported intake identified by comparison with the doubly-labelled water method. *Canadian Journal of Physiology and Pharmacology*, 1990; **68**: 941-949

Scott J. New chapter for the fat controller. *Nature*, 1996; **379**: 113–114

Stubbs RJ. Macronutrient effects on appetite. *International Journal of Obesity*, 1995; **19** (suppl 5): S11–S19

Stubbs RJ, Prentice AM. The effect of covertly manipulating the dietary fat:carbohydrate ratio of isoenergetically dense diets on ad lib food intake in 'free-living' humans. *Proceedings of the Nutrition Society*, 1993; **52**: 351A

Stubbs RJ, Harbron CG, Murgatroyd PR, Prentice AM. Covert manipulation of dietary fat and energy density: effect on substrate flux and food intake in men eating ad libitum. *American Journal of Clinical Nutrition*, 1995a; **62**: 316–329

Stubbs RJ, Ritz P, Coward WA, Prentice AM. Covert manipulation of the dietary fat to carbohydrate ratio and energy density: effect on food intake and energy balance in free-living men, eating ad libitum. *American Journal of Clinical Nutrition*, 1995b; **62**: 330–337

Tartaglia LA, Dembski M, Weng X *et al.* Identification and expression cloning of a leptin receptor. *Cell*, 1995; **83**: 1263–1271

Tremblay A, Lavallee N, Almeras N, Allard L, Despres JP, Bouchard C. Nutritional determinants of the increase in energy intake associated with a high-fat diet. *American Journal of Clinical Nutrition*, 1991; **53**: 1134–1137

van Stratum P, Lussenburg RN, van Wezel LA, Vergroesen AJ, Cremer HD. The effect of dietary carbohydrate:fat ratio on energy intake by adult women. *American Journal of Clinical Nutrition*, 1978; **31**: 206–212

Zhang Y, Proenca R, Maffei M, Barone M, Leopold L, Friedman JM. Positional cloning of the mouse obese gene and its human homologue. *Nature*, 1994; **372**: 425–432

11.3 The problem of obesity and its management

Eric Jéquier

Institute of Physiology, University of Lausanne, Switzerland

Obesity results from a chronic imbalance between energy intake and energy expenditure. The dynamic phase of bodyweight gain, which is due to a positive energy balance, illustrates the fact that energy intake is chronically larger than energy expenditure. Whether a chronic excess in energy intake or a low energy expenditure is the major cause of obesity has been extensively studied. The present concept is that both mechanisms play a role, but it is likely that excess fat intake is the major factor responsible for the development of obesity.

Metabolic predictors of weight gain

In order to improve strategies to prevent the development of obesity, it is important to identify factors predictive of weight gain (Ravussin and Swinburn, 1993). Several longitudinal studies have reported that relatively low rates of energy expenditure predict weight gain in children (Roberts *et al*, 1988; Griffiths *et al*, 1990) and in adults (Ravussin *et al*, 1988). This low rate of energy expenditure may be associated with a low activity of the sympathetic nervous system (Spraul *et al*, 1993). However, a 10-year study of 775 individuals (Seidell *et al*, 1992) has reported no relationship between resting energy expenditure (REE) and long-term weight gain.

When REE is adjusted for differences in fat-free mass, age and sex, the standard deviation of the mean value of REE in a group of adult men or women is about 125 kcal/day (Dériaz *et al*, 1992). The potential effect of a low resting energy expenditure on bodyweight gain can be assessed by the following reasoning. Let us assume that two individuals of similar bodyweight and height have the same energy intake, but energy expenditure of the first is lower by 125 kcal/day than that of the second. While the latter is in energy balance, the former has a positive energy balance of 125 kcal/day. After a weight gain of about 5 kg, the low-REE individual will exhibit an increase in REE until energy balance is reached. This is due to the fact that for each kilogram weight gain, energy expenditure rises by 25 kcal/day (Jéquier and Schutz, 1988). Therefore, a 5-kg weight gain offsets the effect of the 'low metabolic rate'. This example illustrates the fact that 'a low metabolic rate' cannot be responsible for a large weight gain.

Another predictor of subsequent weight gain is a high respiratory quotient (RQ), a reflection of greater carbohydrate and less fat oxidation (Zurlo et al, 1990; Seidell et al, 1992). The development of obesity, which mainly results in an accumulation of fat in adipose tissue, is accompanied by a progressive increase in lipid oxidation (Schutz et al, 1992). The fat mass increases until the expansion of adipose tissue is such that lipolysis provides a sufficiently augmented flux of free fatty acids to stimulate fat oxidation to a level matching fat intake (Flatt, 1987). Thus, the increased fat mass of an obese subject can be considered as an 'adaptation' which is necessary to promote fat balance. In addition, insulin resistance, which is observed in obese individuals, is characterised by a lower uptake and oxidation of glucose in insulin-dependent tissues, and indirectly contributes to enhance fat oxidation (Felber et al, 1987). Insulin resistance has also been reported to contribute to limit weight gain in a weight-gaining population such as the Pima Indians (Swinburn et al, 1991).

A low capacity to oxidise lipids (illustrating a high insulin sensitivity) may have a major influence on bodyweight gain. If an individual has a low 24-h fat oxidation, e.g. a decreased lipid oxidation of 30 g/day, (i.e. 1 standard deviation of the mean lipid oxidation rate of a group of 106 women (Schutz et al, 1992)), a large increase in fat mass will be necessary to reach fat balance, if fat intake is similar to that of individuals who are in fat balance. For each kilogram of fat mass gain, 24-h lipid oxidation increased by 2 g/day (Schutz et al, 1992). Thus, in this individual with a low fat oxidation, fat balance would be reached after a 15-kg fat mass gain ($15 \, \text{kg} \times 2 \, \text{g} \, \text{day}^{-1} \text{kg}^{-1} = 30 \, \text{g/day}$). Since fat mass gain represents about 75% of total bodyweight gain, the expected weight gain is 22.5 kg. This example illustrates the possible weight gain of an individual with a low capacity to oxidise lipids.

Thus, a metabolic disorder characterised by low fat oxidation has a greater impact on bodyweight gain than a low relative energy expenditure. The metabolic origin of a low capacity for lipid oxidation is unknown. It is, however, of interest that individuals with a low resting sympathetic activity may be at risk for bodyweight gain (Spraul et al, 1993). Furthermore, it is well known that insulin indirectly stimulates the activity of the sympathetic nervous system, probably through central mechanisms (Laakso et al, 1990; Anderson et al, 1991; Vollenweider et al, 1993). When hyperinsulinaemia is induced in obese subjects during an euglycaemic clamp, one observes a minor sympathoexcitatory effect, whereas hyperinsulinaemia induces a marked increase in sympathetic activity in lean subjects (Vollenweider et al, 1994). Further investigations are needed to assess whether sympathetic activity may be a mechanism that stimulates whole body lipid oxidation in individuals at rest and that may in part counterbalance the antilipolytic effect of insulin.

Why fat balance is of great importance in bodyweight regulation

There are large differences between the balances of the three macronutrients: proteins, carbohydrates and fats, and this may play an important role in bodyweight regulation (Flatt, 1988; Jéquier, 1995). The mechanisms involved in the regulation of these balances are not completely understood. The ability to achieve protein balance over a wide range of intakes is well documented in humans. Studies on nitrogen balance can be carried out relatively easily, and within a certain range of protein intakes, the maintenance of a constant body protein content is observed. Thus, the regulation of bodyweight is not primarily dependent on protein balance. Before discussing carbohydrate and lipid balances, it is important to assess whether carbohydrate intake can influence lipid balance in humans by stimulating *de novo* lipogenesis. Many clinicians and nutritionists believe that the intake of carbohydrates plays a major role in the development of human obesity. It is often assumed that excess carbohydrate is readily transformed into fat in humans (Masoro, 1962). Liver and adipose tissue contain the enzymes necessary for the conversion of carbohydrate to fat. This metabolic process was extensively studied in young rodents (Assimacopoulos-Jeannet and Jeanrenaud, 1976) and was shown to be an important pathway. Recent evidence, however, has shown that *de novo* lipogenesis does not play an important role in the synthesis and deposition of body fat in humans. Metabolic investigations in humans have demonstrated how dietary carbohydrate decreases fat oxidation and how much carbohydrate needs to be consumed to produce lipogenesis sufficient to induce an increase in the body's fat content. Acheson *et al* (1982) showed that even after a 500 g oral load of carbohydrates, fat synthesis did not exceed fat oxidation in healthy young adult men. Thus it can be concluded that in everyday life, the intake of a normal amount of dietary carbohydrate mainly reduces the rate of fat oxidation, while stimulating glucose oxidation.

When a mixed diet is consumed, RQ measurements indicate that fat synthesis does not exceed fat oxidation. These results support the concept that dietary carbohydrates do not increase an individual's fat content by *de novo* lipogenesis. Using a non-invasive stable-isotope method, Hellerstein *et al* (1991) showed in humans that the fraction of very-low-density-lipoprotein-palmitate derived from *de novo* lipogenesis was only 0.9% in the fasted state and 2% in the fed state after a high-carbohydrate breakfast, and concluded that *de novo* lipogenesis is not an important pathway in humans. Studies on carbohydrate overfeeding (Acheson *et al*, 1982; 1988) show that carbohydrate oxidation is adjusted to carbohydrate intake over a 24-h period. Thus, carbohydrate balance is reached within 24 h under conditions of everyday life. This concept challenges the common perception that conversion of carbohydrate to fat is responsible in part for the accumulation of body fat in adipose tissue.

While carbohydrate and protein balances are under strict metabolic control, this is not the case for fat balance. After a high-fat meal, fat oxidation is not stimulated, and most of the excess fat intake is stored in adipose tissue (Flatt *et al*, 1985; Schutz *et al*, 1989). Comparing a very high-fat meal with a very low-fat meal (less than 1 g fat), Griffiths *et al* (1994) reported an increase of 10 g fat oxidised over the 6-h post-prandial period with a sparing of 20 g CHO. This is a small effect of lipid intake on lipid oxidation. Thus, within a reasonable range of CHO-energy: fat-energy ratio, the addition of fat to a meal does not substantially stimulate fat oxidation.

Another source of dietary energy that has to be considered is alcohol. Ethanol accounts for up to 10% of total energy intake of adult subjects. Ingestion of ethanol with a meal specifically induces a decrease in fat oxidation (Suter *et al*, 1992). Up to 80% of ethanol metabolised in the liver is released as acetate in the circulation, which suppresses fat oxidation in peripheral tissues (Akanji and Hockaday, 1990). When consumed in excess of energy needs, ethanol may favour fat storage and bodyweight gain by inhibiting fat oxidation.

Why obesity management is often unsuccessful

Since obesity results from a chronic imbalance between fat intake and fat oxidation, the obvious management of obesity is to reduce fat intake and to increase fat oxidation. In most developed countries, the percentage of food energy available from fat is 35–45% which is much higher than the upper limit of the recommended fat intake, i.e. 30%. There has been a marked increase in fat consumption during this century; in the early 1900s, people were consuming only about 20% energy as fat. During the thousands of years of human evolution, it is likely that the capacity to store fat has been advantageous for survival when food was limited. Nowadays, this metabolic feature favours bodyweight gain in people living in affluent countries (Lissner and Heitmann, 1995).

Prevention of obesity benefits from a daily moderate fat intake. A decreased proportion of fat-energy and a compensatory increased proportion of CHO-energy in the everyday diet is an effective means of avoiding bodyweight gain. Several randomised clinical trials reporting the effect of a calorically unrestricted low-fat diet on weight change show modest weight reductions in the range of 3–4 kg after six months (Lissner and Heitmann, 1995). The low-fat diet appears to have an interesting therapeutic potential, provided the rate of weight loss can be maintained over longer periods of time than a few months. The available evidence, however, indicates that the weight loss mainly occurs within the first three months of the low-fat diet; thereafter, the subjects are less able to maintain their dietary changes and bodyweight does not decrease further.

Prevention of obesity also benefits from stimulation of fat oxidation. Exercise of low intensity and of long duration mainly stimulates fat oxidation. During exercise, mobilisation of endogenous lipid is increased and muscles utilise fatty acids as substrate. Thus, physical activity may contribute to the everyday fat balance. The duration of low-intensity exercise, however, must be of several hours per day in order to have a significant influence on fat balance. An individual spends about 3 kcal/min while walking at a rapid pace; at rest, energy expenditure is close to 1 kcal/min. Thus, walking induces an increase in energy expenditure by 2 kcal/min; a three-hour walk results in a supplementary energy expenditure of 360 kcal, which corresponds to 40 g of fat. A three-hour exercise period should be carried out each day for 25 days to lose 1 kg of fat. This example illustrates the need for a real change in lifestyle, if a sustained fat loss is to be achieved by exercise. For exercise to be of benefit, the net fat oxidation induced by exercise must be greater than the amount of fat ingested.

The treatment of obesity mainly consists of hypocaloric therapy for prolonged periods of time. In addition, various surgical procedures have been proposed to treat severely obese patients (grade III obesity with a Body Mass Index over 40 kg m^{-2}). The purpose of this short paper is not to describe the various hypocaloric diets or the surgical procedures (see Garrow (1981) for a complete review), but to assess the main reasons which explain why obesity treatment is often unsuccessful.

During a hypocaloric diet, metabolic rate decreases more than could be accounted for by the loss of lean tissue. Several studies in which the resting metabolic rate (RMR) was assessed before and after weight loss show that the decrease in RMR per unit bodyweight loss varies between 9 and 14 kcal/kg/day (Doré et al, 1982; Finer et al, 1986; Froidevaux et al, 1993). This variability in the economy of basal energy expenditure per kilogram of weight loss is accounted for in part by the composition of the tissue lost—usually about 75% fat and 25% fat-free mass (FFM), but this proportion may vary with the rate of weight loss, the duration and the composition of the hypoenergetic diet. A major determinant of the decrease in RMR during weight loss is the reduction in FFM. Furthermore, a decrease in RMR per kilogram of FFM (Apfelbaum et al, 1971; Bessard et al, 1983; Elliot et al, 1989) suggests that other factors, in addition to the loss of FFM, contribute to the reduction in RMR during weight loss. The acute decrease in sympathetic activity assessed by a reduction in urinary norepinephrine excretion (Jung et al, 1979; 1980) and a decrease in plasma triiodothyronine levels are adaptive mechanisms which may explain the lowering in RMR per kilogram of FFM during a hypocaloric diet (Shetty, 1990). It is likely that these metabolic responses do not have a large impact on energy metabolism (Ravussin et al, 1985) and their effects disappear after the end of the hypocaloric diet.

The decrease in the overall energy expenditure during a hypocaloric diet is not only due to a reduction in RMR, but also to a lower thermic effect of food related to the lower energy intake, and to the reduced energy cost of physical activity, due to a lower bodyweight (Ravussin et al, 1985). The decrease in total energy expenditure (TEE) resulting from a weight loss of one kilogram represents about 25 kcal/day (Jéquier and Schutz, 1988). Thus, a weight loss of 20 kg in an obese individual reduces TEE by 500 kcal per day, of which approximately 250 kcal/day are due to a decrease in RMR. Failure to reduce the habitual energy intake by 500 kcal/day after the end of the hypocaloric diet will result in weight gain and the relapse of the obese state.

A second metabolic consequence of bodyweight loss is a decrease in lipid oxidation since the composition of substrate to total energy expenditure changes with weight loss, with a shift from fat to carbohydrate oxidation (Weinsier *et al*, 1995). This lower fat oxidation capacity may contribute to weight gain after weight loss (Zurlo *et al*, 1990; Seidell *et al*, 1992; Astrup, 1993; 1994). Obese subjects express a liking for fatty foods (Drewnowski *et al*, 1985). After weight loss, it is likely that the preference for high-fat foods results in selection of fatty foods; since the capacity to oxidise fat has decreased with weight loss, high fat intake combined with low fat oxidation produces a rapid weight gain. Body fat stores again increase until the expansion of adipose tissue mass induces an increase in plasma concentrations of non-esterified fatty acids (NEFA); the latter results in an increased ratio of lipid to carbohydrate oxidation to a level commensurate with the lipid-to-carbohydrate ratio of the everyday diet. This concept considers the expansion of body fat stores as an adaptation to the high dietary fat content in order to reach fat balance by stimulating lipid oxidation.

In a recent well designed study to increase the understanding of the relationship between various metabolic factors and predisposition to obesity, Weinsier *et al* (1995) concluded that neither resting energy expenditure, the thermic effect of food, nor the patterns of fuel utilisation were predictive of long-term weight regain in previously obese women after reduction to a normal bodyweight. The tendency to regain excess bodyweight among obesity-prone women was more likely to be due to maladaptive responses to the environment in terms of physical inactivity or excess food intake than to reduced energy requirements. Thus the predisposition to obesity, which is in part genetic (Bouchard, 1994), seems to result more from behavioural characteristics, such as the preference for fatty foods and a low level of physical activity, than from reduced energy requirements or abnormalities of resting energy expenditure and fuel utilisation.

References

Acheson KJ, Flatt JP, Jéquier E. Glycogen synthesis versus lipogenesis after a 500 g carbohydrate meal in man. *Metabolism*, 1982; **31**: 1234–1240

Acheson KJ, Schutz Y, Bessard T, Anantharaman K, Flatt JP, Jéquier E. Glycogen storage capacity and de novo lipogenesis during massive carbohydrate overfeeding in man. *American Journal of Clinical Nutrition*, 1988; **48**: 240–247

Akanji AO, Hockaday TDR. Acetate tolerance and the kinetics of acetate utilization in diabetic and nondiabetic subjects. *American Journal of Clinical Nutrition*, 1990; **51**: 112–118

Anderson EA, Hoffman RP, Balon TW, Sinkey CA, Mark AL. Hyperinsulinemia produces both sympathetic neural activation and vasodilation in normal humans. *Journal of Clinical Investigation*, 1991; **87**: 2246–2252

Apfelbaum M, Bostsarron J, Lacatis D. Effect of caloric restriction and excessive caloric intake on energy expenditure. *American Journal of Clinical Nutrition*, 1971; **24**: 1404–1409

Assimacopoulos-Jeannet F, Jeanrenaud B. The hormonal and metabolic basis of experimental obesity. *Clinics in Endocrinology and Metabolism*, 1976; **5**: 337–365

Astrup A. Dietary composition, substrate balances and body fat in subjects with a predisposition to obesity. *International Journal of Obesity*, 1993; **17** (Suppl. 3): S32–S36

Astrup A, Buemann B, Christensen NJ, Toubro S. Failure to increase lipid oxidation in response to increasing dietary fat content in formerly obese women. *American Journal of Physiology*, 1994; **266**: E592–E599

Bessard T, Schutz Y, Jéquier E. Energy expenditure and postprandial thermogenesis in obese women before and after weight loss. *American Journal of Clinical Nutrition*, 1983; **38**: 680–693

Bouchard C. *The Genetics of Obesity*. Boca Raton, FL: CRC Press, 1994

Dériaz O, Fournier G, Tremblay A, Després JP, Bouchard C. Lean-body-mass composition and resting energy expenditure before and after long-term overfeeding. *American Journal of Clinical Nutrition*, 1992; **56**: 840–847

Doré C, Hesp R, Wilkins D, Garrow JS. Prediction of energy requirements of obese patients after massive weight loss. *Human Nutrition: Clinical Nutrition*, 1982; **36C**: 41–48

Drewnowski A, Brunzell JD, Sande K, Iverius PH, Greenwood R. Sweet tooth reconsidered: taste responsiveness in human obesity. *Physiology and Behavior*, 1985; **35**: 617–622

Elliot DL, Goldberg L, Kuehl KS, Bennett WM. Sustained depression of the resting metabolic rate after massive weight loss. *American Journal of Clinical Nutrition*, 1989; **49**: 93–96

Felber JP, Ferrannini E, Golay A *et al.* Role of lipid oxidation in pathogenesis of insulin resistance of obesity and type II diabetes. *Diabetes*, 1987; **36**: 1341–1350

Finer N, Swan PC, Mitchell FT. Metabolic rate after massive weight loss in human obesity. *Clinical Science*, 1986; **70**: 395–398

Flatt JP. Dietary fat, carbohydrate balance, and weight maintenance: effects of exercise. *American Journal of Clinical Nutrition*, 1987; **45**: 296–306

Flatt JP. Importance of nutrient balance in body weight regulation. *Diabetes/Metabolism Reviews*, 1988; **4**: 571–581

Flatt JP, Ravussin E, Acheson KJ, Jéquier E. Effects of dietary fat on postprandial substrate oxidation and on carbohydrate and fat balances. *Journal of Clinical Investigation*, 1985; **76**: 1019–1024

Froidevaux F, Schutz Y, Christin L, Jéquier E. Energy expenditure in obese women before and during weight loss, after refeeding, and in the weight-relapse period. *American Journal of Clinical Nutrition*, 1993; **57**: 35–42

Garrow JS. *Treat Obesity Seriously*. Edinburgh: Churchill Livingstone, 1981

Griffiths AJ, Humphreys SM, Clark ML, Fielding BA, Frayn RK. Immediate metabolic availability of dietary fat in combination with carbohydrate. *American Journal of Clinical Nutrition*, 1994; **59**: 53–59

Griffiths M, Payne PR, Stunkard AJ, Rivers JP, Cox M. Metabolic rate and physical development in children at risk of obesity. *Lancet* 1990; **336**: 76–78

Hellerstein MK, Christiansen M, Kaempfer S *et al.* Measurement of de novo hepatic lipogenesis in humans using stable isotopes. *Journal of Clinical Investigation*, 1991; **87**: 1841–1852

Jéquier E. Nutrient effects: post-absorptive interactions. *Proceedings of the Nutrition Society*, 1995; **54**: 253–265

Jéquier E, Schutz Y. Energy expenditure in obesity and diabetes. *Diabetes/Metabolism Reviews*, 1988; **4**: 583–593

234   E. Jéquier

Jung RT, Shetty PS, Barrand M, Callingham BA, James WPT. Role of catecholamines in hypotensive response to dieting. *British Medical Journal*, 1979; **1**: 12–13

Jung RT, Shetty PS, James WPT. The effect of refeeding after semi-starvation on catecholamine and thyroid metabolism. *International Journal of Obesity*, 1980; **4**: 95–100

Laakso M, Edelman SV, Brechtel G, Baron AD. Decreased effect of insulin to stimulate skeletal muscle blood flow in obese man. A novel mechanism for insulin resistance. *Journal of Clinical Investigation*, 1990; **85**: 1844–1852

Lissner L, Heitmann BL. Dietary fat and obesity: evidence from epidemiology. *European Journal of Clinical Nutrition*, 1995; **49**: 79–90

Masoro EJ. Biochemical mechanisms related to the homeostatic regulation of lipogenesis in animals. *Journal of Lipid Research*, 1962; **3**: 149–164

Ravussin E, Swinburn BA. Metabolic predictors of obesity: cross-sectional versus longitudinal data. *International Journal of Obesity*, 1993; **17** (Suppl. 3): S28–S31

Ravussin E, Burnand B, Schutz Y, Jéquier E. Energy expenditure before and during energy restriction in obese patients. *American Journal of Clinical Nutrition*, 1985; **41**: 753–759

Ravussin E, Lillioja S, Knowler WC et al. Reduced rate of energy expenditure as a risk factor for body-weight gain. *New England Journal of Medicine*, 1988; **318**: 467–472

Roberts SB, Savage J, Coward WA, Chew B, Lucas A. Energy expenditure and intake in infants born to lean and overweight mothers. *New England Journal of Medicine*, 1988; **318**: 461–466

Schutz Y, Flatt JP, Jéquier E. Failure of dietary fat intake to promote fat oxidation: a factor favoring the development of obesity. *American Journal of Clinical Nutrition*, 1989; **50**: 307–314

Schutz Y, Tremblay A, Weinsier RL, Nelson KM. Role of fat oxidation in the long-term stabilization of body weight in obese women. *American Journal of Clinical Nutrition*, 1992; **55**: 670–784

Seidell JC, Muller DC, Sorkin JD, Andres R. Fasting respiratory exchange ratio and resting metabolic rate as predictors of weight gain: the Baltimore Longitudinal Study on Aging. *International Journal of Obesity*, 1992; **16**: 667–674

Shetty PS. Physiological mechanisms in the adaptive response of metabolic rates to energy restriction. *Nutrition Research Reviews*, 1990; **3**: 49–74

Spraul M, Ravussin E, Fontvieille AM, Rising R, Larson DE, Anderson EA. Reduced sympathetic nervous activity. *Journal of Clinical Investigation*, 1993; **92**: 1730–1735

Suter PM, Schutz Y, Jéquier E. The effect of ethanol on fat storage in healthy subjects. *New England Journal of Medicine*, 1992; **326**: 983–987

Swinburn BA, Nyomba BL, Saad MF et al. Insulin resistance associated with lower rates of weight gain in Pima Indians. *Journal of Clinical Investigation*, 1991; **88**: 168–173

Vollenweider P, Tappy L, Randin D et al. Differential effects of hyperinsulinemia and carbohydrate metabolism on sympathetic nerve activity and muscle blood flow in humans. *Journal of Clinical Investigation*, 1993; **92**: 147–154

Vollenweider P, Randin D, Tappy L, Jéquier E, Nicod P, Scherrer U. Impaired insulin-induced sympathetic neural activation and vasodilation in skeletal muscle in obese humans. *Journal of Clinical Investigation*, 1994; **93**: 2365–2371

Weinsier RL, Nelson KM, Hensrud DD, Darnell BE, Hunter GR, Schutz Y. Metabolic predictors of obesity. Contribution of resting energy expenditure, thermic effect of food, and fuel utilization to four-year weight gain of post-obese and never-obese women. *Journal of Clinical Investigation*, 1995; **95**: 980–985

Zurlo F, Lillioja S, Esposito-Del Puente A et al. Low ratio of fat to carbohydrate oxidation as predictor of weight gain: study of 24-h RQ. *American Journal of Physiology*, 1990; **259**: E650–E657

11.4 Obesity and its relationships to other diseases

Lars Sjöström

Department of Medicine, University of Göteborg, Sweden

Obesity is a common disease and its prevalence is increasing in most countries. This is a serious problem, since few, if any, diseases are associated with such a large number of secondary disorders as obesity. These associated disorders include coronary heart disease (CHD), cardiac insufficiency, sleep apnoea, hypoventilation syndrome, cor pulmonale, stroke, gallbladder disease, certain cancers, locomotor dysfunction, various skin diseases, menstrual disorders, infertility, obstetric complications and socio-economic handicaps. Furthermore, obesity is associated with several or all of the aspects of the metabolic syndrome. These aspects comprise insulin resistance, glucose intolerance, non-insulin-dependent diabetes mellitus (NIDDM), visceral adipose tissue accumulation, hypertension, hypertriglyceridaemia, low HDL-cholesterol, decreased fibrinolysis and elevated transaminases. Finally, the visceral fat accumulation causes an increased intra-abdominal pressure which in its turn is an important causal factor in the development of varicose veins, hernias, nephrotic syndrome, increased pleural pressure, reduced venous return from the brain and thus even in the development of pseudo-tumour cerebri.

This brief review will focus on bodyweight and weight changes in relation to cardiovascular morbidity and mortality. Cross-sectional as well as longitudinal observations will be discussed, both by using data from the available literature, and by using data from an ongoing intervention study of obesity in Sweden.

The Swedish Obese Subjects (SOS) study

The SOS Project consists of one registry study and one intervention study. In the registry study, 6000–10 000 severely obese subjects will be examined at the 700 primary health care centres in Sweden. From the registry, patients are recruited into the intervention study, which consists of two groups, one surgically treated group and one conventionally treated control group. Each group will contain 2000 subjects, and the follow-up will be 10 years. The treatments in the surgical group are (variable) banding, vertical banded gastroplasty, or gastric bypass. Operations and follow-up are handled by 30 surgical departments in Sweden. Treatments and follow-up in the control group are handled by the primary health care centres. Treatment consists of traditional advice about caloric restriction and increased physical activity.

In January 1996, SOS had received 7400 applications, 5600 of which were accepted. Nearly 4500 health examinations had been performed, 1300 patients had been operated upon, and the same number of patients had been included in the control group. The follow-up rate at two years was 94% in the surgical group, and 86% in the control group. Of the 700 primary health care centres in Sweden, 480 are connected to SOS. At baseline, BMI was 41 kg/m^2 in the surgical group, and 40 kg/m^2 in the control group. At the two-year follow-up, the weight reduction was on average 28 kg in the surgical group, and 0.6 kg in the conventionally treated control group.

Cardiovascular risk factors in relation to body composition and weight decrease

Ninety-one per cent of the SOS males and 78% of the SOS females had at least one of the traditional risk factors:

- insulin > 20 mU/l
- triglycerides > 2.0 mM
- glucose > 7.1 mM
- systolic blood pressure > 160 mmHg
- diastolic blood pressure > 95 mmHg
- cholesterol > 7.0 mM
- HDL-cholesterol < 1.0 mM.

Except for total cholesterol, average risk factor values were considerably higher among SOS subjects than in age- and gender-matched randomly selected populations (Sjöström et al, 1992). For instance, triglycerides were 50–75% higher than normal among SOS females, and more than twice as high as normal among SOS males. All risk factors were more closely related to the visceral than to the subcutaneous adipose tissue mass (Sjöström et al, 1995). Some risk factors, including insulin, were negatively related to lean body mass (LBM), the non-adipose tissue. When taking these body compartments into account, risk factors were positively related to subcutaneous adipose tissue located in the upper part of the body, and negatively to subcutaneous adipose tissue located in the lower part of the body (Sjöström et al, 1995).

The effects of weight changes on cardiovascular risk factors were examined after pooling the surgical group and control group in order to obtain the largest possible range of weight changes (from −90 to +30 kg) over two years. All risk factor changes were adjusted for initial risk factor value, sex, age and initial BMI

(Sjöström *et al*, submitted). Under these circumstances, a 45 kg weight reduction resulted in 60% reduction in insulin, 40% reduction in triglycerides, 30% reduction in glucose, and blood pressure levels and the total cholesterol decreased by about 10%. HDL-cholesterol increased by 40%. While total cholesterol was reduced only by weight reductions larger than 25 kg, other risk factors changed more or less linearly with the weight change. This implies that substantial risk reductions may require larger weight reductions than can usually be expected from conventional treatment.

The cross-sectional observations on body compartments and subcutaneous adipose tissue distributions (Sjöström *et al*, 1995) were validated by the longitudinal studies (Sjöström *et al*, submitted), since changes in risk factors were related to changes in visceral and subcutaneous adipose tissue mass and to changes in subcutaneous adipose tissue distribution.

Bodyweight, morbidity and mortality

From the literature, it is well known that the prevalent morbidity is markedly elevated in the obese. This has been reconfirmed by the SOS study (Sjöström *et al*, 1992). The prevalence of previously experienced myocardial infarction among the obese SOS males is 6% at the age of 50 and 16% at the age of 55. These figures are five times higher than those observed in a randomly selected population of Swedish males of the same age (Sjöström *et al*, 1992). More than 50 epidemiological studies have shown that a high bodyweight at baseline is associated with an elevated incident morbidity and mortality during follow-up (for details, see Sjöström, 1992). Manson's study of 116 000 US nurses may serve as an illustration of this point (Manson *et al*, 1990). In that study, the endpoints were myocardial infarction plus fatal CHD. With larger BMI at baseline the risk increased, and for non-smokers with a BMI greater than 29, the risk was three times larger than that for women with BMI below 21 at baseline.

Bodyweight increase, morbidity and mortality

A small number of studies have examined the effects of weight increase on incident morbidity and mortality. Again, Manson's study may serve as an example (Manson *et al*, 1990). Subjects with weight increases smaller than 3 kg served as a reference with the relative risk 1.0. Small weight increases tended to be associated with risk decreases (relative risk 0.6, ns) while larger weight increases were associated with risk increases. For weight increases of 10–19.9 kg the relative risk (RR) was 1.7, and for 20–49 kg, the RR increased further to 2.5.

Bodyweight decrease, morbidity and mortality

The observations discussed above indicate that it is dangerous to be obese and to have increases in bodyweight over time. Unfortunately, the situation is more complicated than this. Some 20 carefully performed observational, epidemiological studies have demonstrated that weight reduction in subjects who were obese is also associated with increased mortality risk. This point may be illustrated by Pamuk's study on 2100 middle-aged men followed up for 10 years (Pamuk *et al*, 1992). Mortality occurring during the first five years after inclusion was excluded from analysis in an attempt to get rid of the effects of subclinical mortality at baseline. A weight loss $> 15\%$ was associated with a RR for total mortality of 1.8 (reference: weight loss 5%) among those having a maximum BMI of < 26. For subjects with maximum BMI > 29 and without weight changes, the relative risk was 1.5. This is in keeping with the literature discussed above. Unexpectedly, a weight loss $> 15\%$ among individuals with maximum BMI > 29 was associated with a relative risk of 2.0.

So the literature tells us that it is dangerous *to be* obese, to *decrease* in weight, and to *increase* in weight. This cumbersome situation is probably caused by the fact that studies on effects of weight reduction have not been able to separate intentional from unintentional weight loss in spite of serious attempts to do so. This is an important issue since a recent study on 26 000 women from Iowa showed that unintentional weight losses larger than 20 lbs (approximately 10 kg) were more common (29%) than intentional weight losses of the same magnitude (25%) (French *et al*, 1995).

One single observational epidemiological study has had data available making it tentatively possible to separate obese subjects with intentional weight loss from subjects with unintentional weight loss (Williamson *et al*, 1995). Among those obese subjects with intentional weight loss, there was a significantly reduced lower mortality in patients with obesity-related diseases at baseline, but not in patients without such diseases. With unintentional weight loss and no obesity-associated diseases at baseline, there was a non-statistically significant trend to increased risk in this study. The information used to separate intentional from unintentional weight loss in this study by Williamson and colleagues (1995) can be called into question, and there is a need to separate disease-driven from non-disease-driven weight reductions. There is really only one way to unravel the contradictory situation in the literature, and that is by undertaking controlled intervention studies. SOS is so far the only large-scale intervention study that has been started to address this issue.

It is too early to report on hard endpoints in the SOS study. However, two-year incidence data on cardiovascular risk factors are now available from 712 controls and 767 surgically treated subjects (Sjöström *et al*, submitted). At baseline, the prevalence of diabetes was 14% in both groups. The two-year incidence was 6.5% in the control group, which on average had not reduced bodyweight to any significant degree. In the surgically treated group, the two-year incidence was only 0.2%, that is, a 28 kg weight reduction resulted in a 33-fold risk reduction. The two-year incidences of hypertension, hypertriglyceridaemia and low HDL were of the order of 7–15% in the control group. In the surgical group, 2- to

25-fold risk reductions were seen in these parameters. After pooling the data of the surgical group and the controls, it may be deduced that a 50% risk reduction (in incidence of cardiovascular risk factors) requires a weight reduction of the order of 10%, and to achieve a 75% risk reduction, a 20% weight reduction would be necessary.

Conclusions

Prevalent and incident morbidity as well as total and cardiovascular mortality are dramatically elevated in severe obesity. Both a decrease and increase in bodyweight can increase the risk of morbidity and mortality. It is not yet certain if hard endpoints are reduced by substantial weight reduction, but the two-year incidence of cardiovascular risk factors is markedly reduced by weight reduction. Surgical intervention seems to be more effective than conventional methods to achieve substantial weight reduction.

References

French SA, Jeffery RW, Folsom AR, Williamson DF, Byers T. History of intentional and unintentional weight loss in a population-based sample of women aged 55–69 years. *Obesity Research*, 1995; **3**: 163–170

Manson JE, Colditz GA, Stampfer MJ et al. A prospective study of obesity and risk of coronary heart disease in women. *New England Journal of Medicine*, 1990; **322**: 882–889

Pamuk ER, Williamson DF, Madans J, Serdula MK, Kleinman JC, Byers T. Weight loss and mortality in a national cohort of adults, 1971–1987. *American Journal of Epidemiology*, 1992; **136**: 686–697

Sjöström L. Mortality in severely obese subjects. *American Journal of Clinical Nutrition*, 1992; **55**: 516S–523S

Sjöström L, Larsson B, Backman L et al. Swedish Obese Subjects (SOS). Recruitment for an intervention study and a selected description of the obese state. *International Journal of Obesity*, 1992; **16**: 465–479

Sjöström CD, Håkangård AC, Lissner L, Sjöström L. Body compartment and subcutaneous adipose tissue distribution risk factor patterns in obese subjects. *Obesity Research*, 1995; **3**: 9–22

Sjöström CD, Lissner L, Sjöström L. Relationships between changes in body composition and changes in cardiovascular risk factors: the SOS intervention study. Submitted

Williamson DF, Pamuk E, Thun M, Flanders D, Byers T, Heath C. Prospective study of intentional weight loss and mortality in never-smoking overweight US white women aged 40–60 years. *American Journal of Epidemiology*, 1995; **141**: 1128–1141

11.5 Physical activity, obesity and chronic disease

Anna Ferro-Luzzi

National Institute of Nutrition, Rome, Italy

Modern life is becoming increasingly sedentary. An analysis of time-budget surveys representative of populations reveals that the time needed to earn a living and for domestic work has declined appreciably over recent decades (Ferro-Luzzi and Martino, 1996). This negative secular trend is accompanied by a substantial decline in the energy spent in these activities, given that most modern jobs can be carried out with lower human energy input, due to technical progress, urbanisation, transport, and to the availability of a large range of domestic electrical appliances. The contraction of work time has resulted in a converse increase in free time, but the bulk of this is taken up with leisure activities that do not involve any physical exertion and are carried out at an energy cost just above resting. Watching television for more than three hours a day has been associated with twice the risk of obesity as compared with less than one hour (Tucker and Friedman, 1989) and slimming success was inversely proportional to television watching (Gortmaker *et al*, 1990). In children, television watching has been shown to displace active playing (Buratta and Sabbadini, 1993) and among adolescents, obesity has been found to increase by 2% for each additional hour of television watching per day (Dietz and Gortmaker, 1985). On the other hand, active leisure, such as sports and outdoor activities, often occupies less than 30 minutes per day (Ferro-Luzzi and Martino, 1996). Thus, at least in Western societies, one can reasonably assert that the daily energy expenditure has fallen for some decades, and that the modern style of life is markedly sedentary.

Several authors have highlighted the growing concern of modern affluent societies with the marked positive secular trend of obesity, affecting children (Murata and Hibi, 1992) as much as adults, with a 2–4% increase per decade in mean Body Mass Index (BMI) in most of the countries where repeat surveys have been conducted (Byers and Marshall, 1995). The situation in the Third World is no better, with a precipitous increase of mean BMI in close association with acculturation indices (Byers and Marshall, 1995) and modernity scores (Hodge *et al*, 1995). It is important, therefore, to establish whether this epidemic of obesity is in any way linked to sedentary lifestyles. Much of the evidence that has been gathered in prospective or retrospective case-control type studies over the past two or three decades generally supports this hypothesis. Thus Rissanen et al (1991), crudely classifying subjects on the basis of the frequency of exercise in 'rarely' to 'frequent' leisure-time physical activity categories, found in a cross-sectional study of almost 6000 men and women that those who belonged to the category of rare physical activity were fatter; a follow-up survey indicated that the least active individuals were more likely to gain 5 kg bodyweight over the next five years than their more frequently active counterparts (Relative Risk (RR) = 1.6–1.9). Similar positive results were obtained by DiPietro and colleagues (1993) on 18 000 US subjects attempting to lose weight, where there was an inverse association between selected physical activities and bodyweight, independent of age, sex, race, education, etc. Williamson et al (1993) in their analysis of a 10-year follow-up of more than 9000 men and women in the NHANES-I survey also found that the prevalence of obesity was inversely related to the intensity of recreational physical activity, and that those who were less active had an odds ratio of 3.9 for men and of 7 for women, to gain about 1 kg bodyweight per year if they were inactive at both visits, as compared to those who on the same occasions had reported high levels of physical activity. Free-living energy expenditure of Pima Indians was found by Rising and colleagues (1994) to be significantly correlated ($r = -0.56$, $P < 0.01$) with their body fat. Gardner and Poehlman (1993) calculated that for each 100 kcal increment in physical activity, there would be a 0.16–0.35% decrease in body fat. Romieu et al (1988) showed that in a sub-group of white nurses residing in the Boston area, those in the lowest BMI tertile (< 22.2) had a significantly higher ($r = -0.31$, $P = 0.000$) exercise expenditure (247 kcal/day) than those in the highest BMI tertile (> 24.4). Voorrips and colleagues (1992) in a retrospective study on weight and physical activity of Dutch women found that non-active women had higher BMI and that the differences were already present at the age of 25 years. Similarly, Kromhout and others (1988) found by multivariate analysis that the indicators of body fatness in a group of Dutch men aged 45–64 were inversely related to occupational and leisure time physical activity.

These studies suffer from the fact that they refer exclusively to Northern European and North American populations. This is a limitation that does not allow extrapolation of the findings to many societies who live under profoundly diverse circumstances, such as those encountered in developing countries. To fill this gap, we have recently collated and analysed data extracted from recently published studies (Ferro-Luzzi and Martino, 1996). This analysis also has the advantage that, in these studies, as opposed to the studies cited above, physical activity had been accurately measured by indirect calorimetry or by the stable isotopic doubly labelled water method (DLW). Of the total of approximately 1600 men and women studied in 22 different countries, some 800 are subjects of developing countries. A further 200 represent a special sub-group of Western people engaged in strenuous sports or in other vigorous activities, such as jungle warfare training or mountain climbing. The remainder consist of a miscellaneous group of Western healthy individuals and obese people who have been studied for a variety of reasons. The level of energy expenditure is expressed as PAL (physical activity level) and describes energy expenditure as multiples of Basal Metabolic Rate (BMR).

A multivariate regression analysis of these data with body mass index (BMI) as dependent variable, and PAL and country as independent variables, has yielded a highly significant inverse correlation confirming that physical activity is linked to fatness. However, the main explanatory power is that of the ecological variable, with PAL explaining a much higher proportion of the total variance of BMI. We carried the analysis further and sought to define, using the same database, the existence of a threshold level of energy expenditure below which obesity is more likely to occur. Having taken BMI of 25 as cut-off for overweight and obesity, and adopting a sliding scale of progressively higher PAL values to discriminate between sedentary and active lifestyles, the odds ratios suggest that a PAL of 1.8 might represent the threshold below which the risk of being overweight increases about seven-fold. A PAL of 1.8 corresponds to the energy requirement of an adult man engaged in moderately heavy work (WHO, 1985).

We can thus conclude that the evidence points rather convincingly to lower levels of activity of obese people, as compared to people who are lean and stay lean over the years. However, several studies have also been unable to show any difference in the energy expenditure of obese and lean people (Sallis *et al*, 1985; Paffenbarger *et al*, 1986; Blair and Buskirk, 1987; Leon *et al*, 1987; Prentice *et al*, 1996). The strength of the correlation between physical activity levels and fatness, while statistically significant, is often rather weak, and explains only a small proportion of the total variance in fatness (Folsom *et al*, 1985; Dannenberg *et al*, 1989). This may be due to the crudeness of the methods employed to assess physical activity levels (Baecke *et al*, 1982; Blair *et al*, 1985; Sallis *et al*, 1985; Blair *et al*, 1989; Slattery *et al*, 1990; Haskell *et al*, 1992). Most studies resort to questionnaires, sometimes conducted by telephone interview, although more refined and sophisticated methods have in some instances failed to show any relationship (Hardman *et al*, 1992; Prentice *et al*, 1996). But the weakness of the correlation also suggests that the relationship might be quite complex and that a host of other factors might complicate and confound it.

Physical activity and coronary heart disease (CHD)

Physical activity is thought to influence other possible health outcomes to an appreciable extent. Coronary heart disease (CHD) appears at the top of the list. An inverse relationship has been found between the risk of a first heart attack and engagement in physically strenuous sports or in other physical activities. In a 10-year follow-up of Harvard alumni, the sedentary have a 31% higher risk than the most active (Paffenbarger *et al*, 1978). An estimate of the attributable risk for these men, adjusted for other risk factors, showed that had no man been sedentary, the death rates from all causes would have been reduced by 16%. Paffenbarger *et al* (1986) also estimated that an active lifestyle might have added on an average 2.2 years of life, after adjusting for differences in blood pressure, BMI and other parameters, as compared to those who had maintained very sedentary lifestyles.

A similar inverse relationship was found in San Francisco longshoremen which persisted after accounting for the effect of obesity and other risk factors (Paffenbarger and Hale, 1975). Time dedicated to leisure physical activities categorised as light (2–4 kcal/min), moderate (4.5–5.5 kcal/min) and heavy (> 6 kcal/min), proved to be a good predictor of the risk of CHD morbidity and mortality in the seven-year follow-up of the 12 138 middle-aged men recruited in the MRFIT trial (Multiple Risk Factor Intervention Study) (Leon *et al*, 1987). Less active men (14 minutes per day of activity at an estimated energy expenditure of 74 kcal) had a 27% excess CHD cumulative mortality, as compared to those who were moderately active (48 minutes per day of activity at 224 kcal/day) (Leon and Connett, 1991). That vigorous exercise might be more protective than a similar amount of energy spent in less strenuous activities was first pointed out by Morris *et al* (1973), who hypothesised a dose–response relationship and estimated the threshold level to be about 7.5 kcal/min. Thus, activity might need to be of a certain intensity for a cardiovascular benefit to be accrued (Powell *et al*, 1989).

Several mechanisms have been postulated by which physical activity might afford a protective effect on the heart. The enhancement of triglyceride clearance, the extended half-life of the HDL_2 fraction, the raised circulating levels of specific HDL subclasses, accompanied by a decrease of LDL cholesterol and a more favourable LDL/HDL ratio have all been shown to contribute (Haskell *et al*, 1992; Williams *et al*, 1995). These changes are not a function of dietary factors or weight loss, but rather of the level of exercise achieved, the increase being higher for higher intensity and longer duration and frequency of exercise (Hartung *et al*, 1980). Other suggested mechanisms are the favourable exercise-induced changes of various haemostatic and fibrinolytic parameters (Williams *et al*, 1980). Thus, a 10-week exercise programme significantly enhanced the fibrinolytic response to a standardised thrombotic stress caused by venous occlusion. Promising results were also reported by Folsom *et al* (1993) who showed a decrease of factor VII, PAI-1 and t-PA, while Stratton *et al* (1991) demonstrated an enhanced fibrinolytic activity. Rauramaa *et al* (1986) showed that trained subjects had a decreased platelet aggregability and Sullivan *et al* (1988) showed a raised tissue-type plasminogen activator activity and lower plasma fibrinogen. Endurance-type exercise of low to moderate intensity can protect by lowering by about 10 mmHg both diastolic and systolic pressure of moderately hypertensive subjects (Haskell *et al*, 1992). It can also prevent hypertension developing in subjects at high risk (Paffenbarger and Hale, 1975; Stamler *et al*, 1989). This effect appears to be induced by an attenuation of the sympathetic tone and was independent of BMI, age and insulin resistance. Based on this scientific evidence, WHO issued a consensus statement in 1994 which recognises that the link between sedentary lifestyles and CHD has the requisite attributes to stand as a firm foundation for public health policies in that it is consistent, strong, appropriately sequenced, biologically graded, and plausible and coherent with existing scientific knowledge (Bijnen et al, 1994).

Physical activity and diabetes mellitus

Being physically active has been shown to exert some protection from diabetes, with physically active overweight individuals having somewhat lesser rates of non-insulin-dependent diabetes mellitus (NIDDM) (Helmrich et al, 1991; Manson et al, 1991). The most active, overweight men had risk of NIDDM that was two-thirds that of the least active overweight ones, while risks were similar for active and non-active lean subjects (Blair, 1993). After adjustment for BMI, history of hypertension and parental history of diabetes, it was estimated that each increment of 500 kcal per week in physical activity was associated with a 6% decrease in NIDDM risk. This protection is thought to be mediated by the blunting of insulin secretion, and the lowering of fasting plasma insulin and c-peptide. The reduction of plasma insulin response to a glucose load is an early effect, appearing already after one week of intense daily exercise.

Physical activity and colon cancer

Physical activity is also recognised as an independent and modifiable risk factor for colon cancer, the mechanism in this case being related to an acceleration of the transit time in the left colon and a shorter contact time of the intestinal mucosa with faecal mutagens. For example, Fredriksson and others (1989) found that being employed in a physically demanding job decreased the odds ratio for cancer of the left colon and sigmoid region in both men and women. Similarly, a case-control sample in Sweden found that lack of physical activity caused an excess risk for left colon cancer of about 3.2, the effect persisting even after controlling for BMI and other risk factors, including the diet (Gerhardsson de Verdier et al, 1990). In a Japanese case-control study (Kato et al, 1990) the adjusted RR for male colorectal cancer was 1.89 for proximal colon, 1.59 for distal colon and 1.36 for rectum. A prospective study of over 17 000 Harvard alumni followed up from 1965 to 1988 confirmed physical activity to be protective for colon cancer, the relative risk being halved when activity was maintained at a high level throughout these years (Lee et al, 1991). A sedentary lifestyle was found to compound the effect of diet, the highest risk (odds ratio of 5.2) being observed in sedentary people who consumed more than 20 g of saturated fats per day (Whittemore et al, 1990). In a study by Slattery et al (1988), high levels of physical activity were found to reduce the risk associated with high dietary intakes of fat.

Conclusion

Sufficient evidence exists to prove that physical activity does represent an independent risk factor for a number of health conditions, in particular chronic degenerative diseases, but this association is complicated, modulated, compounded or confounded by many concurrent lifestyle variables. This is essential for translating, in an operational and public health mode, the findings of research into a useful and meaningful message to the public at large, and its implementation in a sustainable manner. Considerations such as how much, how intense, how often and how frequently people should exercise have not been satisfactorily addressed as yet, and need to be seriously considered as a targeted priority for future research.

References

Baecke JA, Burema J, Frijters JE. A short questionnaire for the measurement of habitual physical activity in epidemiological studies. *American Journal of Clinical Nutrition*, 1982; **36**: 936–942

Bijnen FC, Caspersen CJ, Mosterd WL. Physical activity as a risk factor for coronary heart disease: a WHO and International Society and Federation of Cardiology position statement. *Bulletin of the World Health Organization*, 1994; **72**: 1–4

Blair D, Buskirk ER. Habitual daily energy expenditure and activity levels of lean and adult-onset and child-onset obese women. *American Journal of Clinical Nutrition*, 1987; **45**: 540–550

Blair SN. Evidence for success of exercise in weight loss and control. *Annals of Internal Medicine*, 1993; **119**: 702–706

Blair SN, Haskell WL, Ho P et al. Assessment of habitual physical activity by a seven-day recall in a community survey and controlled experiments. *American Journal of Epidemiology*, 1985; **122**: 794–804

Blair SN, Kannel WB, Kohl HW, Goodyear N, Wilson PW. Surrogate measures of physical activity and physical fitness. Evidence for sedentary traits of resting tachycardia, obesity, and low vital capacity. *American Journal of Epidemiology*, 1989; **129**: 1145–1156

Buratta V, Sabbadini LL. Can time use statistics describe the life of children? In: ISTAT, ed. *Time Use Methodology: Towards Consensus*. Rome: ISTAT, 1993: 51–66

Byers T, Marshall JA. The emergence of chronic diseases in developing countries. *SCN News*, 1995; **13**: 14–19

Dannenberg AL, Keller JB, Wilson PW, Castelli WP. Leisure time physical activity in the Framingham offspring study. Description, seasonal variation, and risk factor correlates. *American Journal of Epidemiology*, 1989; **129**: 76–88

Dietz WH, Gortmaker SL. Do we fatten our children at the television set? Obesity and television viewing in children and adolescents. *Pediatrics*, 1985; **75**: 807–812

DiPietro L, Williamson DF, Caspersen CJ, Eaker E. The descriptive epidemiology of selected physical activities and body weight among adults trying to lose weight: the Behavioral Risk Factor Surveillance System survey, 1989. *International Journal of Obesity*, 1993; **17**: 69–76

Ferro-Luzzi A, Martino L. Obesity and physical activity. In: Chadwick DJ, Cardew G, eds. *The Origin and Consequences of Obesity*. Ciba Foundation Symposium 201. Chichester:

John Wiley, 1996: 207–221

Folsom AR, Caspersen CJ, Taylor HL *et al.* Leisure time physical activity and its relationship to coronary risk factors in a population-based sample. The Minnesota Heart Study. *American Journal of Epidemiology,* 1985; **121**: 570–579

Folsom AR, Qamhieh HT, Wing RR *et al.* Impact of weight loss on plasminogen activator inhibitor (PAI-1), factor VII, and other hemostatic factors in moderately overweight adults. *Arteriosclerosis and Thrombosis,* 1993; **13**: 162–169

Fredriksson M, Bengtsson NO, Hardell L, Axelson O. Colon cancer, physical activity and occupational exposures. A case-control study. *Cancer,* 1989; **63**: 1838–1842

Gardner AW, Poehlman ET. Physical activity is a significant predictor of body density in women. *American Journal of Clinical Nutrition,* 1993; **57**: 8–14

Gerhardsson de Verdier M, Steineck G, Hagman U, Rieger A, Norell SE. Physical activity and colon cancer: a case-referent study in Stockholm. *International Journal of Cancer,* 1990; **46**: 985–989

Gortmaker SL, Dietz WH Jr, Cheung LW. Inactivity, diet, and the fattening of America. *Journal of the American Dietetic Association,* 1990; **90**: 1247–1252

Hardman AE, Jones PR, Norgan NG, Hudson A. Brisk walking improves endurance fitness without changing body fatness in previously sedentary women. *European Journal of Applied Physiology,* 1992; **65**: 354–359

Hartung GH, Foreyt JP, Mitchell RE, Vlasek I, Gotto AM Jr. Relation of diet to high-density-lipoprotein cholesterol in middle-aged marathon runners, joggers and inactive men. *New England Journal of Medicine,* 1980; **302**: 357–361

Haskell WL, Leon AS, Caspersen CJ *et al.* Cardiovascular benefits and assessment of physical activity and physical fitness in adults. *Medicine and Science in Sports and Exercise,* 1992; **24**: S201–220

Helmrich SP, Ragland DR, Leung RW, Paffenbarger RS. Physical activity and reduced occurrence of non-insulin-dependent diabetes mellitus. *New England Journal of Medicine,* 1991; **325**: 147–152

Hodge AM, Dowse GK, Koki G, Mavo P, Alpers MP, Zimmet PZ. Modernity and obesity in coastal and Highland Papua New Guinea. *International Journal of Obesity,* 1995; **19**: 154–161

Kato I, Tominaga S, Ikari A. A case-control study of male colorectal cancer in Aichi Prefecture, Japan: with special reference to occupational activity level, drinking habits and family history. *Japanese Journal of Cancer Research,* 1990; **81**: 115–121

Kromhout D, Saris WH, Horst CH. Energy intake, energy expenditure, and smoking in relation to body fatness: the Zutphen Study. *American Journal of Clinical Nutrition,* 1988; **47**: 668–674

Lee IM, Paffenbarger RS Jr, Hsieh C. Physical activity and risk of developing colorectal cancer among college alumni. *Journal of the National Cancer Institute,* 1991; **83**: 1324–1329

Leon AS, Connett J, Jacobs DR Jr, Rauramaa R. Leisure-time physical activity levels and risk of coronary heart disease and death. The Multiple Risk Factors Intervention Trial. *Journal of the American Medical Association,* 1987; **258**: 2388–2395

Leon AS, Connett J. Physical activity and 10.5 year mortality in the multiple risk factor intervention trial (MRFIT). *International Journal of Epidemiology,* 1991; **20**: 690–697

Manson JE, Rimm EB, Stampfer MJ *et al.* Physical activity and incidence of non-insulin-dependent diabetes mellitus in women. *Lancet,* 1991; **338**: 774–778

Morris JN, Adam C, Chave SP, Sirey C, Epstein L, Sheehan DJ. Vigorous exercise in leisure time and the incidence of coronary heart disease. *Lancet,* 1973; **i**: 333–339

Murata M, Hibi I. Nutrition and the secular trend of growth. *Hormone Research,* 1992; **38**: 89–96

Paffenbarger RS, Hale WE. Work, activity and coronary heart mortality. *New England Journal of Medicine*, 1975; **292**: 545–550

Paffenbarger RS, Wing AL, Hyde RT. Physical activity as an index of heart attack risk in college alumni. *American Journal of Epidemiology*, 1978; **108**: 161–175

Paffenbarger RS, Hyde RT, Wing AL, Hsieh C. Physical activity, all-cause mortality, and longevity of college alumni. *New England Journal of Medicine*, 1986; **314**: 605–613

Powell KE, Caspersen CJ, Koplan JP, Ford ES. Physical activity and chronic diseases. *American Journal of Clinical Nutrition*, 1989; **49**: 999–1006

Prentice AM, Black AE, Coward WA, Cole TJ. Energy expenditure in overweight and obese adults in affluent societies: an analysis of 319 doubly-labelled water measurements. *European Journal of Clinical Nutrition*, 1996; **50**: 93–97

Rauramaa R, Salonen JT, Seppanen K *et al.* Inhibition of platelet aggregability by moderate-intensity physical exercise: a randomized clinical trial in overweight men. *Circulation*, 1986; **74**: 939–944

Rising R, Harper IT, Fontvielle AM, Ferraro RT, Spraul M, Ravussin E. Determinants of total daily energy expenditure: variability in physical activity. *American Journal of Clinical Nutrition*, 1994; **59**: 800–804

Rissanen AM, Heliovaara M, Knekt P, Reunanen A, Aromaa A. Determinants of weight gain and overweight in adult Finns. *European Journal of Clinical Nutrition*, 1991; **45**: 419–430

Romieu I, Willett WC, Stampfer MJ *et al.* Energy intake and other determinants of relative weight. *American Journal of Clinical Nutrition*, 1988; **47**: 406–412

Sallis JF, Haskell WL, Wood PD *et al.* Physical activity assessment methodology in the Five-City Project. *American Journal of Epidemiology*, 1985; **121**: 91–106

Slattery ML, Schumacher MC, Smith KR, West DW, Abd-Elghany N. Physical activity, diet and risk of colon cancer in Utah. *American Journal of Epidemiology*, 1988; **128**: 989–999

Slattery ML, Abd-Elghany N, Kerber R, Schumacher MC. Physical activity and colon cancer: a comparison of various indicators of physical activity to evaluate the association. *Epidemiology*, 1990; **1**: 481–485

Stamler R, Stamler J, Gosch FC *et al.* Primary prevention of hypertension by nutritional-hygienic means: final report of a randomized clinical trial. *Journal of the American Medical Association*, 1989; **262**: 1801–1807

Stratton JR, Chandler WL, Schwartz RS *et al.* Effects of physical conditioning on fibrinolytic variables and fibrinogen in young and old healthy adults. *Circulation*, 1991; **83**: 1692–1697

Sullivan MJ, Higginbotham MB, Cobb FR. Exercise training in patients with severe left ventricular disfunction. Hemodynamic and metabolic effects. *Circulation*, 1988; **78**: 506–515

Tucker LA, Friedman GM. Television viewing and obesity in adult males. *American Journal of Public Health*, 1989; **79**: 516–518

Voorrips LE, Meijers HH, Sol P, Seidell JC, van Staveren WA. History of body weight and physical activity of elderly women differing in current physical activity. *International Journal of Obesity*, 1992; **16**: 199–205

Whittemore AS, Wu-Williams AH, Lee M *et al.* Diet, physical activity and colorectal cancer among Chinese in North America and China. *Journal of the National Cancer Institute*, 1990; **82**: 915–926

Williams PT, Haskell WL, Vranizan KM, Krauss RM. The associations of high-density lipoprotein subclasses with insulin and glucose levels, physical activity, resting heart rate, and regional adiposity in men with coronary artery disease: the Stanford Coronary Risk Intervention Project baseline survey. *Metabolism: Clinical and Experimental*, 1995;

44: 106–114

Williams RS, Logue EE, Lewis JG *et al.* Physical conditioning augments fibrinolytic response to venous occlusion in healthy adults. *New England Journal of Medicine*, 1980; **302**: 987–991

Williamson DF, Madans J, Anda RF, Kleinman JC, Kahn HS, Byers T. Recreational physical activity and ten-year weight change in a US national cohort. *International Journal of Obesity*, 1993; **17**: 279–286

World Health Organization (WHO). *Energy and Protein Requirement.* Report of a Joint FAO/WHO/UNU Expert Consultation. World Health Organization Technical Report Series No. 724. Geneva: WHO, 1985

11.6 Methods and paradigms: The basis for new directions in obesity research

George A. Bray

Pennington Biomedical Research Center, Baton Rouge, Louisiana, USA

New directions in obesity research, like those in any field, come from new methods or new paradigms. Over the past 25 years, several new methods have been introduced into the study of obesity which have made possible several important advances. These include techniques for measuring body composition, the application of the psychological techniques called behaviour therapy to the treatment of obesity, refinements in surgical techniques that have significantly improved the treatment of significant obesity, and the use of metabolic chambers, along with doubly labelled isotopic water, for the quantitation of energy expenditure and provision of new insights into the relationship between energy expenditure and food intake. More recently, peptide chemistry of the gastrointestinal tract and brain has identified peptides which provide important signals about the nature of body constituents and their control. Finally, developments in molecular biology have provided major new insights into the causes of obesity. Thus, during the past 25 years, new methods and shifts in the paradigms for conceptualising obesity have provided the impetus for a changing landscape in obesity research. These same forces are likely to be the drivers for new directions in obesity research as they have been in the past.

New methods

Improvements in the methods of measuring body composition have made important contributions in the past 25 years (Lukaski *et al*, 1987; Wang *et al*, 1992). The use of dual energy X-ray absorptiometry (DEXA) or dual photon absorptiometry has largely replaced the use of densitometry as the gold standard for measuring total body fat. With this enhanced ability to measure body compartments have come new models for dividing body components into three, four, five and more compartments. Of equal importance has been the introduction of computed tomographic (CT) scans and magnetic resonance imaging (MRI) scans for measurement of regional fat distribution. The pioneering work of Sjöström and his colleagues (Kvist *et al*, 1988) has shown that the quantity of visceral fat can be accurately measured by using the CT scan.

Following the seminal publication on behavioural control methodology as applied to obesity (Stuart, 1967), a large volume of research has been published demonstrating the importance of behavioural methods in all forms of weight control (Brownell, 1985; Foreyt and Goodrick, 1991; Wing, 1992). These methods of behavioural therapy have improved progressively over the past 20 years (Foreyt and Goodrick, 1991). Added to them have been other treatment modalities, including modest levels of exercise, improved nutritional advice and the introduction of very-low-calorie diets (Blackburn and Bray, 1985). This latter form of treatment began in the early 1970s, and is of benefit largely for individuals with substantial amounts of excess bodyweight.

Another major methodological development has been the shift in the type of surgical treatment used for treatment of individuals with massive obesity (NIH, 1991; Sullivan *et al*, 1993). In the 1970s, jejuno-ileal bypass was widely used, but it was associated with a myriad of complications (Bray *et al*, 1977). As the detrimental impact of these complications became clear, surgeons abandoned the jejuno-ileal bypass in favour of gastric reduction or bypass operations. Two procedures are in current use: gastric partitioning, which produces a small upper pouch attached to the larger lower pouch of the stomach through a narrowed opening, or alternatively, gastric bypass procedures in which a small upper pouch is drained directly into an intestinal loop (Yale, 1989). A Consensus Conference was held by the National Institutes of Health (NIH) in 1991 which recommended that gastric operations be reserved for individuals with a Body Mass Index above 40 kg/m^2 unless there were complications of obesity (NIH, 1991).

The post World War II years have seen the reintroduction of indirect calorimetry and the discovery of doubly labelled water as a technique to measure energy expenditure. With indirect calorimetry, the components of energy expenditure have been quantitatively described (Jéquier and Schutz, 1983). Using this method, Ravussin et al (1988) showed that a low metabolic rate might predict the risk of developing obesity. This is a hypothesis that needs to be tested further. Likewise, the possibility that the rate of fat oxidation might predict the risk for obesity also needs to be tested. With the introduction of doubly labelled water as a technique for assessing energy expenditure in free-living individuals, the way is open for a major expansion in our understanding of human energy expenditure in free-living subjects (Schoeller et al, 1980).

The methods of peptide chemistry have also contributed significantly to new methods in obesity research. As the techniques for isolating peptides and identifying their sequence have increased, the number of peptides identified as present in the gastrointestinal tract and also in the brain has increased. There is now a long list of peptides which increase or decrease food intake when applied to the brain, many of which are also involved as potential signals from peripheral tissues about the adequacy of energy stores.

Molecular biology has provided tools which have radically changed the field of obesity research. With molecular biological techniques it became possible to identify and isolate the genes underlying rare forms of inherited obesity in animals. The first breakthrough came in 1992 with the identification of the genetic defect in the obese 'yellow' mouse. The *agouti* gene which produces this defect provides the information for the cell to make a 133 amino acid peptide (Bultman et al, 1992). In the yellow obese mouse, the *agouti* gene is expressed in many tissues in which it is normally suppressed. The resulting *agouti* protein serves as a competitor for melanocyte stimulating hormone (MSH) and through this mechanism can account for both the yellow coat colour and the hyperphagia present in these animals (Lu et al, 1994).

Shortly after the discovery of the *agouti* gene, the genetic defect in the *ob/ob* mouse was identified (Zhang et al, 1994). The *ob* gene is altered with a stop message (codon) at amino acid 105. This truncates the normal 167 amino acid protein called leptin. Leptin in the normal animal appears to signal the brain about the state of peripheral fat stores and their adequacy for reproduction. Leptin is also involved in modulating a number of other steroid messages. In the obese mouse, leptin will reverse obesity and correct the other defects. A third obesity gene was cloned for the recessively inherited fat (*fa/fa*) mouse (Naggert et al, 1995). The nature of this gene defect was suspected from the high levels of proinsulin in these animals. Cleavage of insulin to proinsulin requires the enzyme carboxypeptidase-E. It was subsequently determined that carboxypeptidase-E was defective, resulting in defective formation of a variety of hormones and neuromodulators from their prohormone and proneuromodulator precursors.

New paradigms in the conception of obesity

In addition to the important advances made possible by new methods, there are new frameworks for thinking about the problem of obesity. Several paradigm shifts in the field of obesity based on new methods, have provided the framework in which new directions for obesity research will come in the ensuing years. The first of these is the recognition of the importance of visceral fat in the syndrome of obesity and its health risks (Bouchard *et al*, 1993; Bray, 1994). A variety of epidemiological and clinical studies have demonstrated that truncal fat and particularly visceral fat are associated with increased risks for mortality, stroke, heart disease, high blood pressure and diabetes (Bjorntorp, 1993) in both men and women. A major challenge for the new millennium will be the elucidation of the mechanisms involved in the detrimental effects of extra-visceral fat and the development of strategies which can reverse fat distribution in local areas, particularly visceral fat. The introduction of CT and MRI scans to quantitate visceral fat has greatly aided research in this area.

Studies of genetic factors in the development of obesity have appeared since 1980 and serve as a major stimulus for basic approaches to obesity in the near future. Using both adoption registries and twins, Bouchard and his colleagues (1988; 1993) and Stunkard and his colleagues (Stunkard *et al*, 1990; Vogler *et al*, 1995) have explored this problem in depth. The range of heritability estimates vary with the model which is used. They go as low as 20% to as high as 90% depending upon the variable and depending on the model in which it is tested. For many of the studies, the heritability estimates of 30–50% of the variance due to genetic and transmissible factors appear to be reasonable. Both genetic and environmental factors thus play a role in the development of obesity (Bray and York, 1979). From the Darwinian perspective (Darwin, 1859), the metabolic systems selected to handle environmental stresses of nutrient abundance and deprivation were developed by natural selection from those variants which had selective advantage (Table 11.3). This framework can help us focus on new directions for obesity research.

The discovery in 1994 of leptin (Zhang *et al*, 1994), which is produced by fat tissue as a signal to the brain and other tissues, was a major breakthrough. Failure to make leptin is associated with massive obesity in the *ob/ob* mouse, and

Table 11.3 Metabolic systems developed by natural selection

Selective pressure	Genetic strategy
1. Periodic surplus of food	1. Thrifty genes for (a) Nutrient choice and intake (b) Nutrient storage
2. Nutrient deprivation	2. Thrifty genes for (a) Energy efficiency (b) Mechanical efficiency
3. Nutrient requirements for reproductive success	3. Information about adequacy of fat stores Fat stores for foetal and lactational needs

this is reversed by treatment with leptin (Halaas *et al*, 1995; Pelleymounter *et al*, 1995; Campfield *et al*, 1995). The fat cell which makes leptin also makes a variety of other peptides in addition to storing and releasing fat. Thus the fat cell appears to be a true endocrine cell. It is worth keeping in mind that, even in the face of these genetic defects, something as simple as adrenalectomy will correct almost all of the defects in these genetically obese animals (Bray and York, 1979).

The tools of molecular biology, the cloning of genes, the expression of genes, the sequencing of the genetic code and the identification of messages produced during the transcription of genes have become tools widely used in biological studies. In the area of obesity, their first application was by Flier and his colleagues (1987) who isolated a peptide called adipsin from adipose tissue during fat cell differentiation. Adipsin is complement D in the indirect pathway for coagulation. Adipsin is one of the many peptides produced by the fat cell and led to the recognition of adipose tissue as an important endocrine organ. The fat cell produces adipsin, tumour necrosis factor-α (TNF-α), angiotensinogen, complement C3, and leptin, among others.

Studies on the genetic susceptibility to obesity have also benefited from advances in genetics and molecular biology. Beginning with the work of Davenport (1923) on the inheritance of Body Mass Index in families and the work of Verschuer on identical twins (1927), a growing body of data argues that important components of total body fat mass and fat distribution are inherited (Bouchard *et al*, 1993; Vogler *et al*, 1995). From this epidemiological data, a search has begun for the genes which are involved in human (Bouchard and Perusse, 1996) and animal forms of obesity. Studies of responsiveness to dietary fat in animals have shown that at least six different genes play a role (West *et al*, 1994; Warden *et al*, 1995). In human beings, a large and growing number of candidate genes have been explored for their possible relationship with the development of obesity, and several have been shown to contribute in small ways to this syndrome (Bouchard and Perusse, 1996).

It is now clear that many forms of experimental obesity are associated with a disturbed function of the autonomic nervous system, with reduced activity of one part of the sympathetic nervous system (SNS) playing a key role (Bray *et al*, 1990). The recognition that overeating by experimental animals was associated with activation of the part of the sympathetic nerves which innervate brown adipose tissue (Rothwell and Stock, 1983), led to the development of drugs which were effective in increasing thermogenesis by acting on β-adrenergic receptors (Arch *et al*, 1984). With the cloning of the β-3 adrenergic receptor in 1989 (Emorine *et al*, 1989) a new tool became available to develop these thermogenic agonists. The adrenergic receptor mechanism is of particular importance as part of a feedback system since it is involved in both regulation of food intake and the partitioning of nutrients in the diet between fat and protein. Destruction of brown adipose tissue which is innervated by the SNS leads to obesity and hyperphagia (Lowell *et al*, 1993).

In addition to the advances in the synthesis of β-adrenergic agonists, serotonergic drugs have been shown to reduce food intake and bodyweights (Guy-Grand et al, 1989; Gray et al, 1991). Fenfluramine was the first serotonergic drug to increase release and partially block re-uptake of the serotonin at nerve terminals. The importance of this drug is its potential for treating obesity and the stimulus it has provided for the evaluation of additional drugs which block serotonin re-uptake. Several of these β-3 adrenergic agonists have had short clinical trials but none has been approved for clinical use (Yen, 1994).

Another area of interest has been the recognition that the SNS and food intake are reciprocally related in many experimental conditions, and that the peptides which increase or decrease food intake may be doing so by acting on specific types of nutrient intake (Bray, 1993a). There are now examples of peptides which increase carbohydrate intake or fat intake and which decrease fat intake and decrease protein intake. It is quite possible that other peptides which affect specific nutrient preferences will also be identified and may serve as the basis for new treatments of obesity.

All the currently available drugs are derivatives of β-phenethylamine, except Mazindol which is a tricyclic compound. Recent studies suggest that the current aversion to the use of these drugs for long-term treatment, and the restrictions which have been placed on their use by many health authorities because of the fear of drug abuse, may be largely unwarranted and the drugs may be potentially more useful than is generally recognised (Bray, 1993b). With drug treatment patients lose weight, but when medications are stopped, weight regain is the rule. This observation proves that drugs work when used but that drugs do not work when not taken.

Since both noradrenergic and serotonergic mechanisms are involved in regulating food intake, Weintraub (1992) reasoned that it might be more productive to combine agents acting on each system than to use agents acting only on one system. In this study patients received fenfluramine and phentermine for periods of up to 3.5 years. With continued treatment by either intermittent or continuous dosage, Weintraub (1992) reported that nearly 50% achieved a significant long-term benefit. For nearly 20%, however, there was little benefit, and for the others the benefit was only modest. The analogy with hypertension is relevant since different patients respond differently to different drugs. Combinations of drugs may prove more effective than single agents for many patients. One of the stimulating new directions is to identify the differences in individual responsiveness to selected agents and to develop algorithms to identify the best long-term treatment for an individual patient. There is thus a great need for development of additional effective therapeutic approaches to obesity. Certainly, pharmacological agents will play a major role in the effective treatment of obesity. With the understanding provided by the feedback approach to regulation of energy expenditure and the growing knowledge of mechanisms for control of nutrient partitioning, the future in this area is bright.

A desirable approach to eliminating obesity would be prevention of the problem before it occurs (Kuczmarski et al, 1994). Although often discussed, there have been few ideas about how this might be accomplished. That it could be accomplished, however, has always been clear from the differences which exist as a function of social and economic class in the prevalence rates of obesity. A recent ray of hope in this area appeared with the publication by Epstein and his colleagues (Epstein et al, 1990) of a 10-year follow-up on a group of children treated by behavioural techniques in three different settings. During the first six months of treatment, all three groups lost weight and there was some regain by all three groups at five years, but a highly significant difference was seen between the three groups. The most effective setting was when the child and parent were treated together. In these children, the relative degree of excess weight at 10 years was lower than when treatment began. In contrast, the two control groups were heavier than at the beginning of treatment. Between five and 10 years, the group of children treated in family units showed no further increase in relative weight. Thus the behavioural techniques introduced by Stuart nearly 30 years ago (Stuart, 1967), when applied to children, can produce long-term effective changes in bodyweight over a 10-year interval. There is thus reason to hope that future research will improve the potential for preventing weight gain in high-risk groups as these groups are identified.

References

Arch JR, Ainsworth AT, Cawthorne MA et al. Atypical beta-adrenoceptor on brown adipocytes as target for anti-obesity drugs. *Nature*, 1984; **309**: 163–165
Bjorntorp P. Visceral obesity: a 'civilization syndrome'. *Obesity Research*, 1993; **1**: 206–222
Blackburn GL, Bray GA. *Management of Obesity by Severe Caloric Restriction*. Littleton, MA: PSG Publishing Co, 1985: 1–396
Bouchard C, Perusse L. Current status of the human obesity gene map. *Obesity Research*, 1996; **4**: 81–90
Bouchard C, Després JP, Mauriege P. Genetic and nongenetic determinants of regional fat distribution. *Endocrine Review*, 1993; **14**: 72–93
Bouchard C, Perusse L, Leblanc C, Tremblay A, Theriault G. Inheritance of the amount and distribution of human body fat. *International Journal of Obesity*, 1988; **12**: 205–215
Bray GA. The nutrient balance hypothesis: Peptides, sympathetic activity and food intake. *Annals of the New York Academy of Sciences*, 1993a; **676**: 223–241
Bray GA. Use and abuse of appetite suppressant drugs in the treatment of obesity. *Annals of Internal Medicine*, 1993b; **119**: 707–713
Bray GA. Topography of body fat. *Advances in Endocrinology Metabolism*, 1994; **5**: 297–322
Bray GA, York DA. Hypothalamic and genetic obesity in experimental animals: an autonomic and endocrine hypothesis. *Physiological Reviews*, 1979; **59**: 719–809
Bray GA, Greenway FL, Barry RE et al. Surgical treatment of obesity: a review of our experience and an analysis of published reports. *International Journal of Obesity*, 1977; **1**: 331–367
Bray GA, Fisler JS, York DA. Neuroendocrine control of the development of obesity:

Understanding gained from studies of experimental animal models. *Frontiers of Neuroendocrinology*, 1990; **11**: 128–181

Brownell KD. *The LEARN Program for Weight Control*. Philadelphia: University of Pennsylvania Press, 1985

Bultman SJ, Michaud EJ, Woychik RP. Molecular characterization of the mouse agouti locus. *Cell*, 1992; **71**: 1195–1204

Campfield LA, Smith FJ, Guisez Y, Devos R, Burn P. Recombinant mouse ob protein: evidence for a peripheral signal linking adiposity and central neural networks. *Science*, 1995; **269**: 546–549

Darwin C. *On the Origin of Species by Means of Natural Selection, or the Preservation of Favoured Races in the Struggle for Life*. London: John Murray, 1859

Davenport CB. Body build and its inheritance. *The Carnegie Institution*, 1923; **329**: 37

Emorine LJ, Marullo S, Briend-Sutren MM *et al*. Molecular characterization of the human β_3-adrenergic receptor. *Science*, 1989; **245**: 1118–1121

Epstein LH, Valoski A, Wing RR, McCurley J. Ten-year follow-up of behavioral, family-based treatment for obese children. *Journal of the American Medical Association*, 1990; **264**: 2519–2523

Flier JS, Cook KS, Usher P, Spiegelman BM. Severely impaired adipsin expression in genetic and acquired obesity. *Science*, 1987; **237**: 405–408

Foreyt JP, Goodrick GK. Factors common to successful therapy for the obese patient. *Medicine and Science in Sports and Exercise*, 1991; **23**: 292–297

Gray DS, Takahashi M, Bauer M, Bray GA. Changes in individual plasma free fatty acids in obese females during fasting and refeeding. *International Journal of Obesity*, 1991; **15**: 163–168

Guy-Grand B, Apfelbaum M, Crepaldi G, Gries A, Lefebvre P, Turner P. International trial of long-term dexfenfluramine in obesity. *Lancet*, 1989; **ii**: 1142–1144

Halaas JL, Gajiwala KS, Maffei M *et al*. Weight-reducing effects of the plasma protein encoded by the obese gene. *Science*, 1995; **269**: 543–546

Jéquier E, Schutz Y. Long-term measurements of energy expenditure in humans using a respiration chamber. *American Journal of Clinical Nutrition*, 1983; **38**: 989–998

Kuczmarski RJ, Flegal KM, Campbell SM, Johnson CL. Increasing prevalence of overweight among US adults: The National Health and Nutrition Examination Surveys, 1960 to 1991. *Journal of the American Medical Association*, 1994; **272**: 205–211

Kvist H, Chowdhury B, Grangard U, Thylen U, Sjöström L. Total and visceral adipose tissue volumes derived from measurements with computed tomography in adult men and women: predictive equations. *American Journal of Clinical Nutrition*, 1988; **48**: 1351–1361

Lowell BB, S-Susulic V, Hamann A *et al*. Development of obesity in transgenic mice after genetic ablation of brown adipose tissue. *Nature*, 1993; **366**: 740–742

Lu D, Willard D, Patel IR *et al*. Agouti protein is an antagonist of the melanocyte-stimulating-hormone receptor. *Nature*, 1994; **371**: 799–802

Lukaski HC. Methods for the assessment of human body composition: traditional and new. *American Journal of Clinical Nutrition*, 1987; **46**: 537–556

Naggert JK, Fricker LD, Varlamov O *et al*. Hyperproinsulinaemia in obese fat/fat mice associated with a carboxypeptidase-E mutation which reduces enzyme-activity. *Nature Genetics*, 1995; **10**: 135–142

NIH, Office of Medical Applications Research. *Gastrointestinal Surgery for Severe Obesity*. NIH Consensus Development Conference, 1991

Pelleymounter MA, Cullen MJ, Baker MB *et al*. Effects of the obese gene product on body weight regulation in ob/ob mice. *Science*, 1995; **269**: 540–543

Ravussin E, Lillioja S, Knowler WC *et al*. Reduced rate of energy expenditure as a risk factor for body-weight gain. *New England Journal of Medicine*, 1988; **318**: 467–472

Rothwell NJ, Stock MJ. Luxuskonsumption, diet-induced thermogenesis and brown fat: the case in favour. *Clinical Science*, 1983; **64**: 19–23

Schoeller DA, Van Santen E, Peterson DW, Dietz W, Jaspan J, Klein PD. Total body water measurement in humans with O and H labeled water. *American Journal of Clinical Nutrition*, 1980; **33**: 2686–2693

Stuart RB. Behavioral control of overeating. *Behavior Research and Therapy*, 1967; **5**: 357–365

Stunkard AJ, Harris JR, Pedersen NL, McClearn GE. The body mass index of twins who have been reared apart. *New England Journal of Medicine*, 1990; **322**: 1483–1487

Sullivan M, Karlsson J, Sjöström L, *et al*. Swedish obese subjects (SOS)—an intervention study of obesity. Baseline evaluation of health and psychosocial functioning in the first 1743 subjects examined. *International Journal of Obesity*, 1993; **17**: 503–512

Verschuer O v. *Die Verebungsbiologische Zwillingsforschung. Ihre Biologischen Grundlagen. Mit 18 Abbildungen. Ergebnisse der Inneren Medizin und Kinderheilkunde*. 31th edn. Berlin: Verlag Von Julius Springer, 1927

Vogler GP, Sorensen TI, Stunkard AJ, Srinivasan MR, Rao DC. Influences of genes and shared family environment on adult body mass index assessed in an adoption study by a comprehensive path model. *International Journal of Obesity*, 1995; **19**: 40–45

Wang ZM, Pierson RN, Heymsfield SB. The five-level model: a new approach to organizing body composition research. *American Journal of Clinical Nutrition*, 1992; **56**: 19–28

Warden CH, Fisler JS, Shoemaker SM *et al*. Identification of 4 chromosomal loci determining obesity in a multifactorial mouse model. *Journal of Clinical Investigation*, 1995; **95**: 1545–1552

Weintraub M. Long-term weight control: The National Heart, Lung and Blood Institute funded multimodal intervention study. *Clinical Pharmacology and Therapeutics*, 1992; **51**: 581–585

West DB, Goudey-Lefevre J, York B, Truett GE. Dietary obesity linked to genetic-loci on chromosomes 9 and 15 in a polygenic mouse model. *Journal of Clinical Investigation*, 1994; **94**: 1410–1416

Wing RR. Behavioral treatment of severe obesity. *American Journal of Clinical Nutrition*, 1992; **55**: 545S–551S

Yale CE. Gastric surgery for morbid obesity. Complications and long-term weight control. *Archives of Surgery*, 1989; **124**: 941–947

Yen TT. Antiobesity and antidiabetic β-agonists: Lessons learned and questions to be answered. *Obesity Research*, 1994; **2**: 472–488

Zhang Y, Proenca R, Maffei M, Barone M, Leopold L, Friedman JM. Positional cloning of the mouse obese gene and its human homolog. *Nature*, 1994; **372**: 425–432

12
Workshop reports

12.1 Diet in early life and chronic disease

David Leon

Epidemiology Unit, London School of Hygiene & Tropical Medicine, UK

There was a consensus in the workshop that the statistical associations between size at birth and blood pressure, non-insulin-dependent diabetes (NIDDM) and coronary heart disease are real. They are unlikely to be due to socio-economic confounding in developed countries, although the potential for socio-economic confounding in studies in developing countries was not as well assessed.

The extent to which these associations between foetal size and adult disease risk could explain disease patterns between populations or over time remains unclear. The fact that time trends in cardiovascular mortality show a pronounced period rather than birth-cohort effect requires further discussion in the context of the foetal origins hypothesis. However, it may be that attempting to project rates of disease in populations from inferred levels of foetal malnourishment in the past ignores the fact that it may be the interaction between foetal growth and factors in adult life such as obesity that is important.

The discussion of potential mechanisms took as its starting point that size at birth was determined by a multitude of factors, of which maternal diet was only one component. However, the workshop expressed a preference to focus on the role of diet and nutrition, reflecting in part the expertise of the participants and because it represented a potential area for public health intervention.

It was the view of the workshop that the association between maternal diet and foetal growth was surprisingly poorly studied. An indication of this was that one of the classic recent works on perinatal epidemiology (Kline *et al*, 1989) has just one of its 400 pages devoted to the effect of nutrition on foetal growth rate and size

Diet, Nutrition and Chronic Disease: Lessons from Contrasting Worlds.
Edited by P. S. Shetty and K. McPherson © 1997 John Wiley & Sons, Ltd.

at birth. It was considered that gross aspects of the maternal diet may not be as important as the balance between various nutrients. Reference was made to animal studies that have highlighted the specificity of effects of different levels of particular amino acids in the maternal diet on the development and function of particular organ systems in the offspring (Snoeck *et al*, 1990; Dahri *et al*, 1991). This was congruent with the consensus in the workshop that, contrary to what was generally believed, it might be the quality and type of protein that was important in human pregnancies.

Although supplementation trials in human pregnancies were ultimately desirable in order to explore these questions fully, it was agreed that what was known was insufficient at the present time to justify such interventions. Instead, it might be worth studying populations such as Papua New Guinea highlanders who traditionally have had a very low animal protein diet, but who are now suffering increasing rates of NIDDM as some move to a more affluent lifestyle.

It was recognised, in more general terms, that the foetal origins hypothesis may be important in understanding the consequences of increased levels of obesity in developing countries, where populations may have undergone very rapid 'acculturation' in the form of a move to a Western diet/lifestyle within one generation. It was suggested that obesity in these populations may be associated with much more severe consequences than in a Western population, because of past and current differences in the prevalence and degree of impaired nutrition *in utero*.

Finally, it was pointed out that pre-pregnancy weight was a very important determinant of size at birth. It was suggested that it may be pre-pregnant nutritional status that might be the crucial influence on the adult physiology and disease susceptibility of a woman's offspring. However, fully characterising pre-pregnancy nutritional status, other than by maternal anthropometry, was a difficult problem, largely because of the paucity of longitudinal data on growth and nutrition in the childhood and adolescence of pregnant women.

In summary, the workshop concluded that:

- research in the field of foetal origins of adult disease should move from questions of 'whether' to questions of 'how' (mechanism);
- diet was likely to play a role, and moves should be made to start to redress the balance of work in this area to investigate in humans and animals the effects of specific dietary components on birth outcome, and the risk of disease in later life, recognising the importance of addressing pre-pregnancy nutritional status of mothers;
- the impact of protein intake in pregnancy, particularly protein type/quality, should be investigated;
- the foetal origins hypothesis might be of particular value in anticipating/explaining the adverse health effects of rapid acculturation in populations where many people had been born to mothers who had lived at a comparatively low plane of nutrition.

References

Dahri S, Snoeck A, Reusens-Billen B, Remacle C, Hoet JJ. Islet function in offspring of mothers on low-protein diet during gestation. *Diabetes*, 1991; **40** (suppl 2): 115–120

Kline J, Stein Z, Susser M. *Conception to Birth: Epidemiology of Prenatal Development.* New York: Oxford University Press, 1989

Snoeck A, Remacle C, Reusens B, Hoet JJ. Effect of a low protein diet during pregnancy on the fetal rat endocrine pancreas. *Biology of the Neonate*, 1990; **57**: 107–118

12.2 Dietary chemoprevention of cancer

Kay Tee Khaw and Sheila Bingham*

*Clinical Gerontology Unit, University of Cambridge, Addenbrooke's Hospital, Cambridge, UK and *MRC Dunn Clinical Nutrition Centre, Cambridge, UK*

While there is substantial evidence to indicate that diet influences risk of many cancers, there are inconsistencies in the epidemiological evidence relating specific dietary factors and cancer at many sites. For example, the strong effects in ecologic and case-control studies contrast with prospective studies and trials, e.g. breast cancer and fat, beta-carotene and cancer. This does not enable incontrovertible dietary or nutritional recommendations for the prevention of cancer, though, for example, there is substantial consensus for alcohol increasing risks for some gastrointestinal cancers, obesity increasing risk of endometrial cancer, and increased fruit and vegetable intake being protective for several cancers. The group discussed limitations of current evidence, and where future research might usefully be focused.

The adverse effect of beta-carotene in intervention trials was discussed in depth at the workshop. When the alpha-tocopherol beta-carotene (ATBC) trial was designed (ATBC Cancer Prevention Study Group, 1994), there was good prospective evidence that smokers with higher beta-carotene blood levels were less likely to develop lung cancer. There was also a good hypothetical reason based on extensive chemoprevention trials in animals to suggest that beta-carotene would be protective in lung cancer. Most importantly, there was no evidence of any adverse effect of beta-carotene. In the ATBC study, which enrolled 29 000 smokers, the risk of lung cancer was significantly increased in the beta-carotene arm as compared to the placebo arm. Similar findings were reported from the CARET study of asbestos workers, with a 28% increase in the active intervention group (Hennekens *et al*, 1996). Reasons for this included confounding with other dietary components, interactions or synergistic activity with other nutrients, isomers with differing activities in food compared to supplements, and dose and duration issues. The results of these two trials had a salutary effect on further trials of supplementation of single nutrients or items of diet. Nevertheless, these trials have been important, for they provided no evidence for any protective effect of beta-carotene supplementation, with even some suggestion that it might be harmful. For the present, any recommendations about the prevention of cancer should be about foods rather than isolated nutrient supplements.

Beta-carotene is found in vegetables, but there are large numbers of other suggested chemopreventive agents present in foods, ranging from essential nutrients such as polysaccharides, folate, vitamins C and E, to metabolically active non-nutrients such as sulphur-containing compounds, other carotenoids and flavonoids. These include lutein, lycopene, quercetin, genistein, daidzein, sulphoraphane (glucoraphanin), and colours such as curcumin. Although the metabolically active compounds are generating a great deal of interest in relation to their possible chemopreventive effects, very little is known about their absorption, physiology, effects on cell biology and metabolism by gastrointestinal flora. There is also likely to be large variation in foods according to cultivar, species, season, growing conditions and cooking practices. As yet, biomarkers to document exposure are poorly developed. More information will contribute to our ability to design better prospective studies and clinical trials. Intervention trials which assess the effect on intermediate biological predictors of cancer such as sex steroid levels, markers of DNA damage such as adducts, or prostate specific antigen are needed.

While there was general consensus, based on current evidence, to recommend increased fruit and vegetable intake, it was recognised that this was based on associations from case-control studies, with their limitations. Prospective studies are weakly consistent that increased fruit and vegetable intake also reduce risk of certain cancers, but most prospective studies have been carried out using relatively crude or inaccurate methodology. The group agreed that future studies should have better characterisation of exposure through improved methods to assess consumption. Future studies need to consider including measures of long-term pattern of exposures, perhaps through repeat measures, methods of cooking, improved food composition tables, and the development of biomarkers for exposure from accessible biological material such as blood and urine. Results need to be considered in relation to different genotypic variations known to confer altered risk of cancer at some sites. Multicentre collaborative studies using standardised methodology are more likely to cover the range of interactions between dietary constituents and cancer, as well as having the statistical power to improve the strength of evidence.

The workshop briefly discussed the lack of information on the effect of diet on survival in patients with cancer and interaction with treatments such as chemotherapy and radiotherapy.

The current recommendations for the dietary prevention of cancer, for example, by a reduction in fat and an increase in polysaccharides and vegetable intakes, do not conflict with the public health recommendations for the prevention of cardiovascular disease, alcohol-related problems, large bowel disorders and obesity.

References

Alpha-Tocopherol Beta Carotene Cancer Prevention Study Group. The effect of vitamin E and beta carotene on the incidence of lung cancer. *New England Journal of Medicine*, 1994; **330**: 1029–1035

Hennekens CH, Buring JE, Manson J *et al.* Lack of effect of long term supplementation with beta carotene on the incidence of malignant neoplasms and cardiovascular disease. *New England Journal of Medicine*, 1996; **334**: 1145

12.3 Vegetarianism and chronic diseases

Jim Mann and Margaret Thorogood*

*Department of Human Nutrition, University of Otago, Dunedin, New Zealand and *Health Promotion Sciences Unit, London School of Hygiene & Tropical Medicine, UK*

There are at least two important reasons for studying the health of vegetarians. There are large numbers of them in both affluent and developing countries, and knowledge of health outcomes amongst the different types of vegetarians may provide further clues concerning the relationship between diet and health. Difficulties of definition present a major problem in interpreting studies of health outcome of those following diets which exclude meat. Vegans are those who consume no meat, fish, animal-derived foods, eggs or dairy products. Lacto-ovovegetarians eat neither meat nor fish but do eat dairy products and eggs. Semi-vegetarians have a wide range of dietary practices including the occasional eating of meat, eating fish but not meat or eating only white but not red meat. The diet of Western vegetarians differs appreciably from that of vegetarians in Asian countries and other less affluent societies. Most studies have not distinguished clearly amongst these different groups.

Three different types of studies have been employed to examine the health effects of vegetarianism in affluent societies: clinical trials of the effects of diet on risk factors, cross-sectional and prospective studies. The health benefits that have been associated with vegetarianism are shown in Table 12.1. Attributes of vegetarians other than their dietary practices could explain some, or all, of these effects. While it is possible to exclude higher socio-economic status and reduced cigarette smoking (both of which characterise vegetarians in affluent societies) as the explanation for these health benefits, it is conceivable that low rates of obesity amongst vegetarians could account in part for these benefits. It is impossible, in the light of current information, to determine whether not eating meat or other characteristics of a vegetarian diet (Table 12.2) might explain the effects.

The EPIC study, and in particular the Oxford cohort which includes an appreciable number of vegetarians, should help to confirm or refute the findings of earlier studies as well as determine whether any particular attribute of the vegetarian diet can explain differences between vegetarians and meat-eaters. A meta-analysis of published studies which is being undertaken may provide information, in particular concerning vegans, who are the most homogeneous group of vegetarians. In India and possibly other Asian countries, religious and cultural factors are the main reasons for following a vegetarian diet, whereas in Western countries, ethical concerns are the most frequently cited reasons for not eating meat. Poverty is another reason why many people in developing countries

Table 12.1   Health implications of vegetarian diets

Possible benefits	Possible risks
Reductions in:	
Total mortality	Iron deficiency
Coronary heart disease	B_{12} deficiency (vegans)
Cancer	Impaired growth (vegans)
Blood pressure	
Glucose, diabetes	
Total and low-density lipoprotein cholesterol	
Diverticular disease	
Gallstones	
Constipation	

Table 12.2   Characteristics of a vegetarian diet compared with an omnivorous diet

Increased	Decreased
Vegetable proteins	Saturated fatty acids
Dietary fibre	Dietary cholesterol
	Haem iron, zinc
Several antioxidant nutrients	Vitamin B_{12} (vegans)
	Energy

do not eat meat. Few formal studies have been undertaken, but much clinical experience in India suggests that vegetarianism amongst the relatively affluent sections of the population is not associated with any health disadvantages and obesity is not uncommon in vegetarians. There are potential problems amongst the less affluent (e.g. deficiency of iron and other micronutrients, inadequate intake of protein and total energy to sustain growth), but these problems can be overcome without the addition of meat. Iron deficiency, one of the most common consequences of an inadequate vegetarian diet, can usually be overcome by the addition of vitamin C to improve bioavailability. Measures to improve the general nutrition status of disadvantaged groups require political and socio-economic change rather than a change in the nature of the diet.

The workshop concluded that there are no general adverse health consequences among those who follow a vegetarian diet. The observed health benefits may not be due to the exclusion of meat from the diet, but to other aspects of a vegetarian diet. Vegans, less affluent groups of vegetarians, and those who have recently changed to a vegetarian diet, may require support to ensure adequate intakes of energy and other nutrients.

The experience of vegetarians is important because it suggests that a global reduction in intake of animal protein would not be detrimental to health. This has implications for overall food policies and nutrition strategies. Conversely, it is important to acknowledge that a vegetarian choice is not always a healthier choice. Vegetarian diets in affluent societies may be high in saturated fatty acids and this may be associated with adverse rather than favourable health outcomes.

12.4 Public health initiatives in obesity

Michael Lean and Prakash S. Shetty*

*Department of Human Nutrition, University of Glasgow, Scotland, UK and *Human Nutrition Unit, London School of Hygiene & Tropical Medicine, UK*

The workshop participants recognised that the prevalence of obesity is increasing at an alarming rate. It was agreed that this increase in obesity has serious implications for health, in particular related to the morbidity and mortality associated with a higher risk of chronic, non-communicable diseases. The requirements for tackling this increasing global problem are:

- A primary prevention approach to make it less likely for the general population to become obese.
- A targeted approach aimed at those sub-population groups at greater risk of becoming obese.
- A therapeutic approach to help those who are already obese.
- Further research and new strategies to address the problem of obesity on an urgent and priority basis.

Is there a need for a public statement on what the consensus is?

At the outset the workshop emphasised the need for a clear and unambiguous public statement on the problem of obesity from an authoritative group of experts. The need is to minimise the impact of erroneous information being delivered to the public by inadequately informed health professionals or members of the media. It was agreed that the following statements should be incorporated in this public statement and would constitute the bedrock of the public health initiatives to reduce the problem of obesity:

- The prevalence of obesity is increasing rapidly world-wide.
- The predisposition to obesity depends on genes and on environmental influences, and also on gene–nutrient interactions; hence everyone is not affected in the same way.
- Obesity affects health, predisposing to and increasing the risk of many chronic diseases, in particular cardiovascular disease, certain cancers, diabetes, gall bladder disease, hypertension, etc.
- Obesity is linked to increased mortality (the question whether this should be publicised widely was debated by the group quite extensively with no consensus opinion emerging).
- Obesity is associated with poor quality of life, stigmatisation and other social problems, and bears a high cost both for the individual and for society.
- The risks associated with obesity can be minimised:

  (i) by restricting weight gain;
  (ii) by weight loss for those overweight; and
  (iii) by other risk-reduction strategies independent of bodyweight, e.g. smoking.

Indicators for the identification of risk and initiation of action at population level

The workshop deliberated at length to arrive at reliable indicators and cut-offs for the identification of risk and for the initiation of action at population level. It was agreed that a BMI > 25.0, waist/hip ratio > 0.95 (for men) or > 0.80 (for women) are good indicators, and that a waist circumference of 94 cm/37 inches (for men) and 80 cm/32 inches (for women) may be considered as a simple measure. It was also agreed that there should be criteria for successful weight loss which confers important and acknowledged health benefits. The emphasis should be on a modest, achievable weight loss of the order of 5–10%/ 5–10 kg/ 5–10 cm waist circumference. Maintenance of an acceptable range of bodyweight and the prevention of the regaining of lost weight, while emphasising the problems associated with weight cycling, were considered as being important public health messages.

Risk reduction strategy for the overweight/obese and restricting weight gain in the community

Recognising the relatively low expectations of weight loss and the problems associated with sustaining weight loss in clinical situations, the workshop emphasised the need for risk-reduction strategies which were not aimed at weight loss alone, and for a holistic approach to health awareness, including tackling smoking (a particular problem among adolescents who choose to smoke to avert weight gain). Issues such as the low self-esteem of obese subjects and their empowerment need to be addressed. The alarming increase in the prevalence of childhood overweight and obesity was considered a priority area that needed urgent attention. Campaigns aimed at increasing the public's awareness of obesity and guidelines for health service management by health professionals should be launched simultaneously.

Integration with other policies: the need for a holistic, preventive approach

The workshop emphasised the need for a holistic approach which involved long-term support to related policies in other sectors. These include: town planning (e.g. location of supermarkets and sports facilities), transport (e.g. bicycle lanes), government regulation and self-regulation of the food industry (e.g. food and alcohol provision, food composition, regulations, food labelling, fiscal policies, food import), advertising and media (e.g. food advertisements aimed at children), sports, leisure and recreation industry and heritage (e.g. ensuring access to public for walks), workplace (e.g. catering, provision for in-house sports facilities) and education (e.g. catering and sports in schools). All this requires a high level of political will, financial commitment and inter-sectoral cooperation.

Conclusion

Hitherto the emphasis on research has been largely aimed at the elucidation of the aetiology of obesity, its links with other chronic diseases and clinical, therapeutic strategies. Research on primary prevention is limited and there is a conspicuous lack of models of success or good practice in the primary prevention of obesity. It is essential that research should be undertaken on health promotion strategies specifically aimed at the problem of obesity and associated chronic diseases. Research is also needed to address topics such as marketing of food, advertising to children, manipulation of portion sizes, and facilitation of increased physical activity, and there should be a review of the psycho-social aspects of obesity. Priority should also be given to research focusing on other sectors and the development of sustainable, feasible and effective programmes to deal with this major public health problem.

12.5 Diet and blood pressure

Diederick Grobbee, Francesco Cappuccio* and Jane Pryer†

Erasmus University Medical School, Rotterdam, The Netherlands, *Department of Medicine, St George's Hospital Medical School, and †Human Nutrition Unit, London School of Tropical Medicine & Hygiene, London, UK

Hypertension is a well established major risk factor for stroke and coronary heart disease. High blood pressure constitutes a global public health problem with a larger burden of fatal and non-fatal disease than, for example, hypercholesterolaemia, the problem of which still remains confined to Westernised societies. Genetic and environmental factors contribute to the occurrence of hypertension, with inter-individual differences in their relative contribution. There are abundant data to relate dietary factors to hypertension, the importance of which is the potential for prevention and intervention. The relation between diet and blood pressure may be viewed from an aetiologic, a therapeutic and a public health perspective. At the workshop the discussion was largely limited to the first and the last areas.

Research on diet and blood pressure has primarily been undertaken in the developed world, and has focused on nutrients, with a major emphasis on the direct association between sodium, alcohol, positive energy balance (obesity) and blood pressure. Sodium intake has been studied most intensively and its relation to blood pressure levels is beyond doubt, although quantitatively modest within the range of sodium intake encountered in most countries. Other nutrients investigated include: potassium (inverse association), calcium (inverse association), and to a lesser extent, magnesium, omega-3 fatty acids, saturated fat, and more recently antioxidant vitamins, protein and fibre. Research on the association between individual nutrients and blood pressure is important in order to delineate the underlying mechanisms. Also, empirical data should direct the most effective preventive measures both at an individual and population level.

However, due to problems of multicolinearity of many nutrients (e.g. potassium, antioxidant vitamins, calcium, magnesium) it is not always possible to disentangle the effects of individual nutrients on blood pressure in observational studies. Randomised intervention trials provide a more direct view on the effects of certain nutrients, but the supplementation dosage or degree of nutrient restriction in some trials has been unrealistic from a practical point of view and of pharmacological rather than physiological significance. Furthermore, it is possible that, due to interactions between nutrients, other lifestyle factors and genes, certain interventions may be more effective in some population groups than others. The latter may have implications for development of interventions aiming to reduce blood pressure in developing countries. American blacks, for example, appear to be more sensitive to sodium intake than whites.

Emphasis for future research on diet and blood pressure includes:

- nutrient–nutrient interaction (for example, sodium and potassium, calcium and alcohol);
- nutrient–lifestyle interactions (e.g. obesity, exercise and alcohol);
- gene–nutrient interactions;
- diet–blood pressure relation in special groups (e.g. newborns, pregnant women, the elderly); and
- effectiveness and efficacy of dietary interventions in different ethnic groups and populations.

From a public health perspective, both the whole population as well as those at high risk need to be targeted for the prevention and control of high blood pressure. The total population approach is natural to public health and aims to influence change at the population rather than the individual level and shift the population distribution of blood pressure downwards. It has been estimated that a reduction of the population blood pressure distribution by 2–3 mmHg would have a greater impact on cardiovascular disease prevention than a near perfect treatment of all subjects with systolic blood pressure levels above 150 mmHg. Empirical data, however, are lacking and unlikely to be generated. Apart from its perceived effectiveness, the approach recognises that individual behaviour is greatly influenced by societal factors, and that individual change is difficult in the absence of socially mediated changes in the determinants of unhealthy behaviours. When safe preventive measures are taken on a population scale, high-risk groups will similarly benefit. In contrast, the high-risk approach focuses on the control of blood pressure in the clinical setting among those already at increased risk. The non-pharmacological management of hypertension in individuals is well described in several national and international guidelines.

At a population level, emphasis should be on a balanced diet, rather than mass administration of pharmacological doses of nutrient supplements. People eat food and not nutrients, and hence nutritional recommendations aimed at the public should focus on food, rather than nutrients. The workshop recognised that current recommendations for a healthy heart (e.g. decrease in saturated fat, increase in polyunsaturated fat, increase in fruit and vegetables) and for a balanced diet are also likely to be beneficial for blood pressure, which is in any case one component of the cardiovascular risk profile. The importance of interaction between cardiovascular risk factors should be recognised. In addition, recommendations to reduce sodium should be included and manufacturers encouraged to substitute potassium for sodium in manufactured products. Current health recommendations to decrease obesity and increase activity are also likely to lead to reductions in blood pressure at the population level. In theory, the population approach to prevention of high blood pressure should be of direct relevance to stem the rise in hypertension and related disorders in many developing countries. However, it should be realised that current recommendations on the prevention of high blood pressure have been developed from a developed country perspective, and may not fit as well in the developing country context. For example, recommendations to increase fruit and vegetable intake may not be successful in a developing country where rural farmers are engaged in cash cropping and export-oriented agriculture. In the light of situations prevailing in individual developing countries, issues such as feasibility and cost-effectiveness of a range of public health interventions to prevent the rise of high blood pressure should be considered by professional groups in developing countries, drawing upon the experience and lessons of population-based interventions in the developed world. Experience from China and India demonstrates the preventive potential when local infrastructures and population attitudes are well appreciated.

13
Diet, lifestyle and chronic disease: lessons from contrasting worlds

Prakash S. Shetty

Human Nutrition Unit, London School of Hygiene & Tropical Medicine, UK

Dietary deficit and excess and the consequent under- and overnutrition along with the lifestyle changes that accompany industrialisation, urbanisation and economic development have significant impact on the health and survival of populations. The usual backdrop to this shift in disease profile is the preceding 'demographic transition' which attributes changes in population structure to a shift from high fertility and high mortality seen in poorer societies to one of low fertility and low mortality typical of modern, industrialised, affluent nations. Abdel Omran (1971) formulated the 'epidemiologic transition' theory which focuses on the complex changes in patterns of health, disease and mortality which result from these demographic changes, and the associated economic and sociological changes. This health and mortality transition entails substitution of chronic diseases for infectious diseases as the primary causes of morbidity and mortality. This transition from a cause of death pattern dominated by infectious diseases with very high mortality, especially at younger ages, to a pattern dominated by chronic diseases and injuries with lower mortality, mostly peaking at older ages, is seen to be responsible for the phenomenal increase in life expectancy. Hence the theory of 'epidemiologic transition' has been popular among demographers and geographers but less familiar to epidemiologists, and according to Mackenbach (1994) 'provides a potentially powerful framework for the study of disease and mortality in populations, especially for the study of historical and international variations'. The theory, while describing and explaining the spectacular fall in mortality and the changes in pattern of morbidity and mortality in industrialised, developed countries, allows us to speculate whether developing countries currently lagging behind those which have already completed the epidemiologic transition will demonstrate a fall in infectious disease mortality and a rise in chronic diseases.

Omran (1971) described three stages of mortality patterns in epidemiological transition: 'the age of pestilence and famine', 'the age of receding pandemics' and 'the age of degenerative and man-made diseases'. The recent significant but unanticipated decline in death rates from degenerative diseases in the USA since the mid-1960s and, more importantly, the redistribution to older age groups of the risk of mortality from these chronic diseases, has resulted in the description of a fourth pattern referred to as 'the age of delayed degenerative diseases' (Olshansky and Ault, 1986). To explain the nature of the mortality and population dynamics among different population groups, three different models of epidemiological transition have been invoked (Omran, 1971; 1983). These are:

1. The Classical or Western Transition model which describes the health and mortality transition in Western societies.
2. The accelerated variant of the classical model which describes the transition seen in countries like Japan, Eastern Europe and the former Soviet Union.
3. The contemporary or delayed model which describes changes that have been observed in developing nations of the Third World.

Rapid, unanticipated changes in this transition are evident even now, typified for instance by the 'reverse transition' seen in countries of the former Soviet Union, with the reappearance of infectious diseases such as diphtheria which had apparently been eradicated. Dynamic changes are also evident in the delayed model typical of developing countries which, apart from a phase shift, show epidemiological changes similar to the accelerated model.

The human diet has changed profoundly over the long and gradual process of human evolution. A long period as hunter-gatherers in pre-agricultural societies associated with variable and uncertain food supplies was followed by a greatly improved food supply during the first agricultural revolution. This led to better nutrition and health and lower mortalities; but as populations increased and the pressure on food supplies rose, this sometimes led to undernutrition and a new rise in mortality. The industrial revolution, second agricultural revolution and the sanitary revolution in Europe over the past 200 or more years contributed to the development of modern industrialised societies. The associated agricultural and technological activities contributed to the modern diet, which is far removed from the diets of hunter-gatherers and peasant agriculture phases of human cultural evolution (Boyden, 1988). In many ways, the differences found between the diets of peasant agriculturists and modern affluent societies are much akin to those between the largely rural majority populations of developing countries, and the people of developed countries or even the urban elites of developing societies. Thus, over the past three centuries, the pace of dietary change appears to have accelerated to varying degrees in different parts of the world.

The modernisation of societies that follows economic development seems to result in a dietary pattern that is high in saturated fats, sugars and refined foods, and low in fibre content. The relationship between these dietary changes and health and mortality transition is probably causal. The replacement of one set of risk factors that predispose to infectious diseases by another set of risk factors that determine the morbidity and mortality patterns typical of degenerative, chronic diseases may be referred to as a 'risk transition'.

Quantifying the burden of chronic disease

Most assessments of the relative importance of different diseases are based on the number of deaths they cause. Death as a measure of disease burden has two advantages: (i) death is an unambiguous event, and (ii) most countries routinely collect data related to death. However, many diseases, including chronic disease, are not always fatal but are responsible for a great loss of healthy life, leading to a significant demand on health systems and adding to the health burdens of society. Measurement of the burden of disease is possible by the use of single or multiple indicators of disease burden, the use of which would depend upon the intended use of such an indicator (Murray, 1994). To quantify the burden of disease and the full loss of healthy life, the World Bank and the WHO have jointly developed a single indicator: disability-adjusted life years (DALYs) for the 1993 World Development Report (World Bank, 1993). DALYs are an indicator of the time lived with a disability and the time lost due to premature mortality. Four general concepts are implicit in the development of DALYs as indicators of disease burden (Murray, 1994):

1. Any health outcome that represents a lost of welfare is included in an indicator of health status.
2. Age and sex would be the only characteristics of the individual which would be considered.
3. Health outcomes will be treated as like wherever they may occur globally.
4. Time is the unit of measure for the burden of disease.

Table 13.1 shows the distribution of DALYs lost globally, by cause and demographic region, for the year 1990 based on the recent World Development Report (World Bank, 1993).

'Programming': prenatal influences on later life chronic disease

Until recently the focus on causes of adult onset chronic non-communicable diseases (NCDs) has been on risk factors—dietary and lifestyle-related—operating in adult life. The 'foetal origins' hypothesis of Barker and his colleagues (Barker et al, 1989; Barker, 1994) drew attention to the important influences on chronic disease risk that are determined prenatally or during infancy. This was considered by some to be an unwelcome diversion that distracted attention and

Table 13.1 Percentage distribution of disability-adjusted life years (DALY) lost by demographic region, 1990

	World	Established market economies	Former socialist economies of Europe	Sub-Saharan Africa	Asia India	Asia China	Asia Far East	Middle Eastern Crescent	Latin America and the Caribbean
Communicable diseases	45.8	9.7	8.6	71.3	50.5	25.3	48.5	51.0	42.2
Non-communicable diseases	42.2	78.4	74.8	19.4	40.4	58.0	40.1	36.0	42.8
Cancer	5.8	19.1	14.8	1.5	4.1	9.2	4.4	3.4	5.2
Ischaemic heart disease	3.1	10.0	13.7	0.4	2.8	2.1	3.5	1.8	2.7
Cerebrovascular disease	3.2	5.3	8.9	1.5	2.1	6.3	2.1	2.4	2.6
Nutritional deficiencies	3.9	1.7	1.4	2.8	6.2	3.3	4.6	3.7	4.6
Injuries	11.9	11.9	16.6	9.3	9.1	16.7	11.3	13.0	15.0
DALYs per 1000 population	259	117	168	575	344	178	260	286	233

Source: Adapted from *World Development Report* (World Bank, 1993)

may possibly lead to the undermining of efforts to reduce the risks by dietary and lifestyle interventions in later life. The significant contribution of the Barker hypothesis is in highlighting the importance of inter-generational and prenatal determinants of birth outcome and the nutritional status and growth during early infancy. Birth outcome and growth during the first years of life programmes to some extent the adult onset of chronic disease. This implies that intervention strategies have to be aimed at a much earlier period, and not just during adulthood. The Barker hypothesis has major implications for the risk of chronic NCDs in developing countries who already bear a heavy burden of low birthweights and poor nutritional status of the child during her/his pre-school years.

There are several issues that need further clarification and elucidation. How does one separate out the role of genetic make-up on the susceptibility to chronic disease from the adverse influences that programme the same during the prenatal period and in early infancy? What is the impact of programming due to prenatal and early infancy nutritional influences on the genetic background? Are the effects additive or multiplicative? Can positive interventions alter programming by influencing pregnancy outcome and infant nutrition? How do the effects of exposure to risk in adult life alter the pathway delineated by programming from prenatal experiences? Does programming influence the effects of later life exposure to risk of adult onset chronic disease?

Recent work by David Leon and his colleagues (1996) shows that impaired foetal growth may lead to substantial increases in blood pressure among only those who become obese or attain relatively increased stature. Those individuals with relatively greater adult heights but lower weights at birth had the highest blood pressures. Does that mean that people who attain full growth potential in adult life but suffered from impaired intrauterine growth are at greater risk of disease in adult life? Does better nutrition in later life that leads to better growth potential (in size and height) have deleterious consequences to a low birthweight infant who is already programmed? The implications in terms of interventions to improve the nutritional status of the child with a low birthweight in developing countries are huge. Should the impact of urbanisation, acculturation and economic development of societies with a high incidence of low birthweights (therefore already programmed) cause further increases in adult onset chronic disease? With increases in life expectancy and better nutrition, will there be a pandemic of degenerative diseases in adulthood even before we have an opportunity to consider the contributions from the negative effects of modern diets and lifestyle changes?

Ethnic variations and socio-economic differentials in chronic disease

Studies on migrants, ethnic differences in the prevalence of diseases within a country and inter-country comparisons provide insights into ethnic variations in the predisposition and the occurrence of chronic disease. Migrant studies demonstrate two characteristic features:

1. *The acquisition of disease patterns of the indigenous population following migration and the consequent adoption of dietary and socio-cultural practices of the indigenous population by the migrants.* The best examples are those seen in the second-generation Japanese immigrants to California who have similar rates of mortality from colon cancer to the native Caucasians but have much lower rates of mortality from stomach cancer than the Japanese resident in Japan (Wynder *et al*, 1981).
2. *The unmasking of a probable genetic predisposition to the risk of early-onset adult disease following migration.* The best examples are the increased risk of non-insulin-dependent diabetes mellitus (NIDDM), X Syndrome and coronary heart disease (CHD) among South Asian migrants to the United Kingdom (McKeigue *et al*, 1991; McKeigue, this volume, Chapter 3).

Other examples in this category include the increased risk of chronic disease and obesity among the original inhabitants of a region on exposure to modern diets and lifestyles as, for example, among the Pima Indians of Arizona (Bennett *et al*, 1971; 1976), the Micronesian community (Zimmet *et al*, 1978) and the Australian Aborigines (O'Dea, 1991). Also in this general category are the rural–urban differences within a country highlighted from India by Gopalan (this volume, Chapter 1.2) suggesting that internal migration, urbanisation and exposure to modern diet and lifestyles increase risk of chronic disease. Both genetic and environmental factors interact here to result in chronic disease, although the exact mechanisms through which genetic factors exert their influence are not clear. The 'thrify genotype' hypothesis (Neel, 1962) postulates that populations exposed to inadequate or fluctuating food supplies are genetically selected for a high level of efficiency in caloric utilisation or for fat storage. When more food becomes available following external or internal migration, this efficiency may lead to an increase in obesity, NIDDM and other metabolic abnormalities that predispose to increased risk of CHD.

There are, however, several issues that remain unresolved with regard to risk among migrant populations and inter-country variations in chronic disease risk. For instance, does the absolute change in a nutritional or metabolic parameter such as blood glucose or lipid profile imply identical risk in different ethnic groups (Reddy, this volume, Chapter 3)? Is change or risk absolute or relative? What about inter-individual variations within a population? In an affluent population with similar socio-economic values and resources, will not genetic factors become relatively more important in determining risk of chronic disease? Do nutritional indicators such as Body Mass Index (BMI) or waist:hip ratio (WHR) have identical biological significance and hence predict risk of chronic disease equally across different ethnic groups in a population within a country, or provide a basis for inter-country comparisons?

Socio-economic variations in chronic disease have been best illustrated by the Whitehall (I and II) studies (Brunner, this volume, Chapter 4) where income distribution is a proxy for a range of factors that predispose to adult onset chronic disease. Is this another illustration of how changes in diet and lifestyle alter the risk of chronic disease, since it has previously been demonstrated that chronic disease first affects the affluent classes within a population and then percolates through to other social classes (Marmot, 1989)? The acquisition of risk seems to depend on the acculturation rate. Ethnic variations and socio-economic differentials in chronic disease risk appear to have one feature in common, and that is the unmasking of the risk of NIDDM and CHD following the onset of obesity. Is this another illustration of genetic factors becoming relatively more important in determining risk in populations when affluence increases and all individuals have similar socio-economic values and resources, at least those related to diet and lifestyles in general?

Socio-economic differentials in health have brought to the fore various non-biological factors that may play an important role in the acquisition of risk. These include factors such as social, geographic, cultural, family structure, social cohesion and psychological determinants. The Roseto effect (Egolf et al, 1992), describes the important role of cultural factors related to a stable family structure, social cohesion, and the supportive nature of the community protecting against risk of heart disease and being conducive to longevity despite similar dietary and lifestyle risk factors. Loosening of family ties and loss of community cohesion predispose to increased risk in the same population. Psychological factors may also play an important role. Lack of control, effort–reward relationship and stress are all now recognised as contributing to increased risk and explaining, if only partially, the socio-economic differentials in chronic disease risk (Brunner, this volume, Chapter 4). This new social dimension has generated terms such as 'mobility', 'access', and 'availability' of resources such as healthy diet and appropriate food choice as being important determinants of social variations in disease (Dowler, this volume, Chapter 4). They have highlighted the importance of non-biological factors such as socialisation, civic cohesion, groupishness and aspiration as being equally important determinants of chronic disease risk. Perhaps these are also common factors that link ethnic variations with socio-economic differentials in the prevalence of chronic disease within a population.

Diet, lifestyle and chronic disease

Obesity

The global burden of obesity is increasing rapidly. Industrialised, developed countries are showing increasing trends in prevalence of obesity over the past two or more decades while developing countries are showing a rise in overweight and obesity among their populations along with economic development and urbanisation (Shetty and Tedstone, this volume). Two critical factors that have influenced the recent explosion in the prevalence of obesity are changes in dietary intake and levels of physical activity. Obesity is the result of energy intake being chronically in excess of energy expenditure, resulting in a positive energy balance and weight gain. In developed countries, despite the steady decline in *per capita* energy intake over the past three to four decades, levels of physical activity have also declined with the move towards more sedentary lifestyles. Occupational activity levels have declined, and in spite of an increased participation in leisure-time activities at most ages, energy expenditure levels have declined.

The growing concern of industrialised affluent societies about secular trends in the prevalence of obesity, particularly among children (Murata and Hibi, 1992) are also mirrored in rapidly industrialising, developing economies. Repeat surveys in developing countries have shown an association between a dramatic increase in mean Body Mass Index of the population and acculturation indices (Byers and Marshall, 1995) or modernity scores (Hodge *et al*, 1995). In these countries the rapid changes in dietary intake have been indicative of an increase in *per capita* availability of food. Countries like China have not only altered overall dietary adequacy but have also seen a marked change in dietary composition, with increasing proportions of the population consuming more than 30% of energy from fat. There has also been a concurrent marked change in physical activity levels and patterns. According to the Chinese Health and Nutrition Surveys of 1989 and 1991 (Popkin, 1994), urban residents have adopted a sedentary lifestyle. Rural–urban dichotomy in dietary and physical activity patterns in China is not only associated with differences in prevalence of overweight and obesity, but also provides evidence that the rate of transition in urban populations is very rapid and dramatic.

Cardiovascular disease

Presentations at this Forum (Willett, this volume, Chapter 5) have attempted to show that an increase in consumption of saturated fat in our diet is not as important a risk factor for CHD and some cancers as hitherto presumed (Keys, 1980). Other fractions of fat in our diet may play an important role both in the increasing risk of CHD as well as some cancers. Should we then abandon the recommendations to reduce total fat intake, and in particular the goals for saturated fat intake? The health gains achieved with regard to CHD, both in the USA and in Finland and Norway, by reducing fat and cholesterol intakes would negate that position. We are also in danger of sending the wrong public health and nutrition messages to countries in Eastern Europe and developing countries where the epidemic of chronic disease has already begun or is beginnning to be manifest. The message should clearly be to reduce intakes of saturated fats and *trans* fats and to moderate the intake of total fat.

Alcohol intake has been demonstrated to reduce the risk of cardiovascular disease (McPherson, this volume, Chapter 8). However, comparison with abstainers is not appropriate (Shaper, this volume, Chapter 8), although the J-shaped relationship of alcohol intake and risk would imply an optimum consumption as having the advantage of lowering risk. There is no basis for encouraging abstainers in an effort to reduce their risk of cardiovascular disease. There are several analytical issues which relate to individual risk as opposed to population risk. One also has to be aware of the problem of heavy drinking and the consequent morbidity and mortality in society when encouraging alcohol intake as a component of health promotion, since shifting the mean intakes would have an adverse impact on the intake levels of the deviant numbers (Rose and Day, 1990).

Cancers

Colorectal cancer is one good illustration of where diet is an important factor in carcinogenesis. The important dietary risk factors are animal fats and meat protein, while there are several protective factors in the diet such as fruits and vegetables, starch, non-starch polysaccharides and oligosaccharides (Bingham and Cummings, this volume, Chapter 6). The direction of dietary changes in developing countries typified by the dietary changes seen in China, for instance, suggest an increase in animal fat and protein, increased intakes of refined cereals with a reduction in intakes of dietary fibre. This trend is disturbing. In most developed countries, however, starch intakes continue to be high (Vorster, this volume) and they may have a more important protective role than non-starch polysaccharide intakes in the diets of Third World countries.

Dietary fat intake has been linearly associated with breast cancer deaths in women (Carroll, 1986). Recent analysis suggests that dietary fat intake provides for only a small risk for breast cancer and that hormonal influences predominate (Riboli, this volume). There is emerging evidence that phyto-oestrogens in the diet may play an important protective role and that obesity may provide an additional risk component for breast cancer. There are several questions that remain unanswered. Do we know enough about populations with low risk of breast cancer? What causes the rapid changes in risk patterns following migration? Since hormonal influences related to reproductive activity predominate, and diet plays a secondary role, is breast cancer a good example for the analysis of gene–nutrient interactions? The evidence presented in this book also suggests that steroid hormone binding globulin (SHBG) may play an important role in breast cancer aetiology (Key, this volume). Is SHBG level likely to emerge as an important advantage marker for breast cancer, like high-density lipoprotein (HDL) cholesterol is for CHD ?

Health impact of globalisation of food trade

The adverse public health impact of the global market in food trade has been ably highlighted by Lang (this volume). He warns us that public health is the lowest priority in influencing global food trade. The main adverse effects are: (1) the global inculcation of imbalanced and calorically excessive Western-type diets; (2) dietary deprivation of the rural poor in developing countries which is likely to increase poverty and malnutrition and widen socio-economic differentials; (3) the health consequences of community disintegration, population displacement and consequent unemployment; and (4) the environmental damage and the 'ecological footprints' left behind. These are important issues that need to be dealt with if we are determined to reduce the 'double whammy' of co-existing problems of undernutrition and overnutrition that face developing countries.

Lessons from population-based intervention studies

Public health intervention strategies are approaches for promoting health, and attempts to reduce adult onset chronic disease and the consequent morbidity and mortality that add to the health burden of a nation. The Norwegian National Nutrition Policy (Norum, this volume) and North Karelia project in Finland (Puska, this volume) are examples of successful intervention strategies to reduce chronic disease in populations. Norway was the first country to merge health and agricultural concerns to forge an effective nutrition policy. The Norwegian National Nutrition Policy formally linked economic and agricultural policies with nutrition and health (Milio, 1990). A systematic nutrition information policy was directed at government, food producers, private organisations and consumers, alongside the significant changes in agricultural and animal husbandry policies which were a key element in the dietary changes that followed in Norway and which resulted in better health outcomes (Milio, 1991). Health promotion and nutrition education and involvement of all the key players and actors thus underpinned the systematic policy changes that were implemented. It demonstrated the importance of political will to change, and the important role of motivation and power of the health professional to bring about better health at the population level. These are good examples of the interaction of the individual and different components of society to reduce the slope of the health burden on the community.

Lessons from contrasting worlds

Developing countries have to learn from the experience of industrialised and affluent countries to tackle the emerging crisis of chronic diseases that they are likely to face in the near future. They have already had to deal with the problems of undernutrition and malnutrition and provide sufficient outlays of resources to tackle this. The emerging health burden of chronic disease affecting mainly the economically productive adult population will consume even more of the scarce resources. However, it is important to realise that the poorer countries will be hurt even further in the long run, if attempts are not made to develop solutions for addressing these emerging issues on an urgent basis.

Developed countries can help this process not only by means of highlighting and underlining the need to tackle these emerging problems, but also by sharing their experiences in dealing with them. The nutrition and public health professions must contribute actively in responding to this crisis. The traditional focus on undernutrition has to be widened to encompass all aspects of malnutrition, including overnutrition. Rather than separate issues of deficit and excess, we need to create health and nutrition messages that broadly address the concerns of unbalanced nutrition in the community—both under- and overnutrition. It is important to emphasise the need for primary prevention of these diet- and lifestyle-determined chronic diseases in countries where resources are scarce and limited. A nutrition-driven policy that encompasses the cooperation of all sectors that influence dietary and food practices is essential to generate changes in health-related behaviour that will address both the problems of dietary deficiency and of dietary excess. The lessons from contrasting worlds are relevant to both developed and developing countries in tackling this major public health problem.

References

Barker DJP. *Mothers, Babies, and Diseases in Later Life Babies.* London: British Medical Journal Publishing Group, 1994

Barker DJP, Osmond C, Golding J, Kuh D, Wadsworth MEJ. Growth *in utero*, blood pressure in childhood and adult life, and mortality from cardiovascular disease. *British Medical Journal*, 1989; **298**: 564–567

Bennett PH, Burch TA, Miller M. Diabetes mellitus in American (Pima) Indians. *Lancet*, 1971; **ii**: 125–128

Bennett PH, Rusforth NB, Miller M, Unger RH. Epidemiologic studies of diabetes in Pima Indians. *Recent Progress in Hormone Research*, 1976; **32**: 333–376

Boyden BM. *Western Civilization in Biological Perspective. Patterns in Biohistory.* Oxford: Oxford University Press, 1988

Byers T, Marshall JA. The emergence of chronic diseases in developing countries. *SCN News*, 1995; **13**: 14–19

Carroll KK. Experimental studies on dietary fat and cancer in relation to epidemiology data. In: Clement IP, Birt D, Rogers D, Mettlin C (eds). *Dietary Fat and Cancer.* New York: Alan R. Liss, 1986, pp 231–298

Egolf B, Lasker J, Wolf S, Potvin L. The Roseto effect: a 50-year comparison of mortality rates. *American Journal of Public Health*, 1992; **82**: 1089–1092

Hodge AM, Dowse GK, Koki G, Mavo B, Alpers MP, Zimmet PZ. Modernity and obesity in coastal and Highland Papua New Guinea. *International Journal of Obesity*, 1995; **19**: 154–161

Keys A. *Seven Countries: A Multivariate Analysis of Death and Coronary Heart Disease.* London: Harvard University Press, 1980

Leon DA, Koupilova I, Lithell HO *et al.* Failure to realise growth potential *in utero* and adult onset obesity in relation to blood pressure in 50 years in Swedish men. *British Medical Journal*, 1996; **312**: 401–406

Mackenbach JP. The epidemiologic transition theory (Editorial). *Journal of Epidemiology and Community Health*, 1994; **48**: 329–331

Marmot M. Socioeconomic determinants of CHD mortality. *International Journal of Epidemiology*, 1989; **18**: S196–202

McKeigue PM, Shah B, Marmot MG. Relationship of central obesity and insulin resistance with high diabetes prevalence and cardiovascular risk in South Asians. *Lancet*, 1991; **337**: 382–386

Milio N. *Nutrition Policy for Food-rich Countries: A Strategic Analysis.* Baltimore, MD: The Johns Hopkins University Press, 1990

Milio N. Toward healthy longevity. *Scandinavian Journal of Social Medicine*, 1991; **19**: 209–217

Murata M, Hibi I. Nutrition and the secular trend of growth. *Hormone Research*, 1992; **38**: S89–96

Murray CJL. Quantifying the burden of disease: the technical basis for disability-adjusted life years. *Bulletin of the World Health Organization*, 1994; **72**: 429–445

Neel JV. Diabetes mellitus: a 'thrifty genotype' rendered detrimental 'by progress'. *American Journal of Human Genetics*, 1962; **14**: 353–362

O'Dea K. Westernisation and non-insulin dependent diabetes in Australian aborigines. *Ethnicity and Disease*, 1991; **1**: 171–187

Olshansky SJ, Ault AB.The fourth stage of epidemiological transition: the age of delayed degenerative diseases. *Milbank Memorial Fund Quarterly*, 1986; **64**: 355–391

Omran AR. The epidemiological transition. A theory of the epidemiology of population change. *Milbank Memorial Fund Quarterly*, 1971; **49**: 509–538

Omran AR. The epidemiological transition theory: A preliminary update. *Journal of Tropical Paediatrics*, 1983; **29**: 305–316

Popkin BM. The nutrition transition in low-income countries: an emerging crisis. *Nutrition Reviews*, 1994; **52**: 285–298

Rose G, Day S. The population mean predicts the number of deviant individuals. *British Medical Journal*, 1990; **301**: 1031–1034

World Bank. *World Development Report 1993. Investing in Health.* Oxford: Oxford University Press, 1993

Wynder EL, McCoy GD, Reddy BS. Nutrition and metabolic epidemiology of cancers of the oral cavity, oesophagus, colon, breast, prostate and stomach. In: Newell GR, Ellison NM (eds). *Nutrition and Cancer: Etiology and Treatment.* New York: Raven Press, 1981, pp 11–48

Zimmet P, Arblaster M, Thoma K. The effect of westernization on native populations. Studies in a Micronesian community with high diabetes prevalence. *Australian and New Zealand Journal of Medicine*, 1978; **8**: 141–146

14
Where do we go from here in public health?

W. Philip T. James

Rowett Research Institute, Aberdeen, UK

We are entering a new period in public health where nutrition-related issues will become ever more prominent. To see this in context, however, we need an historical perspective in both nutrition and public health. In both fields we can discern three major phases or revolutions in thinking during the course of this century, and there is now a need to integrate the two areas as we enter the next millennium: I would claim that nutrition underlies many of the current public health problems and societal challenges in the world today.

The discovery of vitamins and protective foods: implications for social and economic policies

The first part of this century was exciting for biologists because a whole range of fat- and water-soluble micro-components of the diet was being identified; these compounds could prevent several major scourges, such as rickets, scurvy, beriberi and pellagra. New evidence then emerged from Cory Mann and Boyd Orr suggesting that the poor in society were short and sick not because of their poor genetic make-up but because their diet was poor and deficient in protein, energy and a whole range of minerals and in the newly termed vitamins (Boyd Orr, 1936). In Scotland, an ideal recruiting ground for tall, healthy and energetic soldiers in the previous century, recruits were being rejected as too short and puny to bear arms, with great public concern being expressed about the long-term future of Britain as the working class with their poor physique and lack of physical and mental staying power outbred the tall and well built intelligentsia of the aristocracy.

Public health was also increasingly seen as an important societal concern. The scourges of the common infectious diseases could be partially controlled by

Diet, Nutrition and Chronic Disease: Lessons from Contrasting Worlds.
Edited by P. S. Shetty and K. McPherson © 1997 John Wiley & Sons, Ltd.

vaccination for smallpox and BCG for tuberculosis, but careful quarantining, an emphasis on fresh air and reduced crowding were also important preventive strategies. The treatment of these conditions, however, was based on the need to build the patient's resistance with good feeding. This therapeutic concern was then extended to preventive nutrition, with the development of surveillance systems to monitor the growth of babies and schoolchildren. In practice, we can now recognise that the improved conditions of the poor—in terms of hygiene, nutrition and reduced crowding—had a huge impact on public health, with a remarkable decline in maternal and infant mortality rates in the first half of this century, long before antibiotics or modern immunising vaccines became available (McKeown, 1976).

During the economic crises of the mid-1930s, social policies to improve the health of children, pregnant and nursing mothers became the clarion call of doctors and social reformers. They promoted the value of the expensive dietary items, meat and milk, as those foods best able to promote children's growth and contribute to the protein, energy, mineral and vitamin needs of an impoverished population. Boyd Orr, the British Medical Association and others all cooperated with voluntary organisations and the newly formed Milk Marketing Board to promote the provision of milk for all schoolchildren.

Wartime nutrition, public health and agricultural policies

The outbreak of war in 1939 brought rapid changes in public policy and marked the start of the second revolution or phase in our thinking. In 1939, the Government followed expert advice by not only introducing a new form of food rationing with milk, meat and butter as universally available in small amounts, but also stipulating a daily allocation of full-cream milk and school lunch for every schoolchild. In practice the health of the nation during the war improved markedly and did not deteriorate as expected (Acheson, 1986).

With the outbreak of war, British agriculture was exposed as providing only 30% of Britain's food supplies, so agricultural development became a priority. Then, as semi-starvation threatened many millions of European, Middle Eastern and Asian refugees at the end of the war, food supplies became accepted as crucial to national security. The priorities in food policy therefore shifted, as did those in public health. Questions about the adequacy of particular foods for human health were, for practical purposes, solved by the end of the war because the remarkable national experiments in feeding everybody the minimum foods needed for good growth, reasonable adult weights and the ability to work had proved successful. The priority therefore moved from analyses of further nutritional refinements in relation to health to that of research in animal nutrition necessary to help produce enough meat, milk and butter so cheaply that even the poor could afford to purchase these luxuries. This led to the mushrooming of agricultural institutes, and the transfer of most residual interest in human nutritional research to overseas units and food policies geared to the production of cheap food.

Public health also changed. Throughout Europe, after the war, there was acceptance, whether in the new Communist countries or in the West, that universal health care was needed to meet the aspirations of the millions of servicemen and servicewomen who had experienced medical care in the armed forces or as part of the national response under wartime conditions. In Britain a National Health Service (NHS) was introduced with the idea that all that was now required was individual health evaluation of children and pregnant women and good facilities to deal with the burden of illness. The NHS was, in effect, the public health service for Britain, with some community physicians still being retained to deal with any outbreak of food poisoning or other communicable disease. Public health progressively geared itself to helping with analyses of the effectiveness of the NHS, and health services research soon dominated thinking.

The new public health and changes in nutritional perceptions

The third revolution took hold in the US and Scandinavia in the 1970s following the discovery by Keys and his colleagues that the newly recognised epidemic of coronary heart disease had an environmental and behavioural basis linked to smoking and those dietary factors which induced hypertension and elevated blood cholesterol levels (Keys, 1980). We have read of the Scandinavian experience in this volume and of the remarkable success of a range of public health and nutrition policies in transforming the diet of Finns and Norwegians as agricultural practice, urbanisation, transport and pricing policies and guidelines or rules on public sector catering and food formulation all induced changes in dietary patterns.

The US experience has been somewhat different, since the lack of universal health care (given the misinformed US phobia for socialised medicine and for federal provision of tax-dependent services) led to the availability of individual care paid for by customers who relied on information alone to ensure they did not have to pay expensive medical bills. This required the consumer to respond individually; the educated changed as they recognised the value of remaining healthy rather than falling into the clutches of an acquisitive medical profession operating often for financial self-interest. The food industry, operating in a pseudo-free market, then responded so that in the US as well as in Scandinavia there have been substantial reductions in population cholesterol levels, in smoking and in blood pressure levels.

Elsewhere policies have been slow to change. In the post-war European Communist Block there was, and still often is, a huge emphasis on the provision of meat, milk and butter to meet inappropriately high animal protein and animal fat targets for human health, since people were presumed (as elsewhere in the 1930s) to be short of animal protein and energy. Agricultural policies became

W. P. T. James

totally distorted after the war and huge grain imports were needed to feed all the dairy and beef cattle. The claim on the USSR's foreign currency reserve, particularly for grain purchases, from the US, required the additional help of sophisticated intelligence, trade and foreign policies geared to obtaining the cheapest price for the US grain. Huge amounts were needed to sustain a Communist agricultural industry in a grossly inefficient drive to produce meat and dairy products. Elsewhere, the policy-makers' post-war obsession with cheap food to prevent nutritional deficiency led to a hugely subsidised farming and food industry; the new might of these industries has now made change in nutrition and food policies much more difficult.

Our recent analyses suggest that in Western Europe public health initiatives have depended on the efforts of those forceful academic groups or individuals who promote new concepts of nutrition in public health. In countries such as the UK, Sweden and Ireland, where physicians and nutritionists disputed the evidence on diet and health, there was little change in cardiovascular disease rates. This provides a clear example of how conservative thinking can itself be held responsible for thousands of premature deaths! Public opinion had to be mobilised effectively before governmental change was contemplated, and then it might depend, as in Britain, on having the fortunate combination of a sophisticated Chief Medical Officer, Sir Donald Acheson, and a highly intelligent Minister of Health in Mr William Waldegrave to initiate the remarkable proposals seen in *Health of the Nation* (GB Department of Health, 1992). In this governmental initiative at Cabinet level, and without preliminary analyses and formulations by any Advisory Committee such as the Committee on Medical Aspects of Food Policy, nutrition and food relate to nine of the 16 key areas and targets, which ranged from accidents to HIV/AIDS.

The evidence from Norway and Finland of the benefits of new public health policies is clear, but the initiatives stemmed from a coherent and consistent set of policies driven by independent doctors, nutritionists and public health specialists who were able to overcome the conservatism of the farming industry and the antagonism of some food companies. Nutritional research on humans then re-emerged throughout the world as an important priority, with huge functional implications for the food and farming industries. The issue now is how best to move forward into the next phase.

The challenge for nutritional epidemiologists: mechanistic or/and public policy analyses of the changes needed in diet

Epidemiologists now accept that nutrients and other bioactive compounds in the diet are of importance in determining or profoundly modifying cardiovascular disease, cancers, intestinal and respiratory disorders, brain development, resistance to infections and a host of other disabilities. These issues are not only interesting to those of us in public health: they are also considered crucial as a priority for national science. Thus, the recent UK Technology Foresight exercise, which involved 15 expert panels of scientists and industrialists together with widespread consultation, sought to determine what is needed both for the economic rejuvenation of Britain and for the public good. Diet and other lifestyle aspects of health came a close second to biotechnology and bioengineering in the priority listing of all the different options presented. This astonishing emphasis, emerging from proposals which ranged from financial services to clean technologies and sensory information processing, reflects the huge importance attached to society's perceptions of health, to the economic implications of an ageing population as well as to the welfare of the health, food and agricultural industries, which include the pharmaceutical industry. Thus, public health should now be seen in a new light and it is our responsibility to capitalise on this new opportunity. Epidemiologists are in general presented with two possible paths to follow—either a quantitative and mechanistic analysis of the nutritional and other bases of the prevalent diseases, or a route which meshes population analyses of health and disease with other assessments of the basis for behaviour and the socio-economic and societal barriers to lifestyle changes. Both are extremely important and need to interface, but may require very different approaches.

Analytical epidemiology

Epidemiologists have made such progress recently in analytical epidemiology that a tendency has now emerged to disregard the shortcomings of some of the techniques and to ignore the importance of having a biological perspective when designing or interpreting studies. As noted elsewhere in this volume (James, this volume, Chapter 5), we need biomarkers to be included in our studies so that we have a proper appreciation of the errors involved in any dietary survey technique.

We also need to recognise the fundamental limitations of cohort studies and, indeed, their capacity to mislead. Thus, when inter-individual responsiveness to a dietary factor is substantial and further confounded by other biologically relevant factors, then those cohort studies which show no relationship between diet and a disease may be construed as refuting the causal importance of a dietary factor, when in practice it is of fundamental importance. Thus, the cholesterol responses to dietary saturated fatty acids and the confounding effects of antioxidants on the development of heart disease mean that without cholesterol and antioxidant measurements it would be exceptionally difficult to show in cohort studies the importance of saturated fats and fatty acids in the development of CHD. We would then have to rely, except in cross-cultural studies, on animal experiments and clinical trials of secondary prevention. The whole story of CHD has been simplified for us, however, by our having a plausible biological mechanism.

A further example of this problem is the failure of most case-control and cohort studies to show any link between non-starch polysaccharide (NSP) or starch intake and colon cancer. However, metabolic epidemiological studies which we conducted on a cross-cultural basis in the mid-1970s, suggested that carbohy-drate fermentation in the colon could be an important protective factor (IARC, 1977). More recently, cross-cultural studies have extended the concept and shown that an average fecal weight in a population of 300 g/d is associated with a very low risk of colon cancer (Cummings et al, 1992). Thus, it is not surprising to observe a seemingly protective effect of complex carbohydrates including NSP in cross-cultural studies (Cassidy et al, 1994) when in cohort studies their import-ance may well be observed by the very substantial variation in the laxative response to a standard extra intake of NSP and indeed to different types of NSP (Cummings et al, 1978). The inter-individual variation in colonic responses to NSP intakes is as wide-ranging as the cholesterol response to dietary saturated fatty acid intake, so this may be another indicator of risk. Recent studies by Bingham et al (1996) on the basis of nitrosamine production in the colon now allow a completely different biological spectrum to be developed which highlights the promotional effect of red meat intake on colon carcinogenesis and the protective effects of fermentable polysaccharides entering the colon.

The discussion on post-menopausal breast cancer (Riboli, this volume, Chapter 7; Key, this volume, Chapter 7) also suggests that oestradiol and sex hormone binding protein measurements may prove to be equivalent to measur-ing total cholesterol and HDL cholesterol in CHD. We need other indices for such common conditions as pre-menopausal breast, pancreatic and prostatic cancers as well as for the development of other non-cancerous conditions, such as cataract, senile dementia, osteoporosis and arthritis.

The third extension of analytical epidemiology is in the application of gene markers to distinguish individual susceptibility to common public health problems. This is likely to be particularly valuable in relation not only to cancers and CHD but also, for example, to folate metabolism. Dietary folate is likely to prove of crucial importance in future analyses; it is relevant to epidemiological studies of cardiovascular disease as well as to maternal and child health and perhaps to cancer. New data show that > 400 μg folic acid daily is needed to prevent both neural tube defects (GB Department of Health, 1996) and the hyperhomocysteinaemia of those susceptible to cardiovascular disease as adults (Selhub et al, 1993).

Since elevated levels of homocysteine are observed in a majority of the elderly people, this implies an extraordinarily prevalent problem of folate deficiency on a population level. Evidence shows that 43% of the population is carrying, in the heterozygous state, the thermolabile form of 5,10-tetrahydromethylene folic acid reductase with its higher need for folic acid, and that in all populations studied 5–6% have the homozygous condition. Thus we clearly have misunderstood the folate needs of the population. Furthermore, since most neural tube defects are preventable with folic acid but only a fifth of these folate-preventable defects are ascribable to this folate enzyme 'abnormality', we may yet find a series of gene changes in other folic acid-related enzymes, e.g. methionine synthase and cystathione reductase, which would explain the development of birth defects, low birthweights and adult cardiovascular disease on modest folate intakes. This not only portrays Barker's hypothesis (1994) in a different light but implies the need to rethink our nutritional concepts, an issue to which I now turn.

The nutritional biology of *Homo sapiens*

The concept that 400 μg folic acid is needed to avoid hyperhomocysteinaemia suggests that we have an inappropriate perspective on the optimum needs for nutrients. These are at present mostly based on the need to avoid deficiency diseases. Yet recent data from Ames (1989) suggest that to avoid the development of oxidised bases in DNA, measured in practice as $8'$-deoxyguanidine in sperm DNA, we need 100 mg of vitamin C daily. Emerging research also suggests that there is a logarithmic increase in genetic change with age despite the presence of an array of detoxification systems in the liver and several DNA repair enzymes (Cole *et al*, 1991). Smokers have a 50–100% increase in specific DNA changes at any particular age, with new evidence suggesting that diet can modify not only the rate of DNA damage but also the rate of DNA repair. Thus, we may be on the verge of being able to modulate the ageing process by having a much higher micronutrient intake than previously proposed.

These concepts link with Eaton's thesis (1985) that *Homo sapiens* as a hunter-gatherer emerging in Africa was biologically a creature geared to high intakes of tubers, leafy vegetables and fruit as well as meat and fish. This diet provided perhaps two to three times the current specified minimum intakes for health of vitamins and essential amino acids. Crawford's proposal (1989) that humans share with the dolphin the distinction of a disproportionately large brain with its excessive needs for n-3 essential fatty acids again implies the need for ample intakes of fish, vegetables and meat. Thus Crawford highlights the development of most great civilisations around river estuaries where the nutrient-rich effluent supported major fish stocks capable of providing the essential fatty acids needed for the unusual brain biology of man. Cereal growing emerged only 10 000 years ago in the Tigris and Euphrates delta, so the evolutionary experience of *Homo sapiens* has not been conditioned by high-cereal diets at all, let alone modern high-fat diets. McMichael (1995) has recently suggested that with the waves of human migration out of Africa over several millennia there have been subtle evolutionary changes to cope with new environmental conditions. These might include the development of whiter skins and the preservation of intestinal lactase beyond infancy to cope with potential rickets in northern climates, and the change in hepatic acetylation capacity and rates as the high intakes of plant toxicants were reduced; the loss of alcohol-metabolising enzymes in many Oriental groups may be part of the same process.

These evolutionary pressures might explain some of the racial differences in dietary tolerance that are only now becoming clear.

Given our reappraisal of the needs for the carotenoids, found in vegetables, roots and fruit, in limiting oxidative damage to tissues, such as the lens in the eye, in maintaining macular function in the eye, and perhaps gonadal and prostatic function, we may need to reappraise most of our concepts of nutritional physiology and needs as we unravel the biological basis of our most common population problems.

Converting our understanding of the biology of ageing into practical public health policies may not be simply a question of preserving DNA and tissues in non-oxidised states but of how best to prevent a progressive entraining of pathophysiological changes, such as the rise in blood pressure, in serum cholesterol and in bodyweight. All three of these increase with age in Western societies, so we tend to assume that they reflect a progressive change with age in one or more lifestyle conditions, e.g. physical activity. Yet there may be biological mechanisms which entrain a progressive process; Miall and Lovell (1967) made much of the amplifying effect of pre-existing blood pressure on future rises, and there is increasing evidence that obesity leads to adaptive changes in the set-point of appetite, which then defends the new bodyweight, thereby explaining the seemingly powerful physiological process of hyperphagia in the overweight. The age-related rise in lipids is essentially unexplained but could again reflect progressive lipoprotein receptor adaptation. If this concept is sustained, then the preventive implications are profound since childhood, adolescence and early adulthood become the focus for preventive action. Epidemiologists will need to be aware and involved in this reappraisal if we are to move on to the second aspect of epidemiological interactions—those connected with public health policy and with implementing preventive strategies.

Epidemiology and public health

The second major field for applying epidemiological approaches relates to public health and here, in a nutritionist context, we see a plethora of needs. Whilst we have been concerned with the alarming escalation of chronic diseases, we must also recognise the enormous concern about our capacity on a global basis to feed ourselves. The FAO call for a World Summit on Hunger may not be alarmist, because our analyses of food needs are now on a much firmer basis (James and Schofield, 1990). To the population pressure on water resources and food supplies is added the burden of a loss of high-quality, intensively cultivated land. Our recent data currently show that in India and South-East Asia adult malnutrition rates vary from 20 to 50%, with consequent widespread ill-health (Shetty and James, 1994). Yet India's population is not expected to plateau until about 2060, and its land-carrying capacity, particularly in the eastern half of the country, is likely to be at its limit 30 years earlier.

To these problems we need to add the impact of escalating urbanisation with all its demands for water, food resources, transport, sewerage and environmental controls (McMichael, 1993). If current concepts of optimum vegetable and fruit intakes (WHO, 1990) are to be sustained, and if refrigeration is a major requirement for sustaining the nutritional value and microbial safety of foods without the use of salt and other preserving agents, then issues relating to transport policy, city planning and regulation expand the policy implications of public health prevention into economics, social geography, water and energy engineering and social policy to an extraordinary degree.

We have already heard from Tim Lang's remarkable analyses (Lang, this volume) how the almost universal acceptance of free market values has led to an appalling misuse of land in Third World countries, of unsustainable short-term strategies for making food profits at the expense of health and environmental sustainability and how the concentration of power in multinationals is subverting the capacity of the nation state to order its affairs. With the new world trade agreements including food for the first time, despite J. K. Galbraith's long-standing opposition to the inclusion of agriculture in free-trade agreements, we are now embarked on a round with potentially catastrophic implications for public health.

These developments occur at a time when the collapse of the European Communist system has been hailed as a triumph of capitalism and the free market, these views being reiterated constantly by a Western press owned and organised by those who benefit from an unbridled free market. Will Hutton (1996) has recently savaged this view of successful capitalism, and there is a great need to encompass Tim Lang's analysis in the broader canvas of public health policy-making.

Improving public health: the role of the academic

Recently, the Rowett Research Institute, Aberdeen, organised for WHO an international workshop to look at the experience in public health initiatives and how changes in public health have been achieved in different European countries (James et al, 1997). There were representatives from many countries, and personal accounts were heard from Finland and Norway where so much has been achieved. I confidently expected to discover that there were discerning national bodies established for the purpose of promoting public health, and experts who contributed to these centrally organised policy initiatives. To my surprise, the opposite proved to be true. Although some governments, for example in Norway, Belgium, The Netherlands and Finland, did produce coherent programmes, this was in response to independent academic initiatives. The main stimulus for action was the accumulating evidence of the importance of diet in coronary heart disease, but from this disease-specific concern emerged coherent policies on smoking and diet as a whole to combat a range of public health problems.

Clinicians, community leaders and epidemiologists entered the public fray to proclaim the need for societal change and galvanised colleagues to promote coherent strategies. When institutional processes were established they needed stimulus, scrutiny and goading by independent groups operating in the public domain to maintain momentum and to overcome commercial interests.

Where there was academic dispute with readily identifiable and high-profile doctors or nutritionists who debunked the idea that diet had much to do with such complex genetically determined processes as coronary heart disease, death rates continued to rise, as in England and Wales, Scotland and Eire. The doctors and nutritionists who opposed change did so in good faith. They usually considered themselves the guardians of critical thinking and sound judgement who had a responsibility to curb the evangelical call for change by those who were concerned with public health and willing to advocate changes in the whole country without clear proof of their efficacy. These readily identifiable individuals who opposed public health initiatives may find it difficult to fathom the extent of their responsibility for so many tens of thousands of premature deaths, but it is becoming clear that for effective societal action we do need concerted action and a national consensus for change amongst those at the forefront of policy-making.

A new challenge

Given this perspective, where do we go from here? This meeting has highlighted the breathtaking rate of change and the rise of chronic diseases in China (Chen, this volume, Chapter 1.3), in Asia generally (Gopalan, this volume, Chapter 1.2), in the Middle East (Musaiger, this volume, Chapter 1.5), Africa, the Caribbean and the rest of South America (Sinha, this volume, Chapter 1.4). The countries of Central and Eastern Europe with their former command economics also show escalating disease rates and a declining life expectancy (Bobak and Marmot, 1994). Thus something must be done and experience now suggests the need for academic initiatives with community and political involvement.

On a personal note, I know that the global Advisory Council of the World Cancer Research Fund is due to produce its own strategy for preventing cancer, and that this will have a staged launch in different parts of the globe from 1997 onwards. Several contributors to this volume are involved in an International Obesity Task Force designed to promote better societal preventive strategies and obesity management systems, with major links to WHO. Next year, several of us are due to update our original European report on diet and public health for the European region of WHO. What we now need, therefore, is a systematic regional development by WHO, following up on the 1992 World Conference on Nutrition in Rome, of regional nutritional policies. These initiatives would then form the basis for a 10-year follow-up to the WHO Expert Consultation on Nutrition, Diet and the Prevention of Chronic Disease (1990), to which so many of us contributed in 1986–1988. If WHO could take this on board globally, then we would need to see how best to develop effective, nationally relevant but globally coherent strategies to cope with the escalating problems of population pressure, the misuse of land and resources induced by the free market, the pervasive effect of unbridled multinational companies and with the inappropriate environmental development which so concerned Lang (this volume, Chapter 9) and McMichael (Chapter 9).

There could be no greater nor more positively rewarding challenge for the London School of Hygiene & Tropical Medicine as it enters a new era with a new Dean, new Professors of Epidemiology and Nutrition and expanding divisions of Epidemiology and Public Health than to take on a major role in this field. This could be an exciting period to which I am sure we would all be willing to contribute in the hope of improving as well as preventing the mounting public health problem of adult chronic diseases throughout the world.

References

Acheson ED. Tenth Boyd Orr Memorial Lecture. Food policy, nutrition and government. *Proceedings of the Nutrition Society*, 1986; **45**: 131–138

Ames BN. Endogenous oxidative DNA damage, aging and cancer. *Free Radical Research Communications*, 1989; **7**: 121–127

Barker DJP. *Mothers, Babies, and Disease in Later Life*. London: British Medical Journal Publishing Group, 1994

Bingham SA, Pignatelli B, Pollock JRA et al. Does increasing endogenous formation of N-nitroso compounds in the human colon explain the association between red meat and colon cancer? *Carcinogenesis*, 1996; **17**: 515–523

Bobak M, Marmot M. The East–West divide and potential explanations. In: *The European Health Policy Conference: Opportunities for the Future*. Copenhagen: WHO Regional Office for Europe, 1994

Boyd Orr J. *Food, Health and Income: a report on a survey of adequacy of diet in relation to income*. London: Macmillan and Co, 1936

Cassidy A, Bingham SA, Cummings JHC. Starch intake and colorectal cancer risk: an international comparison. *British Journal of Cancer*, 1994; **69**: 937–942

Cole J, Waugh APW, Beare DM et al. HPRT mutant frequencies in circulating lymphocytes: population studies using normal donors, exposed groups and cancer prone syndromes. In: Barton L, Gledhill BL, Mauro F (eds). *New Horizons in Biological Dosimetry: Proceedings of the International Symposium on Trends in Biological Dosimetry, held in Lerici, Italy, October 23–27, 1990*. New York: Wiley-Liss Inc., 1991: 319–328

Crawford M, Marsh D. *The Driving Force: Food, Evolution and the Future*. London: William Heinemann, 1989

Cummings JH, Southgate DAT, Branch WJ et al. Colonic response to dietary fibre from carrot, cabbage, apple, bran. *Lancet*, 1978; **i**: 5–9

Cummings JH, Bingham SA, Heaton KW, Eastwood MA. Fecal weight, colon cancer risk and dietary intake of nonstarch polysaccharides (dietary fiber). *Gastroenterology*, 1992; **103**:1783–1789

Eaton SB, Konner M. Paleolithic nutrition: a consideration of its nature and current implications. *New England Journal of Medicine*, 1985; **312**: 283–290

Great Britain Department of Health. *The Health of the Nation: a Strategy for Health in*

England. London: HMSO, 1992

Great Britain Department of Health. *Folic Acid and the Prevention of Neural Tube Defects.* London: Health Education Authority, 1996

Hutton W. *The State We're In.* London: Vantage, 1996

International Agency for Research on Cancer (IARC), Intestinal Microecology Group. Dietary fibre, transit-time, faecal bacteria, steroids and colon cancer in two Scandinavian populations. *Lancet,* 1977; **2**: 207–211

James WPT, Schofield EC. *Human Energy Requirements: A Manual for Planners and Nutritionists.* Oxford: Oxford University Press, 1990

James WPT, Ralph A, Bellizzi M, Lüthy J. Nutrition policies in Western Europe: National policies in Austria, Belgium, France, Germany, Ireland, Luxembourg, The Netherlands and Switzerland. *Nutrition Review,* 1997 (in press)

Keys A. *Seven Countries: A Multivariate Analysis of Death and Coronary Heart Disease.* Cambridge, MA: Harvard University Press, 1980

McKeown T. *The Modern Rise of Population.* London: Edward Arnold, 1976

McMichael AJ. Beans and genes: source of human metabolic and dietary diversity. Paper presented at the Royal Society of Medicine, London Conference on Food, People and Health: Past, Present and Future, October 1995

McMichael AJ. *Planetary Overload. Global Environmental Change and the Health of the Human Species.* Cambridge: Cambridge University Press, 1993

Miall WE, Lovell HG. Relation between change of blood pressure and age. *British Medical Journal,* 1967; **2**: 660–664

Selhub J, Jacques PF, Wilson PW, Rush D, Rosenberg IH. Vitamin status and intake as primary determinants of homocysteinemia in an elderly population. *Journal of the American Medical Association,* 1993; **270**: 2693–2698

Shetty PS, James WPT. *Body Mass Index. A Measure of Chronic Energy Deficiency in Adults.* FAO Food and Nutrition Paper 56. Rome: Food and Agricultural Organization of the United Nations, 1994

World Health Organization Study Group on Diet, Nutrition and Prevention of Non-Communicable Diseases. *Diet, nutrition and the prevention of chronic diseases: report of a WHO Study Group.* WHO Technical Report Series 797. Geneva: WHO, 1990

Index

isoflavones, 128, 154
isothiocyanates, 128

Japan, ischaemic heart disease in, 7
Japanese migrants, mortality in, 60–1
jejuno-ileal bypass, 249

lacto-ovovegetarians, definition of, 261
Lactobacillus, 140
large bowel cancer, 140–2
    and diet, 121–33
    protective factors in, 127–32
    see also colon cancer; colorectal cancer
Latin America
    mortality patterns, 34(fig.)
    NCDs in, 30–6
LDL (low-density lipoprotein)
    cholesterol, 101, 105, 207, 243
leg length, 86
leptin, 223–4, 250, 251–2
lifestyle, 269–79
lipid disturbance
    in Afro-Caribbeans, 66–7
    and central obesity relationship, 64–5
lipid metabolism, 198
    and short baby, 47–8
lipid oxidation, 232
lipogenesis, 229
lipolysis, 228
liver size, 47–8
low-density lipoprotein (LDL)
    cholesterol, 101, 105, 207, 243
low energy reporting, 87–8
    and BMI, 89(table)
    and relative weight, 88(table)
lung cancer, 25, 161, 259
    AAR (age-adjusted incident rate),
        20(table)
    in Europe, 5–6
lung disease, in Europe, 5–6
lung health, 4

McDonaldization, 177
macronutrient intakes, of South Africans,
    143(table)
magnesium, 266
male mortality, and alcohol, 164–5(fig.)
males, lean, energy balance in, 222(fig.)
malnutrition levels, Caribbean, 35(table)
maternal anaemia, 192
maternal anthropometry, 258

maternal low-protein diets, systolic blood
    pressure, 43(table)
Mazindol, 253
meat consumption, 27
meat industry, 198
meat intakes, and protein, 124–7
menarche, 148, 149, 152
mental subnormality, 121
metabolic predictors, of weight gain,
    227–8
metabolic rate, 228
metabolic syndrome, 72, 235
    obesity, abdominal, 80–2
    variables, occupational status, 82(fig.)
metabolic systems, natural selection,
    251(table)
micronutrient depletion, 12
micronutrients, 20
Middle East countries, NCDs in, 37–40
migrants, 59–68, 71–5
    studies of, 273–4
minerals, 91
molecular biology, 250
    of appetite control, 223–4
monounsaturated fat, 100
    and breast cancer, 107
morbidity
    and alcohol, 171
    and bodyweight, 237–9
mortality
    and alcohol consumption, 157–70,
        171–2
    attributable, 162–8
    and bodyweight, 237–9
    in China, 24(table)
    in England and Wales, 162(table)
mortality patterns
    Caribbean, 31–2, 33(fig.)
    Latin America, 31–2, 34(fig.)
mouth cancer, 157

National Nutrition Council (NNC),
    195–204
natural selection, metabolic systems,
    251(table)
NCDs (diet-related non-communicable
    diseases), in Europe, 2–4
NEFA (non-esterified fatty acids), 65
neoplasms, malignant, death rates,
    19(table)
neural tube defects, 286

Index compiled by A. Campbell Purton